EVALUATION, TREATMENT AND PREVENTION OF MUSCULOSKELETAL DISORDERS

3rd Edition

Volume Two • Extremities

John P. Tomberlin, PT OCS
H. Duane Saunders, MS PT

with guest author and editor

Katherine L. Beissner, PhD PT

Robin Saunders, MS PT, ass't editor

The Saunders Group
4250 Norex Drive
Chaska, Minnesota 55318-3047

Library of Congress Number 84-091301

ISBN 1-879190-07-9

Copyright © 1994 by The Saunders Group
2nd Printing August 1995

Cover Design: Audrey Saunders
Copy Editor and Layout Design: Clarke Stone

Printed in the United States of America

Acknowledgements

I would like to thank the following people:

— H. Duane Saunders, MS PT, for giving me the responsibility of being primary author of this text

— Kathy Beissner, PT PhD, for her patience, dedication, and hard work as editor and as co–author of Chapter 11

— Robin Saunders, MS PT, for her guidance and editing assistance

— Dan Wolfe, PT GDMT, for his friendship and encouragement

— My PT school instructors for instilling the spark to learn

— All of the patients I've seen and the students I've taught for the experience I've gained as I continue to learn

— Dr. Hollis Fritts, Dr. Michael Stuart, and Dr. David Fisher for their help with diagnostic figures.

— Most of all, my family and friends, whose love and support I cherish

John P. Tomberlin, PT OCS

CONTENTS

Section 1: Laying the Foundation

Section 2: The Upper Quarter

Section 3: The Lower Quarter

Chapter 8
The Knee **217**

Chapter 9
The Foot and Ankle **265**

Chapter 10
Gait Evaluation **307**

Section 4: Specific Treatment and Prevention Techniques

Chapter 11
Mobilization Techniques   Katherine L. Beissner, PhD PT **323**

SECTION 1
Laying the Foundation

CHAPTER 1
INTRODUCTION

In the first edition of *Evaluation, Treatment and Prevention of Musculoskeletal Disorders*, the changing role of physical therapy clinicians was emphasized. This text encouraged patients to take an active role in their own treatment and prevention and encouraged physical therapists to become active educators as well as treatment providers.

Eleven years later, physical therapists' professional roles are consistent with these ideas. Managing our patients involves not only the traditional areas of patient evaluation and treatment but also other areas such as prevention, motivation, and creative problem solving. Physical therapists are assuming professional roles as consultants to industry, schools, and sports teams.

As health care reforms take shape, physical therapists must learn to communicate proficiently with all "players" in the system, from the referring physician and rehabilitation case manager to the work supervisor, attorney, sports coach or trainer, family members, and third party payers. More than ever, we must justify our treatment interventions by proving the patient benefited functionally from the treatment given. Cost-effectiveness will be examined more closely in the future.

Cumulative trauma is now recognized as a major cause of musculoskeletal injuries. Although cumulative trauma is usually referred to in the context of the injured worker, it also occurs in sports and leisure activities. Many patients with musculoskeletal disorders may have problems originating from repetitive motions and sustained postures.

Traditional orthopædic physical therapy has always been associated with a management method that emphasizes treatment based on a medical diagnosis. In this role, the therapist is mainly a provider of passive treatments designed to eliminate symptoms. The main tissues considered are the joints and muscles.

This approach has consistently frustrated many physical therapists because it fails to address the *causes* of the patient's symptoms and dysfunctions; thus, the traditional approach usually comes up short for patient and therapist alike.

The methods described in this text emphasize an approach to the management of neuromusculoskeletal disorders based on the evaluation, treatment, and prevention of the *causes* of the symptoms and dysfunctions. The fundamental question that guides this approach is, "What are the problems that prevent the patient from optimal function?"

Our approach also emphasizes teaching patients self–responsibility, which empowers them to learn to manage their own conditions. Even the most skilled physical therapist will not succeed if patients do not learn to manage their own conditions after a course of physical therapy is completed. Fostering dependence on our services is not an ethical goal for our profession and should be discouraged.

In summary, we advocate an integrated management approach. Rather than following a particular evaluation and treatment philosophy, the clinician should strive for a complete understanding of basic physiological and biomechanical sciences. The clinician should remain open minded when performing the evaluation and should consider all structures that *could* contribute to the patient's condition. The treatment scheme should include four main components:

1. controlling symptoms

2. modifying daily stresses

3. restoring function

4. preventing recurrence

Frequent reassessment aids treatment modification and helps measure clinical progress. Figure 1–1 summarizes the main steps of evaluation and treatment.

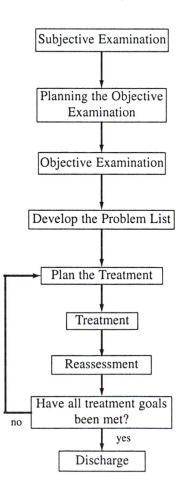

Figure 1–1. The evaluation and treatment process.

ABOUT THE TEXT

This text is intended for physical therapy students and clinicians as an adjunct to Volume I–Spine. It emphasizes the analytical processes and reasoning critical to obtaining a complete history, performing a thorough objective examination, and planning appropriate treatments. Clinicians must use the evaluation process to separate those patients who will not benefit from physical therapy or who need additional medical testing. This is especially important as direct access becomes more common and as the physical therapist's role expands.

Volume II–Extremities consists of thirteen chapters organized into four sections:

Section I, Laying the Foundation, consists of Chapters 1–3, which cover the introductory material and the essential concepts, principles, and guidelines for examination and treatment of neuromusculoskeletal disorders in the peripheral limbs.

Section II, The Upper Quarter, covers the evaluation and treatment of disorders in the upper extremities. The reader will find the principles of Section I expanded and made specific for the joints of the shoulder (Chapter 4), the elbow (Chapter 5), and the wrist and hand (Chapter 6). Each chapter includes examples of clinical problem solving as applied to five common conditions. For example, the conditions lateral epicondylitis, medial epicondylitis, medial collateral ligament sprain, cubital tunnel syndrome, and elbow contracture are discussed in Chapter 5.

Section III, The Lower Quarter, consists of Chapters 7–10, which cover the evaluation and treatment of disorders in the lower extremities. Paralleling Section II, five common clinical conditions are examined in each chapter. Gait analysis is discussed in Chapter 10.

Section IV, Specific Treatment and Prevention Techniques, contains information on mobilization, exercise, and strategies for injury prevention. Chapter 11 includes mobilization of peripheral joints and soft tissues. Chapter 12 discusses and illustrates flexibility, strengthening, and proprioceptive exercises. Chapter 13 contains information about preventing extremity disorders in the worker and the athlete.

Each chapter in Sections II and III addresses a specific anatomical region. These chapters are organized into the following sections:

1. Introduction—general features of the joint and its functional role.

2. Functional Anatomy—the essential anatomical considerations for the joint, muscle, and neural tissues.

3. Evaluation—specific guidelines for the subjective and objective examinations following the general evaluation principles in Chapter 2.

4. Treatment Strategies—general guidelines for treating the region following the general treatment principles in Chapter 3.

5. Common Clinical Conditions—five common clinical conditions are discussed. Each discussion covers introduction, history, signs and symptoms, diagnostics, problem list, and treatment.

The material presented in this text is based on a review of the available literature and on our clinical experience. It is not our intent to teach a specific school of thought; rather, we present material essential to developing the reader's ability to solve problems and make appropriate clinical decisions. Our purpose is to point the student and the clinician toward developing an integrated approach to the management of neuromusculoskeletal disorders of the peripheral limbs.

Physical therapists are entering a period of increasing professional responsibility and liability. The opportunity is at hand for us to assume a leading role in the management of neuromusculoskeletal disorders. It is in the spirit of this opportunity that this text has been written.

CHAPTER 2 PRINCIPLES OF EXTREMITY EVALUATION

INTRODUCTION

Comprehensive, accurate evaluation of patients with musculoskeletal disorders is essential for effective clinical practice. Clinicians cannot assume that patients referred for treatment have been accurately diagnosed. Even with accurate diagnosis, the clinician does not have all the pertinent information about the patient. The purpose of musculoskeletal evaluation is to identify the physical and functional problems that contribute to the patient's complaints. Without a thorough evaluation, some problems may be missed, resulting in ineffective treatment.

Treatments based on "recipes" or protocols for a specific diagnosis are a common frustration for many clinicians. Evaluation and treatment based on a single approach may force us to choose between two extremes (Fig 2–1). Are we more concerned with symptom resolution, or do we focus on biomechanical restoration? Clinically, we should consider both.

Finally, most physical therapists evaluate and treat the muscles and joints. What of the nerves?

Clinical research in Australia suggests we consider three anatomical components for evaluation and treatment—joints, muscles and nerves.[2] Thus we might re–name patients' problems as "neuromusculoskeletal" disorders (Fig 2–2).

Clinicians all have similar goals: to identify and treat patients' neuromusculoskeletal problems to maximize function. Toward this end we must acquire the following information:[5]

- What is the source of the symptoms or dysfunction?

- Are there other contributing factors?

- What is the prognosis?

- What treatment should be selected?

- How should it progress?

- What are the precautions and contradictions to examination and treatment?

These questions are the same, regardless of the patient's complaints, the clinician's treatment style, or the choice of therapy techniques. These questions form the basis for examination, treatment, and

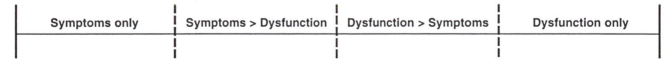

Symptoms only	Symptoms > Dysfunction	Dysfunction > Symptoms	Dysfunction only

Figure 2–1. Continuum of treatment focus, ranging from treatment of symptoms to treatment of dysfunction.

reassessment—the foundations of good physical therapy. Figure 2–3 shows a worksheet that can be used to guide the examination.

SUBJECTIVE EXAMINATION

The subjective examination (patient interview) determines what problems should be evaluated and how they should be evaluated. The clinician may also formulate ideas about what treatment to use and how it will be carried out. The key lies in using a logical thought process to guide the interview. Appropriate questions and active listening are critical during the initial examination and throughout treatment and reassessment.

The subjective examination is guided by four clinical axioms:[5,13]

1. The patient can tell us about the problem or treatment *if* we ask the right questions.

2. The subjective examination should tell us what to expect on the objective examination.

3. If the patient's complaints don't fit with the objective examination, we must be prepared to inquire further.

4. We must identify those patients who will not benefit from treatment or who are inappropriate for physical therapy because of neurogenic disorders, systemic diseases, or other serious pathology.

The main goals of the subjective examination are to obtain information about the patient's main complaints, functional difficulties and pertinent

medical history and to outline the direction and extent of the objective examination. The subjective examination will also help clarify the patient's most significant functional complaints; these can be used to measure treatment effectiveness in reassessments. Finally, with a thorough subjective examination the clinician can begin to identify those problems that can be helped by physical therapy and those problems that are not appropriate for physical therapy.

The subjective examination can be divided into nine steps:

1. Identify the patient's main complaint.

2. Identify the nature of the complaint.

3. Identify the location of symptoms.

4. Identify the problem onset.

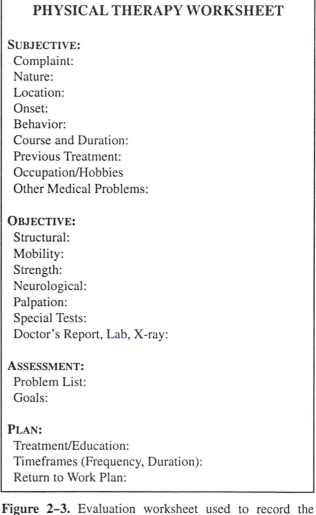

PHYSICAL THERAPY WORKSHEET

SUBJECTIVE:
Complaint:
Nature:
Location:
Onset:
Behavior:
Course and Duration:
Previous Treatment:
Occupation/Hobbies
Other Medical Problems:

OBJECTIVE:
Structural:
Mobility:
Strength:
Neurological:
Palpation:
Special Tests:
Doctor's Report, Lab, X-ray:

ASSESSMENT:
Problem List:
Goals:

PLAN:
Treatment/Education:
Timeframes (Frequency, Duration):
Return to Work Plan:

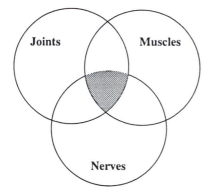

Figure 2–2. Patient's problems can originate from joints, muscles and nerves.

Figure 2–3. Evaluation worksheet used to record the results of the exam.

5. Describe the behavior of symptoms.

6. Determine the course and duration of symptoms.

7. Identify previous treatments and outcomes.

8. Describe work, home and recreation demands.

9. Note pertinent medical history.

The following sections will discuss the issues that should be addressed at each step of the subjective examination.

Patient Complaint

It is critical to establish exactly what is bothering the patient. When taking the history, the first question to ask is simply, "What is your main complaint?" This gives patients a chance to tell in their own words anything that they believe is important. It lets patients say why they are seeking physical therapy, including functional complaints and expectations from physical therapy. This first question facilitates the rest of the interview by placing both the clinician and the patient at ease. Common complaints include:

- pain

- decreased range of motion

- swelling

- weakness

- loss of function

- apprehension in movement

It can help to ask patients to rate their symptoms on a 1–10 scale to get an idea of the intensity of their pain or the severity of their functional problems. The symptoms may differ from day to day; therefore it is important to find out how the patient's complaints on the day of the examination compare with other typical days.

Nature

The clinician often has to ask more detailed questions about the patient's complaint. Pain, weakness, numbness, stiffness, and hypersensitivity are common symptoms. The clinician should ask for a specific description of the symptoms such as a "constant deep ache," "intermittent pain," or "sharp stab of pain." *The clinician should not lead the patient by suggesting descriptions.*

It is also important to differentiate between "pins and needles" sensations and "numbness." The patient should be asked if there is an area of skin that can be pinched or pricked with a pin and not be felt. If this is the case, nerve root impingement or peripheral nerve injury is likely. "Pins and needles" and "tingling" are non–specific descriptions and do not indicate a specific type of pathology.

Weakness without pain suggests either a neurological deficit or prolonged disuse. Painless weakness associated with a peripheral nerve entrapment or spinal nerve root compression often follows a specific dermatome or myotome distribution. Weakness associated with a neurological disease or disuse will typically be more generalized. If weakness is present with pain, it is sometimes difficult to determine if the pain alone is causing the weakness or if there is also an underlying neurological deficit. This will be clarified in the objective examination.

The patient will describe often slipping, popping or clicking sensations associated with certain movements. It is important to determine if this sensation occurs every time the particular movement is repeated. Many joint noises result from carbon dioxide formed by decreased pressure that occurs when joint surfaces are suddenly separated. This is a normal phenomenon. When this type of pop occurs, it cannot be repeated immediately. If a joint cannot be popped, the joint may be hypomobile. If a joint can be popped easily, it may be hypermobile.

If a patient reports a joint noise that can be repeated over and over, it indicates either A) an unstable joint that may be subluxing or partially subluxing with certain movements; B) a mechanical roughness or abnormality of the joint surfaces such as a meniscus tear or osteophytosis; or C) thickening and scarring of the ligaments and the capsule surrounding the joint.

Location

The patient should be asked to identify the location of the symptoms, but the clinician should remember that the location the patient describes is not necessarily a reliable indicator of the actual site of pathology.[3] Patients often have referred pain—pain or tenderness felt away from the site of pathology. Pain that migrates from one joint to another suggests a systemic disease rather than a neuromusculoskeletal disorder. Pain that spreads from the original site to the surrounding tissues can be caused by inflammation or muscle spasm, both of which are often secondary reactions to the primary disorder.

It can help to use body diagrams to document the nature and location of the patient's complaints. Body diagrams can include a list of important questions, such as those shown in Figure 2–4. The diagrams aid the clinician two ways: first, they help keep the evaluation organized and decrease the likelihood the clinician will forget to ask important questions; second, they help the clinician remember details of the patient's original complaint so the patient can be specifically questioned about his or her status during reassessments. The body diagram is kept as a part of the patient's permanent medical record.

Onset of Symptoms

The patient should be asked about the original onset of symptoms and the onset of the most recent episode. Specific movements, activities, or postures that could have contributed to the onset of symptoms should be identified. It can help to know the mechanism of injury. For example, sprains and strains usually involve an identifiable overuse or a specific incident of onset. Inflammatory and systemic disorders may have a more subtle onset.

It is important to realize that the patient may not be able to describe an exact mechanism of injury. It is often misleading to place too great an emphasis on the patient's description of onset. The patient may also try to relate current complaints to old injuries.

Many neuromusculoskeletal disorders can be caused by the cumulative effects of faulty body mechanics; repetitive or stressful activities; loss of flexibility and strength; and a general state of poor physical condition. The clinician must sometimes ask comprehensive and detailed questions to identify the events leading to cumulative trauma injuries; therefore, it is important to question the patient about common postures or movement patterns.

The answers to both the cause and the treatment of the problem are frequently found in this line of questioning. In fact, when considering a corrective or preventive exercise program, it sometimes helps more to understand the patient's occupation, life-style, and hobbies than it does to know about the incident that led to the current episode of symptoms.

Behavior of Symptoms

The effects of activity, movement, positions, and rest should be identified. The aim is to determine the severity, irritability and nature (SIN) of the problems. Severity and irritability are subjective measures of symptoms. The symptoms are *severe* if the patient cannot maintain a position or posture due to the intensity of the symptoms. A problem is *irritable* if symptoms are easily provoked and take a long time to resolve. The *nature* of a problem is either mechanical or inflammatory. Generally, mechanical symptoms are changed by movement or positioning. Inflammatory conditions remain unchanged by these factors. Unremitting symptoms, especially at night, are consistent with an active inflammatory condition or other sinister pathology.

In addition to SIN, it is important to know what makes the symptoms worse. Knowing the *aggravating factors*—the positions, movements, or activities that increase the patient's symptoms—is the key to understanding the patient's functional complaints. For future comparison, it helps to list and remember the factors that give the most information about the patient's function. Determining the aggravating factors during the subjective examination also gives the clinician clues about which movements or positions to focus on in the objective examination. *Easing factors* refer to those activities, movements, and positions that have helped at home. Easing factors may give clues to the diagnosis and treatment approach. Obtaining information about *24 Hour Behavior* is important because it reveals the daily pattern of symptoms. The clinician should ask how the symptoms behave on awakening, with daily activities, at the end of the day, and at night. Waking features help identify the effects of sleep postures and rest on the patient's symptoms. The times of day symptoms occur or change can give clues about aggravating and easing factors that can be used to plan treatment. Symptoms that increase at the end of the day may be cumulative in nature. Night–time pain that has no mechanical feature may indicate an inflammatory process or sinister pathology. Daily patterns of symptoms can be reassessed to measure treatment effectiveness.

an acute, subacute, or chronic state. Acuteness or chronicity will influence treatment. The clinician should also "stage" the disorder by determining whether the problem is resolving, worsening, or remaining about the same.

Course and Duration of Symptoms

The clinician should consider the time since onset of symptoms to determine whether the condition is in

The natural progression of the condition should be considered, too. Was the pain greatest when the injury first occurred, or did it worsen on subsequent

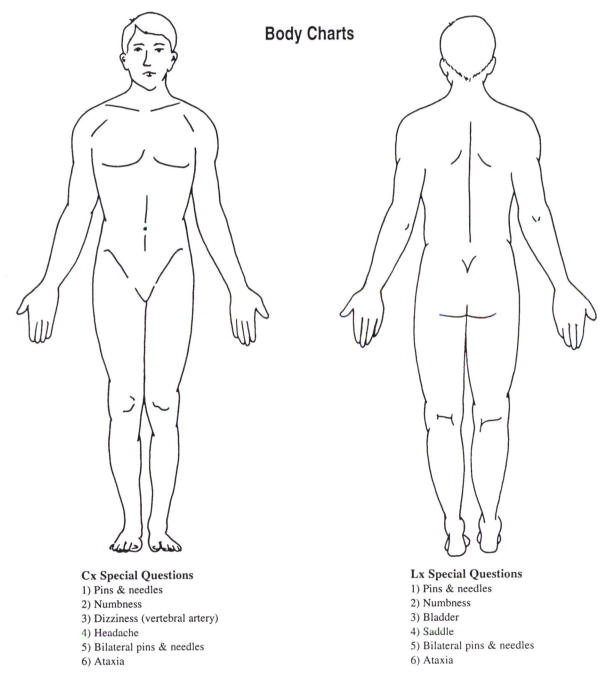

Body Charts

Cx Special Questions
1) Pins & needles
2) Numbness
3) Dizziness (vertebral artery)
4) Headache
5) Bilateral pins & needles
6) Ataxia

Lx Special Questions
1) Pins & needles
2) Numbness
3) Bladder
4) Saddle
5) Bilateral pins & needles
6) Ataxia

Figure 2–4. Body diagram used to document patient's symptoms. Special questions are included on the diagram as reminders to the clinician.

days? Has the patient continued to work or play sports since the onset of symptoms? Is this the patient's first injury, or have there been previous episodes? In the case of multiple episodes, how does this episode differ from previous ones?

Effect of Previous Treatment

It is important to determine what treatments have been tried, whether they have been helpful, and whether concurrent treatment is being carried out by other health care professionals. It is particularly important to know the specific effect of any previous treatment. This may help the clinician narrow treatment options and rule out those that have not helped.

Occupation/Hobbies

The patient's occupation and hobbies are very important, even in a non–work related injury. Functional goal–setting depends on this often neglected area of the subjective examination.

For a work–related injury, the clinician needs to know any current work restrictions set by the physician. The patient also should be asked to describe current duties at work if he or she is on light or modified duty. Often, a patient may not be working at the level allowed by the physician because there is no work available at that level. An astute clinician will supplement the patient's work activities and prevent deconditioning by having the patient practice work activities as a part of the rehabilitation. As the patient improves, the clinician can add more resistance or repetitions to functional activities and can give the physician information about appropriate changes in the patient's work restrictions.

The clinician needs to understand the patient's regular job duties to set functional goals. For example, if a patient with wrist tendinitis is a typist who cannot type because of the injury, the clinician will identify *improved typing tolerance* as a specific goal of therapy. The exercises and functional activities chosen for treatment will be oriented, in part, toward achieving this goal.

All patients should be asked about their hobbies and sports, just as they are asked about their work

duties. If the patient's problems prevent participation in sports or hobbies, goals can be set for return to these activities, and sports or hobby simulation can be incorporated into the treatment program.

Other Related Medical Problems

General medical problems should be identified, including their treatments and outcomes. To avoid omitting information pertinent to patient management, it helps to ask the patient about common medical disorders, including:

- Arthritis (rheumatoid arthritis [RA], degenerative joint disease [DJD])
- Neurological disorders
- Cardiopulmonary problems (myocardial infarction [MI], hypertension, angina, asthma, chronic obstructive pulmonary disease [COPD], etc.)
- Disease (osteoporosis, diabetes mellitus, etc.)
- Cancer
- Trauma
- Relevant orthopædic problems
- Surgeries and medications
- Current medications

Any other conditions that would interfere with the patient's ability to tolerate treatment should be noted. The patient's physician should be consulted as needed to obtain a more extensive medical history.

The patient should also be asked about the results of any tests performed and about the physician's diagnosis. This gives the clinician information about the patient's understanding of the condition. The clinician may need to explain the diagnosis further or clarify misconceptions about the patient's condition. The tests performed and the patient's report of the diagnosis should always be confirmed with the physician's office.

Summary of Subjective Examination

The patient interview sets the stage for the remainder of the examination. The way the patient responds to the clinician's questions should be noted.

What kind of attitude does the patient seem to have toward the condition? Some patients present with positive attitudes, consulting the clinician to help resolve problems. Others may seem more negative about the potential benefits of therapy. Since the patient's attitude often affects treatment success, the clinician should consider this important aspect of the patient's condition.

After the subjective examination, the clinician should have an initial impression of the potential sources of the patient's symptoms and have some ideas of what tests need to be performed to clarify the problem. The functional goals of treatment are based in part on the limitations described in the interview. Most importantly, the objective examination is based on clues from the subjective examination.

PLANNING THE OBJECTIVE EXAMINATION

When planning the objective examination, the clinician should consider these questions:

1. What are the main problems?

2. What are the probable sources of the symptoms?

3. What are the qualities of the symptoms?

4. What will be the focus of the objective examination?

What are the main problems?

Based on information and clues provided by the patient in the subjective examination, the clinician should have some expectations about what will be found in the objective examination. If, for example, the patient says that he or she can no longer reach the top shelf in the kitchen, the clinician would expect to find decreased range of motion at the shoulder during the objective examination.

While the patient will usually have one main complaint, there may be several other problems that could eventually be addressed in treatment. All these problems should be kept in mind during the objective examination as the clinician looks for links between the problems.

What are the probable sources of the symptoms?

The clinician should consider all structures (joint, muscle, nerve, etc.) that could contribute to the symptoms. This includes anatomical structures underlying the area of symptoms and those that may refer symptoms to the areas of complaints. For example, a patient may be unable to reach overhead because of shoulder pain. The clinician should recognize this complaint is consistent with impingement syndrome but it may also be caused by adhesive capsulitis or a problem in the cervical spine.

During the objective examination, *differentiation tests* are useful when symptoms are provoked during mobility or posture examinations, but it is not clear what aspect of the movement or posture causes the symptoms. With differentiation tests, the movement or posture is analyzed to identify the structures that are stressed. Then the movement or posture is reproduced gradually, adding one element at a time to stress the various structures in isolation. Based on the patient's symptomatic response, it is possible to determine what aspect of the movement or posture causes the symptoms.

What are the qualities of symptoms?

The clinician should be aware of the SIN of the symptoms.

Severity may limit:

- the depth of palpation

- the range of motion of passive movements

- the overpressure applied to the end range of active or passive movements.

Irritability may limit:

- the number of motions tested

- the specific motions or postures examined

- the extent of examination

Nature may limit:

- the type and extent of examination based on known or suspected pathology (i.e., inflammatory conditions, systemic disorders, surgical procedures, etc.)

What will be the focus of the objective examination?

When determining the focus of the examination, the clinician must realize that it may not be appropriate to perform every test on every structure on the first day of examination. The subjective examination is used to prioritize A) the structures to examine and B) the extent to which these structures will be provoked. The clinician should ask:

- Which positions, postures, and motions will be examined, avoided, deferred?

- What are the apparent relationships between pain and dysfunction?

The subjective examination also guides the clinician to screen for medical disease. This will become more important with direct access to physical therapy. Symptoms may be referred from the lumbar spine or the hip joint. The screening examination should be a quick survey of several areas and should provide the clinician with enough information to decide which specific areas must be examined in detail. The aim is to help clear specific joints as contributors to the patient's problem.

Screening exams are typically performed when the patient's primary complaint is extremity symptoms. It is important to remember that extremity symptoms may be related to spinal pathology, even in the absence of spinal symptoms. The cervical and thoracic spine should always be examined if the patient is complaining of an upper extremity symptom. Similarly, the lumbar spine and pelvis should always be examined if the patient is complaining of a lower extremity symptom. Furthermore, symptoms in a distal joint, e.g., the elbow, may originate in a more proximal joint, e.g., the shoulder. The screening examination helps the clinician sort the location of the symptoms from the location of the pathology.

For example, consider the patient with shoulder pain. The quadrant test in the cervical spine (combined extension, rotation and ipsilateral sidebending with overpressure—see Figure 2–5) effectively determines whether the cervical spine is contributing to the shoulder symptoms. If the quadrant test reproduces the patient's shoulder symptoms, the cervical spine is implicated as a potential contributor, and it should be examined further. The upper and lower quarter screening tests are summarized in Figure 2–6 and Figure 2–7. Boissenault has developed more extensive exams to screen for medical diseases. These expanded screenings are particularly useful for those clinicians working without a physician's referral.[1]

Clearing Tests

Clearing tests are used to assess the potential contribution of a related joint complex to the patient's main joint complaints. The following are examples of tests to clear (rule out or implicate) a joint.

1. *Cervical Spine*—Quadrant test (Fig 2–5)

2. *Shoulder*—Overpressure applied to active flexion, abduction, and the hands–behind–the–back position (Fig 2–8).

3. *Elbow*—Overpressure applied to active flexion, extension, pronation, and supination.

4. *Wrist and Hand*—Overpressure applied to active wrist flexion, extension, radial deviation, ulnar deviation, pronation, and supination.

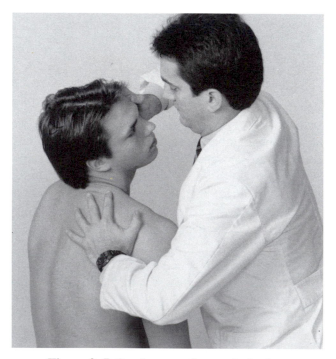

Figure 2–5. Quadrant test for cervical spine.

1. Postural assessment
2. Active range of motion of cervical spine
3. Passive overpressures if symptom free
4. Vertebral artery test
5. Quadrant test
6. Resisted muscle tests cervical spine (rotation C-1)
7. Resisted shoulder elevation (C-2, 3, 4)
8. Resisted shoulder abduction (C-5)
9. Active shoulder flexion and rotations
10. Resisted elbow flexion (C-6)
11. Resisted elbow extension (C-7)
12. Active range of motion of elbow
13. Resisted wrist flexion (C-7)
14. Resisted wrist extension (C-6)
15. Resisted thumb extension (C-8)
16. Resisted finger abduction (T-1)
17. Babinski's reflex test (UMN)

Figure 2–6. Upper quarter screening exam.

1. Postural assessment
2. Active forward, backward and lateral bending of lumbar spine
3. Standing flexion test/Gillet's test
4. Toe raises (S-1)
5. Heel walking (L-4, 5)
6. Sitting flexion test
7. Active rotation of lumbar spine
8. Overpressures if symptom free
9. Straight leg raise (L-4, 5; S-1)
10. Resisted hip flexion (L-1, 2)
11. Passive range of motion to hip
12. Resisted knee extension (L-3, 4)
13. Knee flexion, extension, medial and lateral tilt
14. Femoral nerve stretch
15. Babinski's reflex test (UMN)

Figure 2–7. Lower quarter screening exam.

5. *Lumbar Spine*—Quadrant test (Fig 2–9)

6. *Hip*—Full squat in standing, overpressure to hip flexion in supine.

7. *Knee*—Full squat in standing, duck walk (walking in squatted position), single limb half squat.

8. *Ankle*—Full squat in standing with heels up and with heels down, heel walk, toe walk.

If any of these tests reproduce the patient's symptoms, a more detailed evaluation of the corresponding area is warranted.

Structural Examination

The structural examination involves a closer, more specific inspection of the area of complaint. Inspection involves observing the structure of the bones, the joints, and the muscles in the areas involved. It is essential for the parts to be examined to be adequately free of clothing.

The structural examination begins with general observation of the patient. How does the patient walk and sit? Does the patient seem to be in pain? If so, how intense? Are there any obvious abnormalities in the way he or she moves about? Such observations are important for the clinician to note, as they may tell more about the patient's progress than direct questioning does.

The symmetry of the patient's body contours should be examined. Limb size, shape, color, atrophy, and hypertrophy should be compared bilaterally. Edema should be noted. A baseline measurement of limb volume or joint circumference can be used for bilateral limb comparison and reassessment.

Any incisions, wounds, abscesses, sores, or ecchymosis should be inspected carefully. Signs of

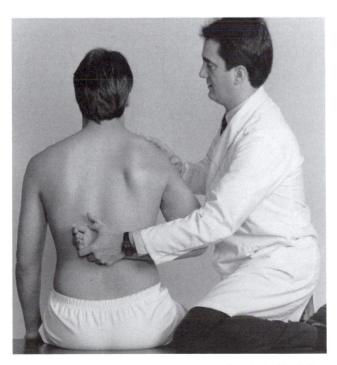

Figure 2–8. Shoulder clearing test—hands-behind-the-back position

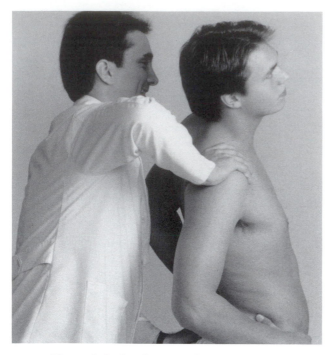

Figure 2–9. Quadrant test for lumbar spine.

infection or inflammation such as skin redness or red streaks; diffuse limb edema; or excessive warmth should be noted and relayed to the referring physician. Any special assistive devices or supports used by the patient should be examined, assessing whether the device has been properly fitted and if it is being used correctly.

In summary, the clinician should look for the following in the structural examination:

- general body alignment

- quality of movement

- postures maintained or avoided

- presence of muscle guarding or spasm

- symmetry of soft tissue contours

- bilateral limb size, shape, symmetry, color, atrophy, hypertrophy

- presence of edema

- presence of open wounds, abscesses, sores, ecchymosis

- incisions from surgeries or injuries

- signs of inflammation or infection

- use of assistive devices, splints, supports, and braces

Mobility Examination

The mobility examination consists of active, passive, and accessory mobility tests. Active and passive mobility are types of physiological mobility. Physiological mobility is movement in standard planes (e.g., flexion, abduction, rotation) and combined functional movements (e.g., diagonal patterns of movement). Accessory mobility is the small movement within the joints and surrounding tissues that is necessary for normal physiological movements. While physiological movements can be performed voluntarily by the patient, accessory movements cannot.

The mobility examination helps determine the structures involved and the extent to which they are involved. When performing any mobility test—active, passive or accessory—the clinician should ask two main questions:

1. What is the effect of the test on the patient's symptoms?

2. Is the amount of movement normal, hypomobile (restricted) or hypermobile (excessive)?

The findings of the mobility examination are significant if the test changes the patient's symptoms, or the amount of movement seen or felt is abnormal. To perform a thorough mobility examination, the clinician must include in the examination all tissues from which the patient's symptoms might arise, including the joints, muscles, and neural tissues.

Since posture often plays an important role in both the cause and the treatment of neuromusculoskeletal disorders, an important part of the mobility examination involves observing the effects of correcting postural abnormalities. Posture correction is done to determine if return to normal posture is possible and if the patient's symptoms are altered when posture is corrected. This may help find the structures at fault and may help the clinician decide to what extent the postural deformity contributes to the patient's current complaint.

The tissues to examine are divided into two groups: non–contractile and contractile. Non–contractile tissues include joint capsules, ligaments, bursæ, cartilage, and nerves. Contractile tissues include muscles and their tendon attachments. To differentiate between contractile and non–contractile tissue as the cause of the patient's symptoms, the clinician considers the results of mobility and strength testing.

Active Mobility

Active movements provide general information about the patient's functional abilities, including the patient's willingness and ability to move the joint. Since active mobility testing assesses function, movements in functional patterns will often yield more information than straight planar motions. The following should be noted during active mobility testing:

1. *The range of motion* obtained when the patient is asked to perform a movement.

2. *The quality of the motion* being evaluated. Note any substitution patterns, apprehension, guarding, catching, or giving way.

3. *Symptoms associated with movement.* Note when the symptoms start or change in the range of motion; where they were felt by the patient; and what happens to the symptoms when movement stops and the limb is returned to neutral.
   Remember, the patient may have a delayed symptom response (a "latent response"), so a short pause is necessary between testing motions.

4. *Crepitus or joint noise.* Joint noise can indicate roughening of cartilage surfaces or tendons moving within sheaths or over bony prominences. Specific types of joint crepitus may indicate the source of noise and the type of problem.[14] Crepitus is discussed further in the "Palpation" section of this chapter.

5. *Response to overpressure.* Overpressure is applied to gain information about the quantity, quality, symptom response and end–feel of the motion limitation. The clinician must consider the SIN of the problem when deciding whether to apply

overpressure. Overpressure should be avoided if the symptoms are severe or irritable or if the known or suspected pathology would contraindicate overpressure. The patient should be asked whether he or she can go any further after reaching voluntary, available end range. The clinician then applies overpressure by pushing further into the range of motion.

Passive Mobility

Passive mobility tests differentiate between contractile and non–contractile structures. These tests determine if the joint range is restricted (hypomobile), excessive (hypermobile) or normal. If passive range of motion is greater than active range of motion, this implies contractile tissue is at least partly responsible for the patient's symptoms. If active range of motion is greater than passive range of motion, the patient is probably unable to relax enough to let the clinician complete the passive range of motion testing.

The joint or limb being examined should be taken through passive functional movements as appropriate (based on SIN), beginning with straight planar motions, then combining movements to mimic functional movement patterns.

When assessing passive joint mobility, the following should be considered:

A. *The range of motion available.* Is the range of motion symmetrical? Is it normal, restricted, or excessive?

1. If limited motion is present, what is the source of limitation (pain, muscle spasm, or connective tissue tightness)?

2. If excessive motion is present, are any symptoms provoked with movement (Pain, spasm, apprehension, guarding)?

3. What is the response to overpressure applied at available end range?

B. *Symptoms associated with movement.* As the limb is moved through the range of motion and into resistance, are any symptoms produced? The symptom behavior should be documented. Symptoms presenting early in the range of motion may need to be treated before the clinician can perform treatments in the range of motion restriction.

C. *End–feel.* End–feel describes the quality of resistance to motion the clinician feels at the end of available range. There are three normal and five abnormal end–feels.[4]

Normal End–Feels

1. *Soft tissue approximation.* The range is limited by soft tissue being compressed (i.e., the calf pressing against the posterior thigh during knee flexion).

2. *Tissue stretch.* This is a firm but springy end–feel that comes on toward the end of available range and has "give" to it. The limiting factors are the soft tissues being stretched (e.g., the rotator cuff muscles and glenohumeral capsule stretching at the end range of shoulder internal rotation, or the finger flexors and anterior capsule stretching with metacarpophalangeal (MCP) joint extension).

3. *Bone–on–bone.* This is a hard and usually painless end–feel at the end of available range. The limiting factor is bony approximation (e.g., the olecranon in the fossa with full elbow extension).

Abnormal End–feels

1. *Capsular.* The motion limitations at a joint occur in a predictable pattern. The pattern is different for each joint. A capsular pattern indicates the joint capsule is the limiting structure. The end–feel is firmer than the normal "tissue stretch" end–feel and occurs earlier in the range than expected.

2. *Bone–on–bone.* Bone–on–bone end–feel is abnormal when it occurs sooner than expected in the range of motion or in joints that normally have a different end–feel. The limiting factor is usually joint hypertrophy secondary to trauma or DJD.

3. *Muscle guarding.* The clinician will feel a sudden, guarding restriction that firmly limits the motion. Muscle guarding is often associated with pain. The limiting factor is a muscle contraction by the patient that prevents further movement into the range of motion. Muscle guarding end–feels often

accompany internal derangement, instability, fracture, or other serious pathology.

4. *Springy.* The springy end–feel is similar to the normal tissue stretch end–feel, but it occurs sooner than expected in the range of motion. It can be felt either suddenly or gradually.

If there is a quick, springy feel on stretch, the limiting factor is usually an internal derangement of cartilage. If the clinician detects a slowly building springy feel, the limiting factor is probably intra–articular edema.

5. *Empty.* The clinician is sometimes unable to achieve enough motion to evaluate the quality of the end–feel. This is called an empty end–feel, and it is associated with one of two situations: pain or other symptoms limit the range of motion before the clinician feels resistance, or the joint is grossly unstable.

Accessory Mobility

The passive mobility tests give the clinician a general picture of the patient's joint mobility, and the accessory mobility tests help find the origin of the abnormal motion. Although it is quite easy to observe loss of functional (physiological) motion, it is more difficult to determine accessory mobility limitations.

There are two types of accessory mobility. *Component motions* occur with normal active motions but are not under voluntary control. The upward rotation of the scapula that accompanies shoulder flexion is an example of a component motion. *Joint play* motions are intra–articular motions that occur between joint surfaces during normal physiological movement. Joint play motions are necessary for normal movement, but they cannot be performed voluntarily in isolation from physiological movement. For example, the tibia glides forward on the femur during knee extension. This forward (anterior) glide is the normal joint play, and it must occur with extension. The patient cannot anteriorly glide the tibia voluntarily, but the clinician can passively move the tibia in an anterior glide.

Even if the patient has normal passive range of motion, the accessory mobility tests can still be useful because abnormal joint mechanics may still be present. For example, the glenohumeral joint may be extremely stiff, but the clinician may not be able to detect any stiffness in the passive mobility examination because excess mobility in the scapulothoracic joint gives the appearance of full range of motion. Accessory mobility tests may also be performed to see if the structure being tested provokes symptoms.

Accessory mobility testing can be a difficult part of the objective examination for many clinicians. Developing a feel for subtle differences in joint mobility requires experience. Initially, the clinician should not be concerned about detecting these very subtle differences. It helps to perform the accessory mobility testing procedures on as many patients as possible. The clinician will soon be able to determine that a certain joint "feels abnormal" or "is definitely stiff" when compared to the hundreds of other joints examined in the past. Eventually, the clinician will be able to detect very subtle differences. Intra–rater reliability for detecting joint feel in accessory mobility testing is high.[7,10] The mistake most inexperienced clinicians make is avoiding testing accessory mobility for fear of not understanding the results.

Traditionally, accessory mobility is tested with the joint in the loose–packed position. This is the position in the physiological range of motion at which the joint capsule is most relaxed. Clinically, it is also useful to test accessory mobility at the restricted range of motion. A working knowledge of each joint's normal accessory mobility is necessary when examining joint function.

Many clinicians use the following scale to grade accessory mobility:[6]

0 – Ankylosed joint

1 – Considerable limitation

2 – Slight limitation

3 – Normal mobility

4 – Slight hypermobility

5 – Considerable hypermobility

6 – Pathologically unstable

This scale is not universal. It is better to use the words than the numbers when reporting accessory mobility.

Strength Examination

The strength examination is performed to rule out muscles as the source of symptoms, to decide if muscle imbalances are a source of the problem, and to provide a baseline for any strengthening that will be part of the treatment. Specific muscles are tested with manual muscle tests (MMT). These tests are usually done in a comfortable neutral position in the midrange of motion available at that joint. The clinician gradually elicits a strong contraction with little or no joint movement and grades the strength of the contraction. A common system of grading MMT is shown in Table 2–1. Any muscle acting on, acting across, or influencing the joint being examined should be tested. The clinician should compare bilateral joints in all extremity strength testing.

The SIN of the condition should be considered when deciding how strongly to resist the patient's muscular contraction. For example, a person with a Grade II hamstring strain may have pain with active knee flexion. Based on the severity (pain with knee flexion) and nature (hamstring tear) of the problem, a maximal resistance to isometric knee flexion is not advisable during examination—it will not provide any more information than already available and may increase pain. In this case, a sub–maximal resistance should be applied and the symptom response noted.

If resisted muscle contraction produces pain, there may be pathology within the muscle, the tendon, or the tendon attachment. If no pain or weakness is observed, the contractile tissues being tested can be ruled out as a source of the symptoms. Weak and painful muscle contractions do not necessarily indicate true weakness, since the pain may be interfering with the patient's ability to contract. A weak and painless contraction, on the other hand, suggests neurological involvement or weakness due to inactivity.

Cyriax has identified four possible findings with resisted muscle testing.[3] They are:

I.   *Strong and Painless*

In this case, there is no apparent pathology to either the contractile or the nervous tissues.

II.   Strong and Painful

Usually a minor structural lesion of the muscle–tendon unit is at fault. The problem is not neurological.

III.   Weak and Painless

There are two interpretations of a weak and painless contraction:

1. Complete rupture of the muscle–tendon unit has occurred. The clinician can confirm this with other testing such as palpation or muscle squeezing, which produces motion at the distal joint insertion of the muscle/tendon unit if it is intact (e.g., the Thompson Test for gastrocnemius–soleus tendon rupture— see Chapter 9, The Foot and Ankle).

2. Neurological deficit is present. Further testing is necessary to determine whether the deficit has central or peripheral origins.

IV.   Weak and Painful

There are three interpretations of a weak and painful contraction:

1. Partial disruption of the muscle–tendon unit.

2. Pain inhibition secondary to serious pathology (inflammatory process, neoplasm, or fracture).

3. Concurrent neurological deficit.

The results of resisted muscle testing add to the emerging clinical picture. They must be correlated to the subjective findings and to the rest of the objective examination.

Neurological Examination

The neurological portion of a neuromusculoskeletal evaluation consists of a series of tests to determine if the patient's problem is caused by spinal nerve root involvement, peripheral nerve pathology, or a central nervous system lesion. Although it is an important part of any objective examination, the neurological examination is not always indicated on the initial evaluation. The clinician should look for certain clues in the subjective examination to decide if a comprehensive neurological examination is warranted.

The three most commonly used neurological tests are resisted muscle tests, light touch sensation, and deep tendon reflexes (DTR's).[1] We will also discuss

Table 2–1. Grades of Muscle Testing[8]

Name	Numerical Equivalent	Description
Normal	5	Can move the limb into the test position against gravity and resist maximal pressure
Good	4	Same as 5 but can only resist moderate pressure
Fair+	3+	Same as 4 but can only resist minimal pressure
Fair	3	Can only move the limb into the test position against gravity and hold
Fair–	3–	Same as 3 but gradual release against gravity
Poor+	2+	Can move the limb against gravity in a small ROM
Poor	2	Can move the limb in full ROM with gravity eliminated
Poor–	2–	Can only initiate ROM with gravity eliminated
Trace	1	Fasiculating or palpable muscle contraction but unable to move limb
Zero	0	No visible or palpable muscle contraction

neural tension tests, tests of spinal cord function, and nerve tissue palpation.

A neurological examination should be carried out during the initial evaluation for any patient who describes any of the following complaints:

- pain following a nerve path (radicular pain)

- numbness (loss of sensation)

- paresthesia (abnormal sensation)

- weakness (decrease or loss of muscle function)

- ataxia (poor coordination).

If neurological signs are detected during the initial evaluation, neurological testing should be performed before and after treatment during subsequent visits. Changes should be carefully documented. Progressive worsening of neurologic signs indicates serious pathology, and the patient's physician should be notified.

Neurological test findings can provide more information than which nerve or spinal level is involved.[2, 11] The present stage of the problem can be assessed by the types of sensory and motor impairment found in the objective examination (Fig 2–10). In the early stages of neurological impairment, vibration sensation is altered. As the condition progresses, there is a cutaneous hypersensitivity, followed by decreased light touch sensation. With motor testing, the initial changes will be muscle weakness and diminished reflexes, followed by muscle atrophy.

All neurological tests should be carried out completely and consistently each time to ensure their reliability and validity. This includes the position of the patient, the patient's posture, and the joint position.

Resisted Muscle Tests

Resisted muscle testing, as described in the "Strength Examination" section of this chapter, can give information about the status of a given spinal or cranial nerve. Muscles or muscle groups associated with a certain spinal or cranial nerve are commonly called myotomes (Table 2–2). In the neurological exam, muscles in each cervical myotome are tested if the patient has upper extremity symptoms; all lumbosacral myotomes are tested if the patient has lower extremity symptoms. Specific myotome testing procedures are shown in Figure 2–11.

Resisted muscle testing requires good handling skills and concise communication between clinician and patient, and the results may need interpretation. For example, pain can inhibit the generation of a strong muscle contraction, giving a false sense of muscle weakness; therefore, results of myotome tests should be correlated to other neurological examination findings and to other findings in the subjective and objective examinations.

Sensory Testing

Light touch sensation is tested to identify nervous system involvement and to help determine which nerve roots or peripheral nerves may be involved. *Dermatome* refers to the area of skin innervated by a spinal nerve. *Cutaneous nerve fields* are the areas of skin innervated by peripheral nerves. The cutaneous nerve fields and dermatome areas may contain overlapping nerve supplies (Figure 2–12). *Sclerotomes* refer to the areas of fascia or bone innervated by a specific nerve root. Neuroanatomical anomalies are common,[2] and the literature contains

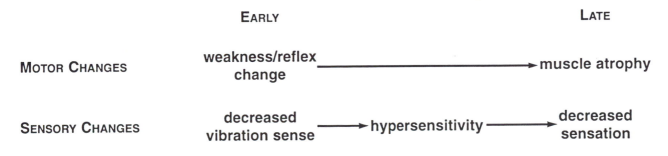

Figure 2–10. The progression of sensory and motor neurological impairment.

Table 2–2. Extremity Myotomes

Upper Limb		Lower Limb	
C1–2	cervical spine flexors	L1–2	hip flexors
C3	cervical spine side flexors	L3	knee extensors
C4	scapular elevators	L4	ankle dorsiflexors
C5	shoulder abductors	L5	great toe extensors
C6	elbow flexors and wrist extensors	S1	ankle plantar flexors/evertors knee flexors hip extensors
C7	elbow extensors and wrist flexors	S2	toe and knee flexors
C8	thumb extensors		
T1	hand intrinsics		

references to variations in dermatomal and cutaneous innervation fields; however, there are reasonable and consistent patterns that are clinically useful.

Light touch sensation is tested manually by stroking a finger over the patient's skin, or by stroking the skin with an object such as a cotton ball. The patient should be asked to state when and where the skin is being touched. The examination should be done with the patient's eyes closed, and differences should be noted when comparing A) one limb to the other; and B) different innervation fields on the same limb. These findings can be used as the basis for reassessment on follow–up examination and may help determine if the condition is worsening or improving.

It can be useful to further test the sensation component of the nerve system. This may include pin prick (superficial pain), vibration, two–point discrimination, and proprioception. These tests are

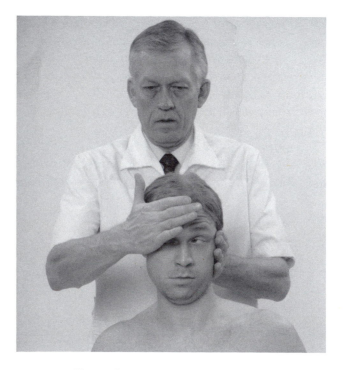

Figure 2–11A. C1: cervical rotation.

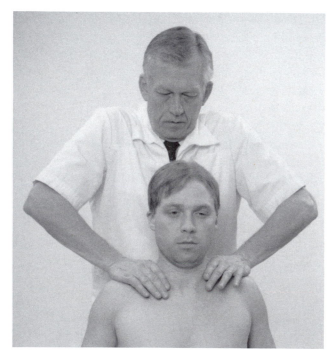

Figure 2–11B. C2–3–4: shoulder elevation.

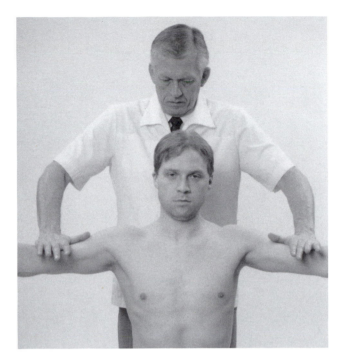

Figure 2–11C. C5: shoulder abduction.

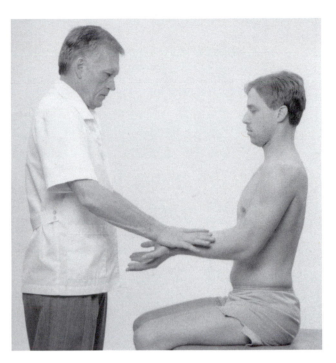

Figure 2–11D. C6: elbow flexion.

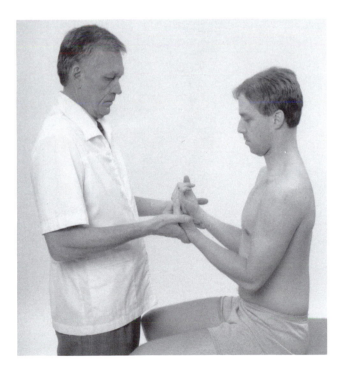

Figure 2–11E. C7: elbow extension.

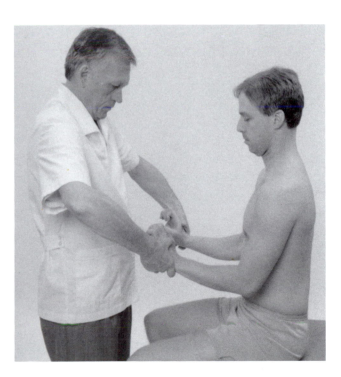

Figure 2–11F. C6: wrist extension.

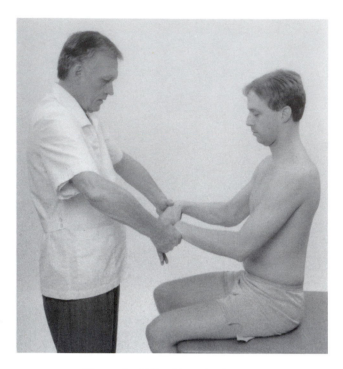

Figure 2–11G. C7: wrist flexion.

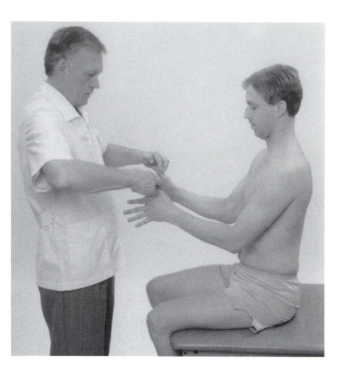

Figure 2–11H. C8: thumb extension.

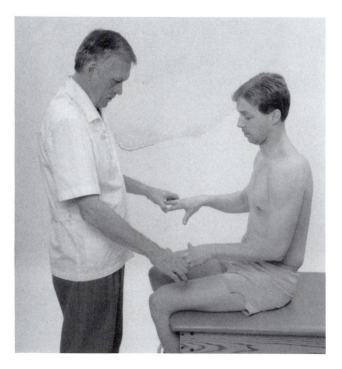

Figure 2–11I. T1: resisted finger abduction.

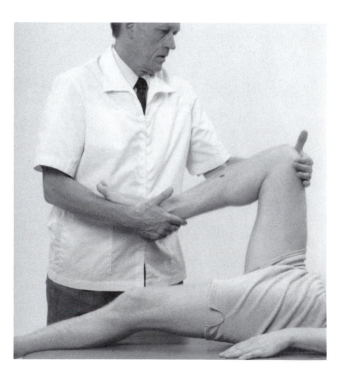

Figure 2–11J. L1–2: hip flexion.

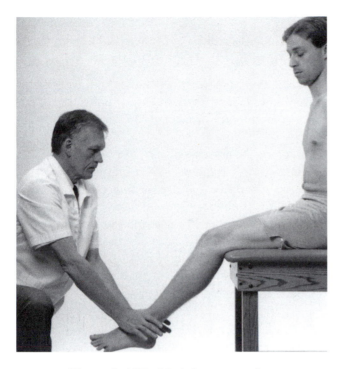

Figure 2–11K. L3–4: knee extension.

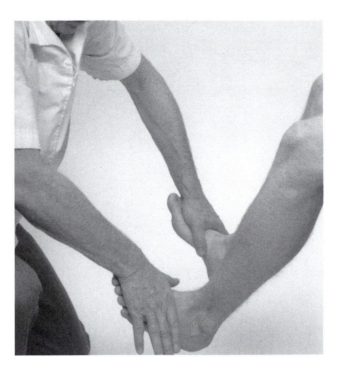

Figure 2–11L. L4–5: ankle dorsiflexion.

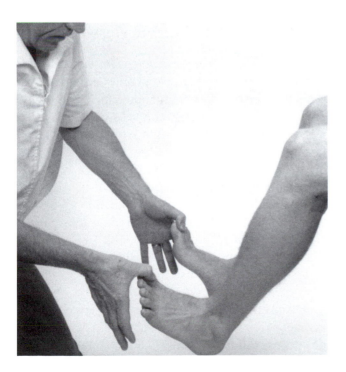

Figure 2–11M. L5: great toe extension.

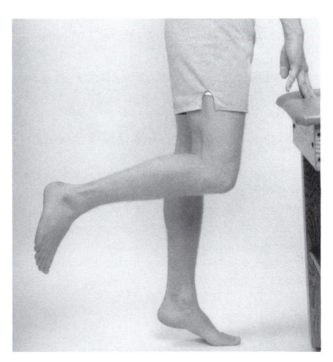

Figure 2–11N. S1–2: ankle plantar flexion.

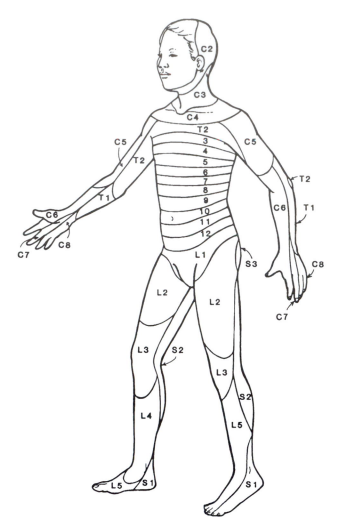

Figure 2–12A. Sensory distributions: dermatomes

- loss of reflex response – areflexia (absent)
- increased reflex response – hyperreflexia (brisk).

Generally, hyporeflexia indicates lower motor neuron injury, and hyperreflexia indicates upper motor neuron injury or disease.[2]

Bilateral comparison is also important in unilateral limb problems, and asymmetrical reflex responses should be correlated with other objective examination findings, especially other neurological examination findings. For example, weak quadriceps should be correlated with decreased knee jerk; both indicate involvement at the L3–4 spinal levels. Any significant findings should be noted and can be used as a basis for reassessment comparison.

Reliable reflex testing requires adequate patient relaxation and adequate stimulus by the clinician. The tendon to be tested should be placed in a slight stretch position. If the clinician is unable to elicit DTR's, the Jendrassik Maneuver can be used sensitize the nervous system. In the Jendrassik Maneuver, the patient is instructed to clasp the hands as shown in Figure 2–13 and pull outward while the clinician tests the reflexes. Reflex testing for the upper and lower extremities is shown in Figure 2–14.

Neural Tension Tests

Although the term "neural tension test" may be new, clinicians often perform neural tension tests to clear the neural tissues for potential pathology. Examples of the most common tests include passive neck flexion (PNF), the straight leg raise (SLR), and the prone knee bend (PKB). More recently, however, researchers have recognized the greater role that adverse mechanical neural tension (AMNT) may play in a patient's symptoms or dysfunction. Recently developed tests include the upper limb tension test (ULTT) and the Slump test. The ULTT is generally for the upper limbs and the Slump test is generally for the lower limbs and trunk.

Given that the human nervous system is a continuous tissue tract,[2] any peripheral limb movement will mechanically affect the peripheral nerve tissues and possibly the central nerve tissues. For example, the ulnar nerve is stretched when the

used at the clinician's discretion. Other texts have useful guidelines for specific neurological testing.[2]

Deep Tendon Reflex (DTR) Tests

DTR testing gives the clinician information about the integrity of the nerve roots and nerves that supply the tendon being tested. The tendon should be tapped six times to establish response reliability.[2] This repeated tapping lets the clinician detect a fading reflex response, which may indicate a developing nerve root lesion.

Common findings include:

- decreased reflex response – hyporeflexia (sluggish)

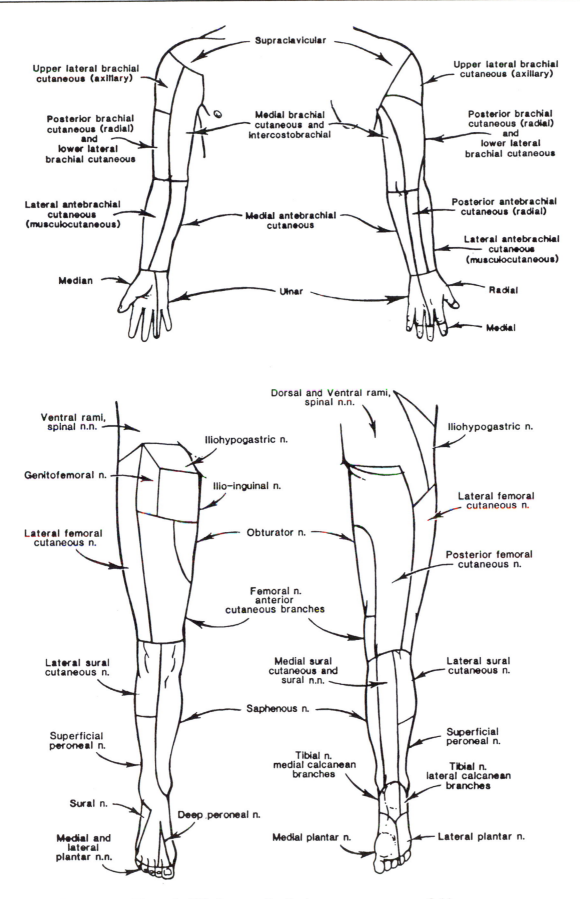

Figure 2–12B. Sensory distributions: cutaneous nerve fields

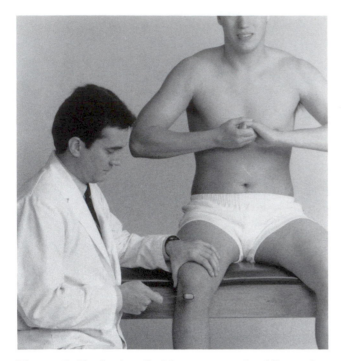

Figure 2–13. Jendrassik Maneuver used while testing knee jerk.

elbow is flexed, while the median and radial nerves are shortened. Apparently the human body normally provides built–in protection for the neural tissues during movement to ensure continued chemical and electrical neural conduction. It seems appropriate, then, that an examination of the response of the neural

tissues to mechanical stresses should be included in a complete examination of the spine or extremities.

Symptoms related to mechanical deformation of the nervous system can result from three processes:[2]

1. Interruption of blood supply to neural tissues.

2. Interruption of axonal transport systems.

3. Irritation of the connective tissues of the nervous system.

There are also many mechanical tissue interfaces where neural tissue mobility may be affected. These may be myofascial, bony, or ligamentous. For example, the posterior interosseus branch of the radial nerve pierces the supinator muscle (myofascial), the ulnar nerve rests in the ulnar groove (bony), and the median nerve lies under the transverse carpal ligament (ligamentous). The clinician should consider these interfaces as possible causes of decreased neural tissue mobility and as possibly related to symptom provocation in the peripheral limbs.

Research is implicating AMNT in many neuromusculoskeletal disorders. Recent clinical studies have linked positive neural tension tests to various peripheral limb symptoms,[2] so any patient

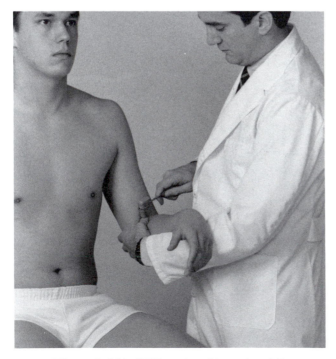

Figure 2–14A. DTR testing: biceps brachii.

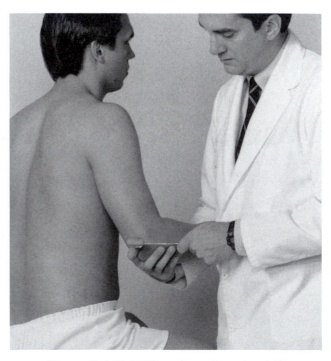

Figure 2–14B. DTR testing: triceps brachii.

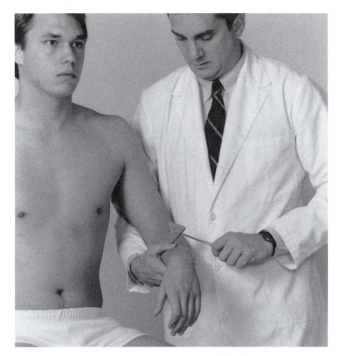

Figure 2–14C. DTR testing: brachioradialis.

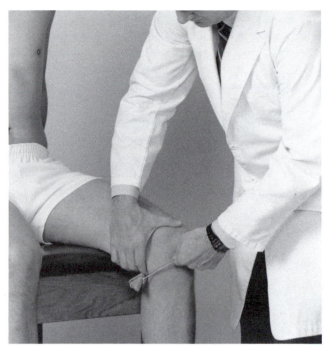

Figure 2–14D. DTR testing: medial hamstring.

presenting with non–irritable symptoms where there may be a potential neural tension component should be examined for AMNT. This includes any patient complaining of central or peripheral symptoms where the symptoms cannot be clearly traced to a non–AMNT source.

Administration of, contraindications to, normal responses to, and interpretation of neural tension tests are at the end of this chapter in an addendum (see "Addendum: Neural Tension Testing," on page 32). The definitive resource on this subject: *Mobilization of the Nervous System* by David S. Butler.[2]

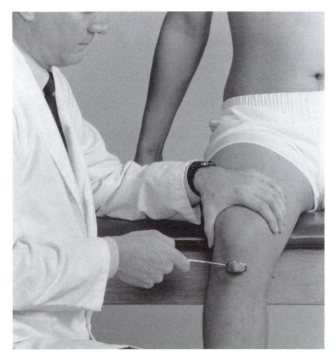

Figure 2–14E. DTR testing: knee jerk.

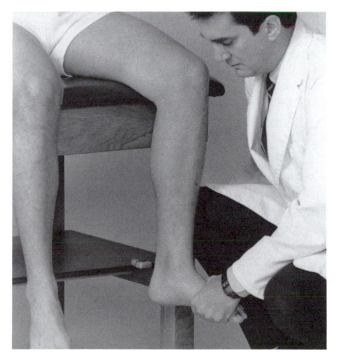

Figure 2–14F. DTR testing: ankle jerk.

In summary, neural tension disorders should be considered a potential contributing factor in the patient's complete clinical picture. Neural tension testing is included in this text because it is an exciting area of clinical research and a potential factor in many clinical disorders the clinician sees. Knowledge in this area is evolving; scientifically designed clinical and anatomical studies should provide valuable information about AMNT.

Spinal Cord Function (Upper Motor Neuron Testing)

Two essential tests to screen for spinal cord signs are ankle clonus and Babinski's Test.

Ankle clonus is tested by positioning the leg in mild knee flexion and rapidly dorsiflexing the ankle. The normal response to this movement is no response. The test is positive if there is cogwheel rigidity (clonus).

Babinski's Test is performed by stroking the plantar aspect of the foot with a blunt instrument. The stroke is begun at the heel, moves along the lateral border of the foot, and crosses over the ball of the foot to the base of the great toe. The test is positive if there is dorsiflexion of the great toe and fanning of the other toes (Fig 2–15). A normal finding is either an absent response or flexion of all toes.

A positive Ankle Clonus Test or Babinski's Test indicates possible upper motor neuron impairment.

Palpation and Tapping

Tinel describes tapping a superficial peripheral nerve to identify nerve involvement (Fig 2–16).[18] A "tingling" sensation is often reproduced in the distribution of the nerve being tapped. Direct palpation of a superficial nerve can also be useful. Nerve tenderness is common at a site of entrapment,[16] and enlargement or thickening can often be palpated in entrapped nerves.[17] Results should be interpreted carefully, as positive tests can sometimes be found in normal subjects.[12]

The peripheral nerves can be palpated to implicate nerve system injury, entrapment, or AMNT.[2] The nerves are susceptible to trauma at these sites. Palpation may provide information about the

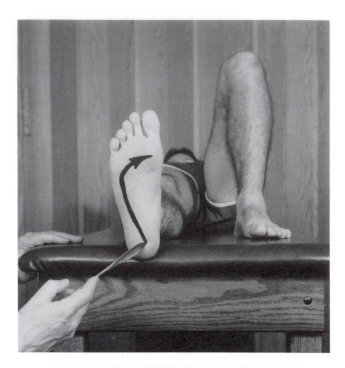

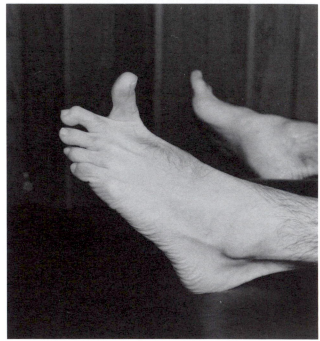

Figure 2–15. Babinski's Test. A positive result is great toe extension with fanning (abduction and slight flexion) of the other toes.

nerve's contribution to the patient's signs and symptoms.

Palpation Examination

Pain or tenderness felt on palpation can often be misleading. Palpation findings must be correlated

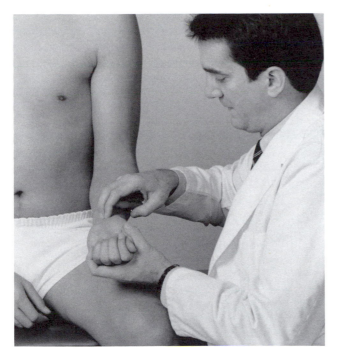

Figure 2–16. Testing for Tinel's Sign over the median nerve.

with the rest of the examination. The clinician should not overemphasize the significance of palpation, tenderness, or crepitus.

Palpation should be performed using the "layered" approach. With layered palpation, the clinician assesses the joint or limb starting with the skin, then moving deeper to the fascia, muscle, and joint. The clinician's overall goal is to gain a "feel" for the tissues for comparison to the uninvolved joint or limbs he or she has palpated. Palpation can also elicit a symptom response. Generally, the uninvolved joint or limb is palpated first for comparison to the involved side. Palpation depth is guided by the SIN noted in the subjective examination. The following is a guide to performing and interpreting layered palpation.

Skin

The patient's sensitivity to light touch should be checked first. Symptoms provoked by light stroking may indicate dysesthesia. Any changes in *moisture* and *texture* should be noted, whether moist and smooth or dry and scaly. Findings here may reflect changes in sympathetic activity consistent with a reflex sympathetic dystrophy (RSD). *Temperature* changes should also be noted. Elevated temperatures

may indicate reduced sympathetic activity, an inflammatory process, or an infection in a post–operative incision or post–traumatic wound. A reduction in skin temperature may reflect problems with increased sympathetic activity or vascular insufficiency. Finally, the clinician should feel for skin *mobility*. Incisions and post–traumatic wounds commonly develop adhesions during healing and should always be checked.

Myofascial Soft Tissues

Benign fatty tumors or lipomas are common. The clinician can often feel myofascial restriction that can be correlated with the patient's problems and symptoms.[14] Soft tissue mobility can be assessed with skin–rolling—picking up the skin and rolling it between the fingers and the thumb (Fig 2–17). Any symptom provocation or lack of mobility may indicate an underlying myofascial lesion. A working knowledge of the underlying tissue structure and direction of muscle fibers is necessary to fully appreciate this level of palpation.

In cases of traumatic injury, it may be possible to palpate the effects of trauma (e.g., ruptured tendon, torn muscle belly). The clinician may detect tendon thickening—often a response to chronic stress, inflammation, or edema. Pain to touch in the muscle

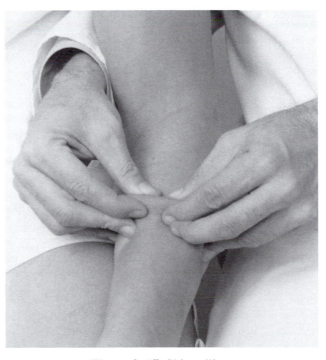

Figure 2–17. Skin rolling.

itself can indicate a muscle strain or contusion. Hypersensitive areas palpated in the muscle may correlate with "trigger points" or "muscle hardenings" that give rise to pain in specific patterns when the areas are palpated. [19, 20, 21]

Other Soft Tissues

Bursæ should be palpated to determine their responses to touch. Palpation may provoke pain, but it must be correlated to the patient's problems and symptoms. Bursæ can sometimes refer pain.

Joints

The structures attaching to and surrounding specific joints should be palpated. The capsule and its normal thickenings (such as ligaments or a retinaculum) should be felt and distinguished from abnormal thickenings (e.g., plicæ). Joint palpation findings are especially important in the acute injury, where pain and tenderness can be caused by ligament sprain or capsule injury. These findings should correlate with passive mobility testing and ligamentous stress testing for signs of instability.

Joint effusion should be palpated and compared to the uninvolved side. Swelling can be measured volumetrically or circumferentially to assess treatment effectiveness.

It is important to distinguish between localized edema and a more generalized swelling. General limb edema can indicate vascular insufficiency secondary to lymphatic blockage or a blood clot. Chronic edema feels firmer and thicker than acute edema, sometimes being described as a "woody" feeling.

Lastly, the bony structures should be palpated. The attachments of ligaments and tendons to the bones should be palpated, as should the bone itself. The bone should be percussed, noting any focal tenderness. Bony enlargements may be caused by DJD or may accompany fracture healing. Post–traumatic deformities in the bone itself or at the joint should be documented and correlated with the medical history. Focal tenderness to palpation or sensitivity to vibration can indicate a stress fracture. [15]

Crepitus

The significance of palpable crepitus and audible joint noise is not readily agreed on. Clinically, two conditions should be noted.

1. *Joint crepitus palpated in an acute injury.* A fracture must be ruled out.

2. *Joint noise associated with increasing symptoms.* This should not be ignored because it may represent serious pathology.

Sources of joint crepitus may be:

- Movement of tendons or sheaths against other anatomical structures

- Roughness or thickening of tendons or tendon sheaths

- Calcification in tendons

- Articular cartilage degeneration

- Cartilage tears or internal derangement

Special Tests

This last section of the examination can be considered a catch–basin of neuromusculoskeletal tests. Special tests are used to differentiate between possible causes of the patient's symptoms.

The specific special tests for each joint will be discussed in its corresponding chapter. With the special tests, it is sometimes possible to determine which structure causes the patient's problem. For example, a runner with complaints of pain at the lateral knee could have iliotibial band (ITB) syndrome or a problem with the lateral collateral ligament (LCL). Special tests for each of these structures help the clinician distinguish between these conditions.

Doctor's Report, Lab, and X–ray

On completion of the evaluation, the clinician correlates the subjective and objective findings with other information that is available, such as the doctor's reports, x–rays, lab and other tests. To ensure the evaluation is done without bias, this correlation should be done at the conclusion of the evaluation instead of at the beginning. Knowledge of any severe pathology is, of course, important and should be considered immediately.

PROBLEM LIST

Based on the subjective and objective examination findings, the clinician develops an initial problem list. The problem list helps the clinician in three ways: 1) it reminds the clinician of the patient's problems so that each is addressed in treatment; 2) it is used to prioritize treatment; and 3) it aids goal setting and treatment planning. The problem list bridges the gap between the patient's subjective complaints and the objective examination findings. Based on the problems identified, the clinician develops goals for therapy, and plans treatments to reach those goals. Goal setting and treatment planning are addressed in Chapter 3, <u>Pathology and Treatment Principles</u>.

Physical therapy problems can be of three types: symptomatic, physical, and functional. *Symptomatic* problems are the symptoms identified in the subjective examination and provoked during the objective examination. *Physical* problems are objective findings that are abnormal and problematic for the patient. A physical problem might be decreased range of motion, or muscle weakness. *Functional* problems are the work or leisure limitations the patient experiences as a result of the physical problem. Functional problems are very specific to the patient's work and recreational demands and are stated in terms of activities meaningful to the patient. For example, a teacher with limited shoulder flexion may be unable to write on the chalkboard—a functional problem. A soccer player with weakness in the anterior tibialis may be unable to run or kick. A secretary with carpal tunnel syndrome (CTS) may have pain or numbness brought on by finger movements, leading to an inability to tolerate typing.

SYMPTOM MAGNIFICATION

It should be noted that physical therapists as a group sometimes fall victim to manipulative patients who have secondary gain, conversion syndromes, or other psychophysiologic reasons for their complaints. While no one can deny that psychological and emotional factors can significantly influence a

patient's perception of pain and actually increase muscular tension, the clinician must be aware that these factors can influence a patient's response to treatment.

The "M–A–D–I–S–O–N" mnemonic provides a guide for identifying psychophysiologic factors:

M Multiplicity. When one symptom goes, another one comes. The patient presents a history of bizarre or non–organic symptoms in multiplicity.

A Authenticity. The patient seems more concerned with convincing the clinician that the symptoms are real than with the symptoms themselves.

D Denial. The patient refuses to consider the possibility that these symptoms may be psychogenic.

I Interpersonal variation. Symptoms get better when the patient is having fun and worse when a professional is around.

S Strangeness. No one else has ever had anything exactly like this patient has.

O Only you can help! Patients are setting the clinician up for a fall. "All those other doctors before you were incompetent, but you'll figure out what it is."

N Never varies. Symptoms are always terrible and are theatrically described with superlatives.

When psychophysiological factors are suspected or when the patient appears to be magnifying symptoms, treatment should still be initiated if the patient has objective physical findings that correlate with his or her complaints. But the clinician should beware of a prolonged course of passive treatments with such a patient, especially when the patient's condition is not improving. Treatment that emphasizes self–responsibility and functional restoration is most appropriate.

SUMMARY

This chapter has presented the general features of subjective and objective examinations. An integrated approach to patient evaluation, as presented here, lets the clinician apply the examination appropriately to each patient's unique clinical picture of presenting signs and symptoms.

Objective examination findings should confirm subjective examination findings. If the signs and symptoms don't "fit," then there are several questions to be asked:

- Were the right questions asked?

- Was the objective examination thorough and appropriate?

- Were screens for serious pathology (medical disease, non–mechanical features, inflammatory processes, etc.) performed?

- Are symptom magnification or unexplained inconsistencies in the patient's examination present?

After common sense and clinical reasoning have been applied to the information obtained, the clinician can decide on the appropriate therapeutic intervention.

ADDENDUM:
NEURAL TENSION TESTING

Contraindications to Neural Tension Testing

Neural tissue is by nature highly irritable; therefore, neural tension testing is usually not indicated for severe, irritable, inflammatory, or pathological disorders. The tests should be performed carefully.

Contraindications to neural tension testing and treatment include:

1. Irritable conditions

2. Inflammatory conditions

3. Spinal cord signs

4. Malignancy

5. Nerve root compression signs

6. Severe, unremitting night pain

7. Neurological signs (including weakness, reflex changes, or true numbness)

8. Recent paresthesia or anesthesia

9. Active spinal motions that easily provoke distal symptoms, paresthesia, or anesthesia

10. Reflex sympathetic dystrophy

Performance of Neural Tension Tests

- Before beginning, carefully identify all the patient's symptoms.

- Note which symptoms are present in the starting position.

- Carefully note any *onset or change* of symptoms at each step of the test.

- Move the patient's limb in each step to the point of *onset or change* of symptoms.

As with any neuromusculoskeletal test, reassessment will help the clinician decide if treatment is effective. To compare later findings, the clinician must document the following thoroughly:

- the range of motion at which the symptoms first appear

- the nature and location of the symptoms

- any abnormal resistance felt during the test

Passive Neck Flexion (PNF)

The PNF test is indicated for all spinal disorders and any headaches or extremity complaints that may be of spinal origin. To perform the test, the patient can be supine, sitting, or standing. The clinician passively induces neck flexion. Symptom response, range of motion, and any resistance to movement should be noted (Fig 2–18).

PNF should be painless, although occasionally there is a "pulling" sensation in the cervicothoracic junction. PNF can be combined with other tension tests such as the SLR to reproduce functional postures

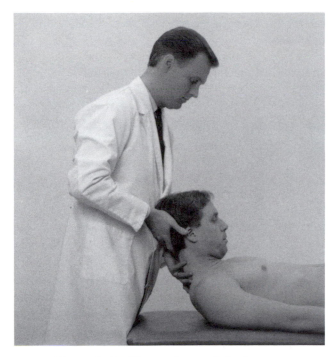

Figure 2–18. The passive neck flexion test.

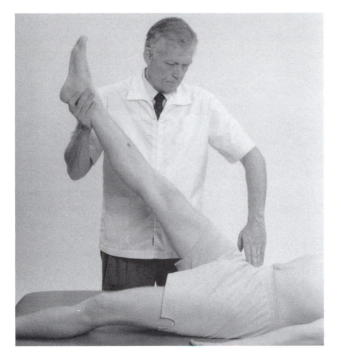

Figure 2–19. The straight leg raise test.

and to assess the effect of combined neural tension on symptoms.

Straight Leg Raise (SLR)

The SLR is the most neural common tension test. It is indicated for patients presenting with any spinal or lower limb complaints.

The SLR is traditionally performed to determine if there is compromise of the nerve roots or irritation of the sciatic nerve (radiculitis). The clinician must be aware that *any* acute, painful condition in the lumbar spine or sacroiliac may be irritated by the SLR. Tight hamstring muscles, hip joint pathology, or sacroiliac joint pathology also can cause a painful response to the SLR. An adherent nerve root will cause a positive SLR. Piriformis syndrome also can be irritated by the SLR. Considering all the variables associated with this test, the clinician must interpret findings carefully. Differentiation tests can help the clinician distinguish true radiculitis from other neuromusculoskeletal conditions.

The patient is supine for the SLR. The clinician raises the patient's leg while making sure the knee remains straight (Fig 2–19). As the straight leg is raised, progressive tension is applied to the sciatic

nerve, which in turn places tension on the nerve roots. If there is compromise or irritation of the nerve roots, symptoms will be exacerbated. If the test increases pain in the posterior thigh, it may not be a positive neurological sign but may still be a significant clinical finding.

The clinician should palpate the anterior superior iliac spine (ASIS) for the first sign of movement into posterior rotation. Posterior rotation of the pelvis is caused by hamstring tension. It helps to do hold-relax stretching of the hamstring muscle to distinguish between true nerve root signs and tight hamstrings. If hold-relax stretching seems to increase the range of motion, the pain and restriction are probably in the hamstring. If the hold-relax technique does not seem to change the pain or restriction, spinal nerve root impingement or irritation may be involved. The hold-relax technique is not advised for patients presenting with a positive SLR at <30° hip flexion as it may provoke an irritable condition.

The bowstring test is a useful variation of the SLR. The clinician flexes the patient's hip and knee to 90°. With one hand, the clinician palpates the sciatic nerve in the popliteal fossa. When the nerve is located, the clinician extends the knee to the point of hamstring tightness and then presses the sciatic nerve with the other hand, which causes increased neural tissue tension (Fig 2–20). If pain is produced proximally, this may be a sign of nerve root irritation.

Lasegue's sign helps further differentiate true nerve root signs. After the clinician raises the leg to the point of symptom onset, the leg is lowered 1/2 to 1 inch. The stress to all structures, including the nerve roots, should be relieved. With the leg stationary, the foot is then dorsiflexed. This applies tension to the nerve roots without affecting the other structures (hamstring, sacroiliac joint, and hip joint). Exacerbation of pain on foot dorsiflexion is the Lasegue's sign of true radiculitis.[15]

Other differentiation tests can be useful. Adding neck flexion, ankle dorsiflexion, hip rotation, or hip adduction can alter the tension applied and the symptom response. When the head is flexed, the dura is pulled superiorly, putting an added tension on the spinal nerve root, which may increase a positive sign of the SLR.

Normally, the positive SLR suggests more severe pathology when positive at 20°-40° of hip flexion and less severe pathology if positive at 50°-70°. It is difficult to interpret an SLR >70° as positive for radiculitis. The degree of hip flexion present when the symptoms occur should be recorded so the clinician can decide during reassessment whether progress has been made.

Raising the opposite leg occasionally provokes symptoms. This may suggest a disc herniation with protrusion medial to the nerve root. If raising the opposite leg relieves symptoms, a bulge lateral to the nerve root may be present.

Prone Knee Bend (PKB)

The PKB is akin to the SLR, with the PKB putting selective tension on the upper lumbar segments. If the patient has complaints in the upper lumbar spine or in the L1-4 dermatomal region, a femoral nerve stretch test (PKB) should be done. As the femoral nerve is stretched by flexing the knee and hyperextending the hip, the nerve roots L1, 2, and 3 are stretched across their respective intervertebral foramen. If there is reduced mobility or impingement of one of these spinal nerve roots, the symptoms will increase as this test is done. The clinician must distinguish between a painful quadriceps muscle and a true nerve root sign. If nerve root impingement is present, the symptoms may extend into the lateral aspect of the hip, into the upper lumbar spine, or into the anterior thigh.

The PKB is simply passive knee flexion with the patient lying prone (Fig 2–21). Symptom response,

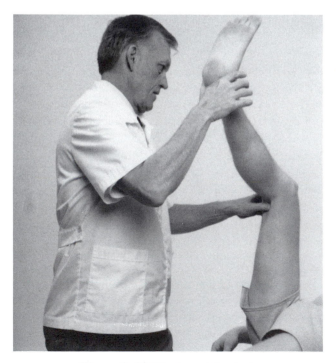

Figure 2–20. The bowstring test.

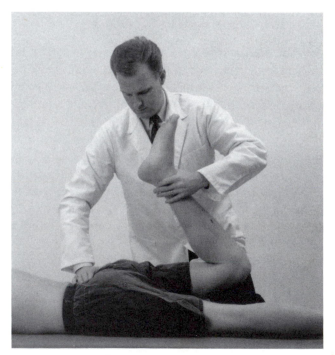

Figure 2–21. The prone knee bend test.

range of motion, and resistance to movement should be noted and compared to the contralateral side. The normal response for the PKB is not well documented; however, common clinical findings include a "stretching" sensation in the rectus femoris and an anterior pelvic tilt with an increase in lumbar lordosis.

Upper Limb Tension Test (ULTT)

Base ULTT

The basic ULTT is performed as follows:[2]

1.   Cervical spine neutral. The patient lies supine on the treatment table, close to the edge of the side being tested, with the cervical spine in neutral. The clinician faces the patient and supports the upper extremity at the wrist.

2.   Shoulder girdle depression. The clinician depresses the shoulder girdle by reaching under the scapula and pulling it caudally. This position is sustained throughout the rest of the procedure. Any change or onset in symptoms should be noted (Fig 2–22).

3.   Glenohumeral abduction. The clinician grasps the patient's elbow and abducts the shoulder.

The patient's upper arm should be supported on the clinician's thigh (Fig 2–23).

4.   Wrist and finger extension, forearm supination. Maintaining the position in step three, wrist and finger extension are added (Fig 2–24).

5.   Glenohumeral external rotation. While steps 1-4 are maintained, the clinician externally rotates the glenohumeral joint to ≈60° (Fig 2–25).

6.   Elbow extension. The clinician extends the patient's elbow to the point of resistance or symptom onset (Fig 2–26).

7.   Cervical sidebending. The patient is then asked to sidebend the cervical spine away from the limb being examined (Fig 2–27). This is followed by sidebending to the same side.

Each step must be maintained during the test as steps are added. The onset or change of symptoms or resistance should be identified and recorded after each step. Both upper limbs should be examined.

Other ULTT's increase tension in a selected upper extremity nerve. These tests include the median nerve, radial nerve, and ulnar nerve bias tests.

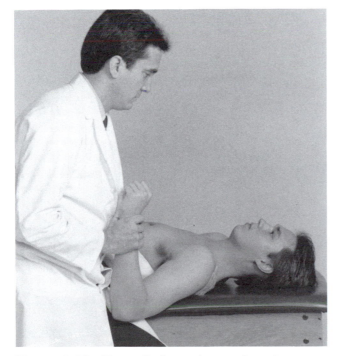

Figure 2–22. Upper limb tension testing—base test. Shoulder girdle depression.

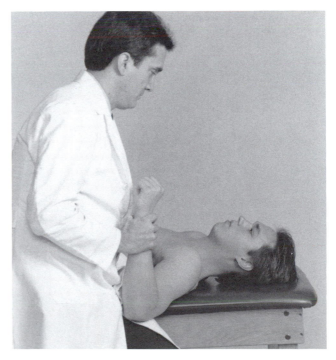

Figure 2–23. Upper limb tension testing—base test. Glenohumeral abduction.

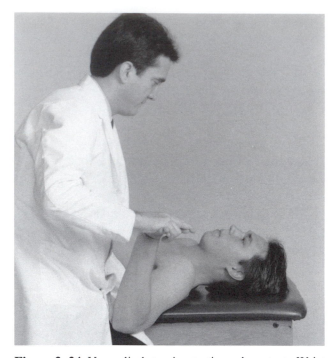

Figure 2–24. Upper limb tension testing—base test. Wrist and finger extension, forearm supination.

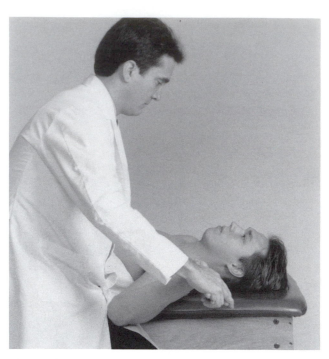

Figure 2–25. Upper limb tension testing—base test. Glenohumeral external rotation.

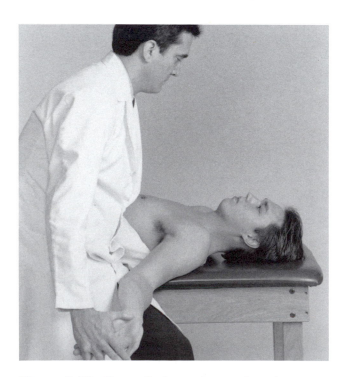

Figure 2–26. Upper limb tension testing—base test. Elbow extension.

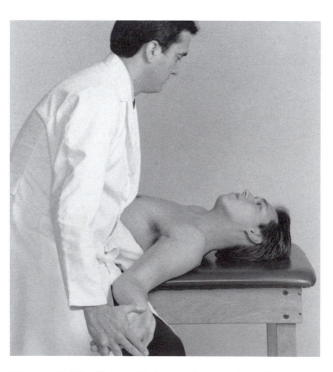

Figure 2–27. Upper limb tension testing—base test. Cervical sidebending.

Median Nerve Bias ULTT

1. Cervical spine neutral. The patient lies diagonally across the table with the scapula free (off the table) and the cervical spine in neutral. The clinician's thigh rests on the examination table, just above the shoulder being tested. The clinician supports the patient's elbow and wrist (Fig 2–28).

2. Shoulder girdle depression. The clinician uses the thigh to gently depress the shoulder girdle, maintaining the arm in about 10° abduction (Fig 2–29).

3. Elbow extension. The clinician maintains shoulder depression while extending the elbow.

4. Glenohumeral external rotation. The clinician externally rotates the shoulder (Fig 2–30).

5. Wrist and finger extension. Maintaining the position in step four, wrist and finger extension are added.

6. Glenohumeral Abduction. The shoulder is moved into abduction to the point of resistance (Fig 2–31).

7. Cervical sidebending. The patient is then asked to sidebend away from the limb being examined.

Radial Nerve Bias ULTT

1. Cervical spine neutral. The patient lies diagonally across the table with the scapula free (off the table) and the cervical spine in neutral. The clinician's thigh rests on the examination table, just above the shoulder being tested. The clinician supports the patient's elbow and wrist as shown (Fig 2–28).

2. Shoulder girdle depression. Testing, the clinician uses the thigh to gently depress the shoulder girdle, maintaining the arm in about 10° abduction (Figure 2–29).

3. Glenohumeral internal rotation. The arm is internally rotated and the forearm pronated.

4. Wrist and finger flexion. Maintaining the position in step three, the wrist and fingers are flexed (Fig 2–32).

5. Glenohumeral abduction. Maintaining the position in step four, the shoulder is abducted (Fig 2–33).

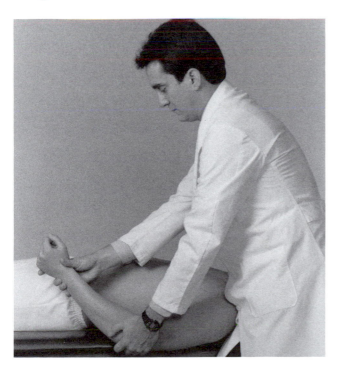

Figure 2–28. Upper limb tension testing—median and radial nerve bias. Start position.

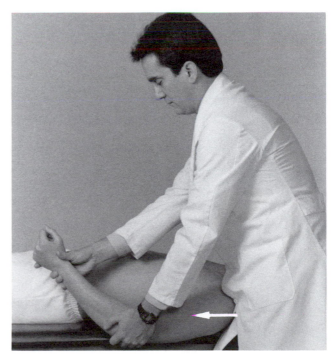

Figure 2–29. Upper limb tension testing—Median and Radial Nerve Bias. Shoulder girdle depression.

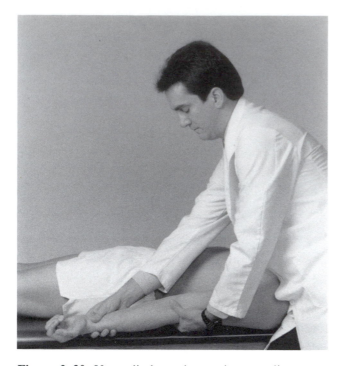

Figure 2–30. Upper limb tension testing—median nerve bias. Elbow extension; glenohumeral external rotation.

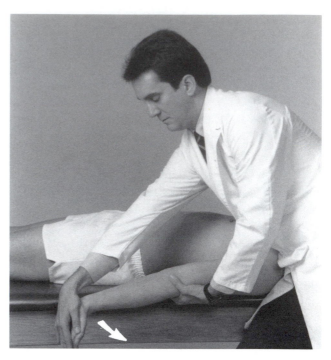

Figure 2–31. Upper limb tension testing—median nerve bias. Wrist and finger extension; glenohumeral abduction.

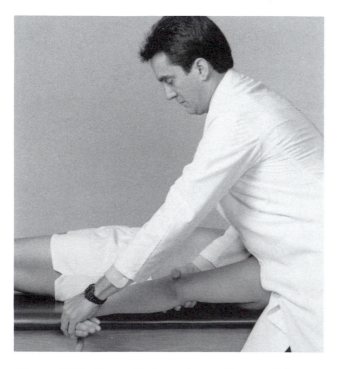

Figure 2–32. Upper limb tension testing—radial nerve bias. Glenohumeral internal rotation; wrist and finger flexion.

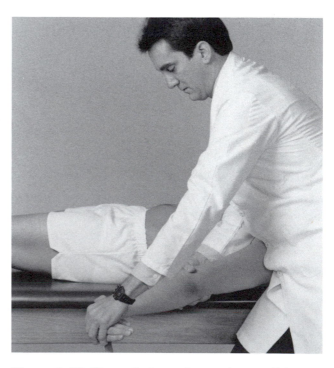

Figure 2–33. Upper limb tension testing—radial nerve bias. Glenohumeral abduction.

6. Cervical sidebending. Maintaining the position in step five, contralateral cervical sidebending is added.

Ulnar Nerve Bias ULTT

1. Cervical spine neutral. The patient lies supine on the treatment table, close to the edge of the side being tested, with the cervical spine in neutral. The clinician faces the patient, supporting the upper extremity at the wrist.

2. Wrist extension and forearm supination. The clinician extends the wrist and supinates the forearm (NOTE: research suggests pronation may be more sensitive than supination).[22]

3. Elbow flexion. The elbow is flexed while maintaining the wrist and forearm position (Fig 2–34).

4. Shoulder girdle depression. Maintaining the position in step 3, the clinician uses the opposite hand to depress the shoulder.

5. Glenohumeral external rotation. Maintaining the position in step four, the shoulder is externally rotated (Fig 2–35).

6. Glenohumeral Abduction. Maintaining the position in step five, the arm is moved into abduction (Fig 2–36).

7. Cervical sidebending. Maintaining the position in step six, the patient is asked to sidebend the cervical spine away from the side being tested.

Slump Test

The Slump test is a relatively new neural tension test. It combines the sitting SLR, the PNF, and a slump or slouch of the lumbar spine in sitting. This test was first developed and researched by Maitland in 1979.[12] The test is indicated for patients with low back pain or lower limb complaints.

The Slump test is performed as follows:

1. The patient sits comfortably at the end of an examination table.

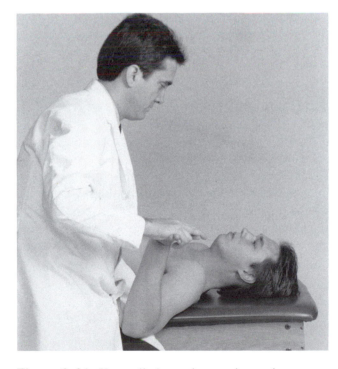

Figure 2–34. Upper limb tension testing—ulnar nerve bias. Wrist extension and forearm supination; elbow flexion.

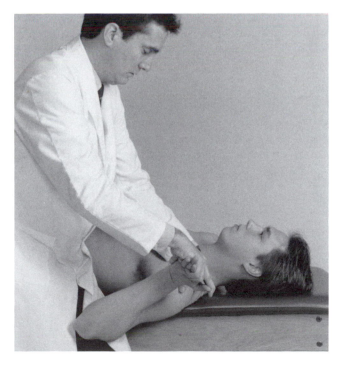

Figure 2–35. Upper limb tension testing—ulnar nerve bias. Shoulder girdle depression; glenohumeral external rotation.

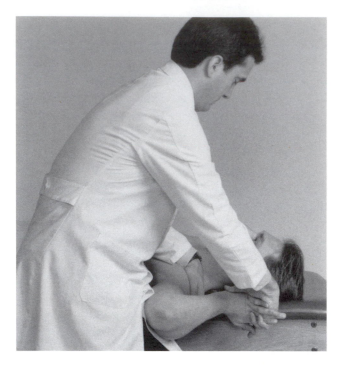

Figure 2–36. Upper limb tension testing—ulnar nerve bias. Glenohumeral abduction.

2.   The clinician asks the patient to slump or slouch. This is sustained by the clinician (Fig 2–37).

3.   The patient performs neck flexion (Fig 2–37B).

4.   While sustaining neck flexion, the clinician asks the patient to straighten either leg (Fig 2–37C).

5.   The clinician then asks the patient to dorsiflex the ankle of the straight leg (Fig 2–37D).

6.   The neck flexion is released to neutral, and any change in symptoms is noted (Fig 2–37E).

7.   The test is repeated with the opposite leg.

8.   The test is repeated with both legs at once (Fig 2–37F).

Normal Responses to the ULTT and Slump Tests

Normal responses for the ULTT base test have been identified in a recent study of 400 subjects without pathology or complaints.[9]

- deep ache or stretch in the cubital fossa (99% of subjects) extending down the anterior and radial forearm into the radial hand (80% of subjects)

- a definite tingling in the thumb and first three fingers

- a stretch feeling in the anterior shoulder area (small percentage of subjects)

- increased responses with cervical sidebending away from the tested side (90% of subjects)

- decreased responses with cervical sidebending toward the tested side (70% of subjects)

Normal responses to the Slump test are:

- When the patient initially slumps, no complaints are usually offered.

- When the neck is passively flexed, 50% of subjects report a stretch in the T8-T9 area.

- When the leg is straightened, there is a symmetrical limitation of range bilaterally and a stretch feeling in the posterior hamstring and knee.

- A symmetrical restriction of dorsiflexion is normal.

- A release of the neck flexion may increase the available range of dorsiflexion at the ankle.

Interpreting Results of Neural Tension Tests

Normal responses to the ULTT and Slump tests should be reviewed to avoid false positives. The clinician must be careful when deciding whether the results of neural tension tests are positive or whether they are a normal response to stretching neural tissues. Bilateral results should always be compared.

Generally, a neural tension test is positive if:

- it reproduces the patient's symptoms

- the test response can be altered by moving distant body parts that alter neural tissue tension alone. For example, when the patient is in the ULTT position, the symptoms are

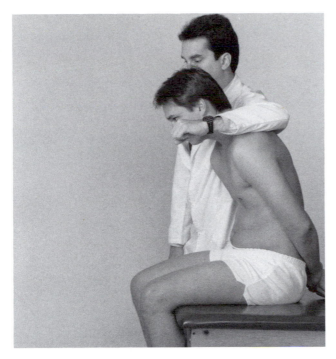

Figure 2–37A. The Slump test. Slump sitting with overpressure.

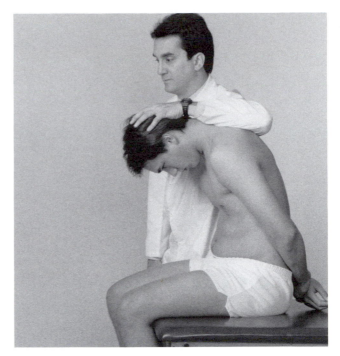

Figure 2–37B. The Slump test. Passive neck flexion.

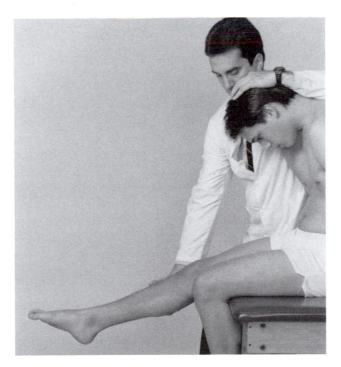

Figure 2–37C. The Slump test. Knee extension.

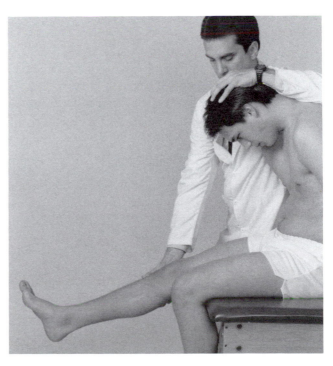

Figure 2–37D. The Slump test. Ankle dorsiflexion.

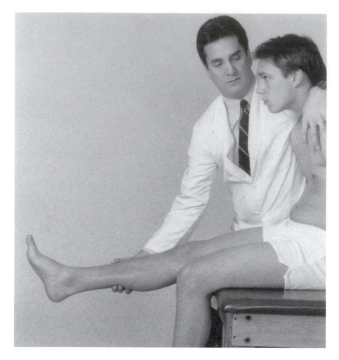

Figure 2–37E. The Slump test. Cervical release.

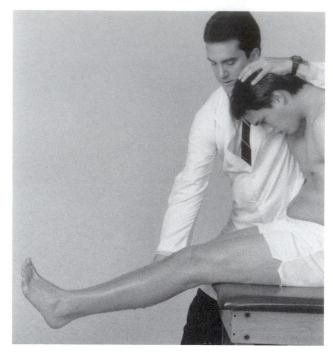

Figure 2–37F. The Slump test. Bilateral Slump test.

changed by isolated movement of the wrist or cervical spine

• the test response differs from side to side

Any symptoms or decreased mobility findings should fit with other clinical findings. Any pathological process that causes less space for neural tissue to slide freely will produce an earlier onset of symptoms with the neural tension tests.

REFERENCES

1. Boissonnault W, Janos S: Screening For Medical Disease: Physical Therapy Assessment and Treatment Principles. Examination in Physical Therapy Practice: Screening For Medical Disease. Churchill-Livingstone, New York NY 1991.

2. Butler D: Mobilisation of the Nervous System. Churchill-Livingstone, Melbourne Australia 1991.

3. Cyriax J: Diagnosis of Soft Tissue Lesions. Textbook of Orthopædic Medicine, Vol 1, 8th edition. Bailliere-Tindall, London 1982.

4. Hertling D and Kessler RM: Management of Common Musculoskeletal Disorders, 2nd ed. JB Lippincott, Philadelphia PA 1990.

5. Jones M, Butler D: Clinical Reasoning. Mobilisation of the Nervous System. D Butler, ed. Churchill-Livingstone, Melbourne Australia 1991.

6. Kaltenborn F: Manual Therapy of the Extremity Joints, 4th ed. Olaf Norlis Bokhandel, Oslo 1989.

7. Keating J, Matyas T, Bach T: The Effect of Training on Physical Therapists' Ability to Apply Specific Forces of Palpation. Physical Therapy 73(1):38-45, 1993.

8. Kendall F and McCreary E: Muscles: Testing and Function. Williams and Wilkins, Baltimore MD 1983.

9. Kenneally M, et al: "The Upper Limb Tension Test: The Straight Leg Raise Test of the Arm." In Physical Therapy of the Cervical and Thoracic Spine, Vol 17 of Clinics in Physical Therapy. R Grant, ed. Churchill-Livingstone, Edinburgh 1989.

10. Lee M, Mosely A, Refshauge K: Effect of Feedback on Learning a Vertebral Joint Mobilization Skill. Physical Therapy 70:97-104, 1990.

11. MacKinnon SE, Dellon AL: Surgery of the Peripheral Nerve. Thieme, New York NY 1988.

12. Maitland GD: Negative Disc Exploration: Positive Canal Signs. Australian Journal of Physiotherapy 25:129-134, 1979.

13. Maitland G: Vertebral Manipulation, 5th edition. Butterworth, London 1986.

14. Manheim CJ, Lavett D: The Myofascial Release Manual. Slack, Thorofare NJ 1989.

15. Roy S, Irving R: Sports Medicine: Prevention, Evaluation, Management, and Rehabilitation. Prentice Hall, Englewood Cliffs NJ 1983.

16. Saal JA, et al: The Pseudoradicular Syndrome. Spine 13:926-930, 1988.

17. Thomas PK: Clinical Features and Differential Diagnosis. In Peripheral Neuropathy, Vol 2, 2nd ed. PJ Dyck, et al (ed). WB Saunders, Philadelphia PA 1984.

18. Tinel J: Le signe du fourmillent dans les lesions des nerfs peripheriques. La Presse Medicale 47: 388-389, 1915

19. Travell J and Rinzler S: The Myofascial Genesis of Pain. Postgrad Med 11:425, 1952.

20. Travell JG: Myofascial Trigger Points: Clinical View. Advances in Pain Research and Therapy, Volume I. JJ Bonica and D Albe-Fessard, ed. Raven Press, New York NY 1976.

21. Tsujii Y, Gould J: Myotherapy: Treatment of Muscle Hardenings. University of Wisconsin–LaCrosse, February 27-29, 1992. Continuing education seminar.

22. Yaxley GA, Jull GA: A Modified Upper Limb Tension Test: An Investigation of Responses in Normal Subjects. Australian Journal of Physiotherapy, 27:143-152, 1991.

CHAPTER 3 PATHOLOGY AND TREATMENT PRINCIPLES

INTRODUCTION

The bases for developing an effective treatment plan are comprehensive subjective and objective examinations. Interpretation of the objective examination findings and correlation of the objective findings with the patient's main complaints help the clinician make a list of the patient's problems (see Chapter 2, <u>Principles of Extremity Evaluation</u>). To choose a therapeutic intervention, the clinician must A) determine the nature and extent of each pathological process present; B) determine the severity and irritability of the problems present; and C) apply clinical knowledge and experience to the patient's problems. This chapter will discuss the body's response to trauma and immobilization, the development of treatment plans, and the treatment of common neuromusculoskeletal pathologies.

THE BODY'S RESPONSE TO TRAUMA

Cellular Response to Tissue Injury

After tissues are injured, whether by an acute injury or by repetitive stresses, the body responds by removing damaged tissues and replacing them with healthy ones. The inflammation and repair process proceeds through three phases: acute inflammation, proliferation, and remodeling (Fig 3–1).

Acute Inflammation

This stage of repair is characterized by removing tissue debris and pathogens from the injured area. The inflammatory phase usually lasts 2–3 days but may persist longer if tissue damage was severe.

Soft tissue injury activates platelets and mast cells, which release chemotactic agents. These agents attract polymorphonuclear leukocytes (PML's) and monocytes to the area. Monocytes develop into phagocytic macrophages, which help the PML's remove debris. As mast cells degrade, histamine is released, which dilates the capillaries in the tissues surrounding the injury. The local increase in blood flow facilitates the influx of phagocytic cells.

Proliferation

The proliferation phase is characterized by an influx of new cells, development of granulation tissue, and revascularization. Proliferation overlaps acute inflammation, usually beginning about three days after injury.

As removal of damaged tissues is completed, the phagocytic macrophages release chemotactic agents and growth factors to promote healing. These agents attract fibroblasts and endothelial cells. Fibroblasts produce the collagen that serves as the connective tissue matrix. Some fibroblasts differentiate into myofibroblasts. Myofibroblasts help decrease the size

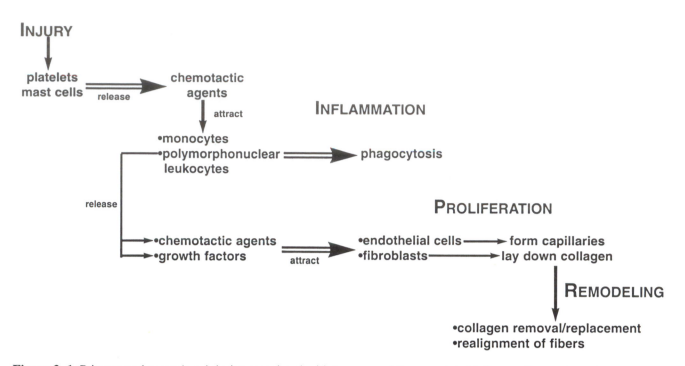

Figure 3–1. Primary and secondary injuries associated with trauma and the associated inflammation and repair processes

of the wound. This is referred to as wound contraction. Endothelial cells help develop new capillaries.

Remodeling

The remodeling phase can persist for months. In the proliferation stage, collagen fibers were laid down haphazardly. During remodeling, malaligned fibers are gradually removed and replaced. The new alignment of collagen conforms to the mechanical stresses applied to the tissues.

Inflammation Signs and Symptoms

When soft tissues are injured, there are three common signs of inflammation—swelling, redness, and warmth; and one symptom—pain.

Swelling

After neuromusculoskeletal trauma, intracellular fluid from the damaged cells moves into the extracellular space. This increases the protein in the extracellular fluid and raises the osmotic pressure surrounding the injury site. The pressure gradient draws more fluid out of the cells and blood vessels and into the extracellular space, causing swelling.

Redness and Warmth

Skin redness and warmth indicate increased blood flow to the injured area. Histamine and other vasodilators are released in response to tissue injury, resulting in a local increase in blood flow.

Pain

The original trauma can stimulate pain receptors in the injured tissues. If capillaries are damaged, the blood supply to tissues distal to the injury site will be decreased, causing ischemic pain. Anoxia (lack of oxygen) stimulates the release of bradykinin and prostaglandin, which cause pain.

Response of Joints to Trauma

Joint trauma can affect each structure of a joint. The synovial membrane reacts to injury with a proliferation of surface cells and an increase in synovial blood flow. There can also be a gradual fibrosis of the subsynovial tissues, termed post–traumatic synovitis. Continued mechanical irritation can result in chronic synovitis, which can be perpetuated by an inflammatory cycle.

The joint capsule reacts similarly. Continued mechanical irritation perpetuates the inflammatory response, and the capsule becomes more fibrous in nature. Chronic effusion can lead to stretching of the capsule and associated ligaments.

The articular cartilage is susceptible to enzymatic degradation by proteolytic enzymes that are released in response to trauma. The enzymes also affect the collagen fibers of the cartilage, making them susceptible to mechanical damage and degeneration. Erosion of the articular cartilage can result in early degenerative joint disease (DJD) that is irreversible. The process of cartilage degeneration is outlined in Figure 3–2.

Joint effusion—the accumulation of fluid within the joint capsule—is concurrent with the damage caused by proteolytic enzymes. Prolonged effusion can cause chronic synovitis and fibrous thickening of the joint capsule. Continued effusion into the joint cavity can lead to stretching of the capsule and associated ligaments.[29]

Joint effusion can also inhibit muscle function. A knee distended with effusion results in quadriceps weakness in normal individuals, even without pain.[17,33,36] Injecting 20–30 ml of liquid into normal knees results in a 60% quadricep inhibition, with the inhibition increasing as infusion increases.[36,65] It is

unclear whether this inhibition is mediated by the central or peripheral nervous system.

Controlling and eventually eliminating post–traumatic joint effusion is critical to the rehabilitation process. Prolonged effusion can result in reactive synovitis, joint capsule changes, and degradation of articular cartilage and lead to early degenerative joint changes. Joint effusion also can inhibit muscle function and deter muscle strength development. Pain is thought to inhibit muscle contraction and joint function; therefore, early treatment and continued monitoring of joint effusion and pain is paramount to improving and restoring joint function in the rehabilitation process.

Effects of Immobilization

It is common practice to immobilize an injured area to allow healing and to prevent further trauma. Even if the body part is not immobilized with external supports like a cast or splint, it may be immobilized by muscle guarding or a conscious decision not to move the part (e.g., due to fear of pain on movement). The effects of prolonged immobilization can be devastating.[31,38] The proper use of exercise can speed healing, while the lack of exercise during the early stages of rehabilitation can result in permanent disability.[28] Immobilization initially causes a loss of tissue substrate, and continued immobilization contributes to tissue degradation and atrophy. These losses occur in muscles and within the joints (bones, cartilage and connective tissues). The reversibility of these changes appears to depend on the length of immobilization.[28]

Effects of Immobilization on Muscles

Loss of muscle strength is one of the first and more obvious changes resulting from immobilization. Strength loss can be profound. Immobilizing an elbow in a cast for six weeks can result in a >40% decrease in the strength of the muscles surrounding the joint.[41] The other changes include a reduction in muscle size and a decease in tension per unit of muscle cross–sectional area.[4,41,42]

Immobilization can also affect muscle fatigue, probably as the result of decreased oxidative capacity. Reductions in maximum O_2 consumption, glycogen levels, high–energy phosphate levels, and

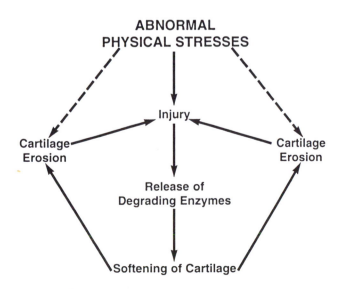

ABNORMAL PHYSICAL STRESSES

Injury

Cartilage Erosion

Cartilage Erosion

Release of Degrading Enzymes

Softening of Cartilage

Figure 3–2. The process of cartilage degeneration

mitochondrial activity are secondary to immobilization.[3,4,11,42,43,53] Loss of muscle strength occurs rapidly in the initial days of immobilization (24–72 hours).[40] After 5–7 days, the loss of muscle mass slows considerably.[4] The question of whether fast or slow twitch muscle fiber atrophy predominates with immobilization has not been answered. Research results have been contradictory, and the issue appears unclear.[18,23]

Muscle atrophy can also occur from reflex inhibition caused by joint injury or inflammation. This type of atrophy—termed "arthrogenic muscle wasting"—commonly occurs in the quadriceps muscles after an injury to the knee (Fig 3–3).[56] While joint pain and effusion may contribute to this problem, the exact causes of the muscle inhibition are unclear.

Effects of Immobilization on Joints

Joints consist of connective tissue, cartilage, and bones. While ligaments are connective tissue, they will be considered as a separate joint structure because of their critical function in limiting movement and controlling stability.

Connective Tissue

Immobilization can lead to arthrofibrosis–fibrotic tissue proliferation and tightening of the connective tissues around the joint (Fig 3–4). The tissues involved include the joint capsule, synovial membrane, fascia, tendons, and ligaments.

The primary mechanism for arthrofibrosis is the loss of ground–substance. Ground–substance is primarily composed of glycoaminoglycans and water. With immobilization, there is a loss of glycoaminoglycans, leading to abnormal collagen cross–link formation and subsequent joint restriction. Immobilization may also produce excessive connective tissue in the joint space. These later mature to scar tissue that may adhere to intra–articular surfaces and further restrict joint motion.[20]

Articular Cartilage

The effects of immobilization on articular cartilage appear to depend on the length of immobilization, the position maintained, and joint weightbearing.[28] Articular cartilage is avascular, receiving its nutrition through diffusion and osmosis. Joint nutrition is facilitated by loading and unloading the joint; therefore, immobilization that reduces joint loading may negatively affect cartilage integrity. Cartilage degeneration can begin as early as the first week of immobilization[9] and gradually progress as immobilization continues.[58] Prolonged knee joint immobilization in forced full extension may result in full–thickness loss of articular cartilage.[55] Even short–term immobilization can result in cumulative and harmful joint effects,[62] and repeated periods of immobilization longer than 30 days can eventually lead to progressive osteoarthritic joint changes.[61] The changes in cartilage caused by immobilization are

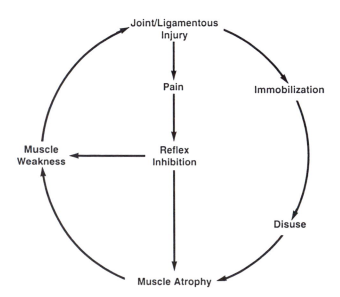

Figure 3–3. Arthrogenic muscle wasting.[7]

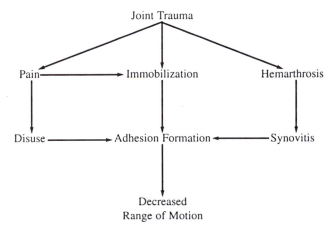

Figure 3–4. Trauma and immobilization can lead to adhesion formation and decreased range of motion.

generally irreversible, but it may depend on the length of immobilization.

Bone

Bone loss occurs in response to diminished weightbearing and diminished muscle contractions. These changes can be detected as early as two weeks after immobilization. [23,46,60) The exact pathogenesis of immobilization–induced osteoporosis is unclear, but animal [5,21,24] and human studies [19,24,27] have shown decreased bone formation and increased resorption after immobilization.

Ligaments

Ligaments undergo the same changes in structure as other connective tissues. They remodel in response to the mechanical demands placed on them, just as bones remodel to adapt to stresses (Wolfe's Law). Immobilization reduces glycoaminoglycans levels in ligaments, resulting in decreased compliance and early ligament failure if overstretched. [1,22,50] This decrease in ligamentous strength and resistance to stress can reduce a ligament's ability to stabilize a joint.

Summary of Effects of Immobilization

The more obvious changes occur with the loss of muscle strength and endurance. Changes in periarticular tissues can result in arthrofibrosis and joint restriction. Immobilization can weaken ligaments, decreasing functional joint stability. Bone loss results from diminished weightbearing and diminished muscle contractions. To avoid deleterious immobilization, early protected motion and controlled weightbearing are recommended for successful rehabilitation.

TREATMENT

The foundations for treatment are the patient's presenting signs and symptoms, which were clarified in the initial examination. The primary question for developing a treatment plan is: "What is preventing the patient from normal function?" This helps prioritize the problems identified in the patient's problem list. These goals should reflect the patient's functional problems and expectations and should be attainable. Finally, the treatments should be individually designed to address each patient's functional problems, complaints, and clinical signs and symptoms.

The treatment planning process can be broken into eight steps:

1. Develop the problem list (see Chapter 2, Principles of Extremity Evaluation).

2. List the goals for the patient. Generally, there should be a goal for each problem identified. Goals should address both the specific clinical problems (e.g., decreased range of motion), and the patient's functional problems (e.g., inability to lift loads overhead at work).

3. Identify structures contributing to the disorder (nerve, muscle, joint, etc.) and identify possible therapeutic interventions to address each structure.

4. Estimate the degree of patient compliance that can be expected.

5. Plan realistic and practical guidelines to reduce the effects of daily physical stresses.

6. Estimate the current prognosis of the problem. The prognosis is the clinician's educated judgment of treatment's potential success. It is based on the severity, irritability, and nature (SIN) of the problem, the estimated patient compliance, and the goals of treatment.

7. Predict the duration of treatment. This will depend on the SIN of the patient's problem, the treatment goals, and the prognosis.

8. Prioritize therapeutic intervention and develop an initial treatment plan.

When planning a treatment program, it is important to remember that neuromusculoskeletal disorders of the extremities can be caused by many factors. Extremity symptoms can be caused by underlying neuromusculoskeletal tissue pathology, or they may have visceral, systemic, or spinal origins. It is imperative for the clinician to have a working knowledge of the potential sources of the problems. Clinicians must understand that most neuromusculoskeletal disorders have several contributing sources of symptoms—not a single cause or a single pathology. Thus, a single treatment for a single problem does not exist, except in theory.

Treatment programs should not be "written in stone." Frequent reassessments are necessary to see if the initial plan is still working. The treatment program should be continually modified as the rehabilitation progresses, depending on the patient's response to prior treatments.

The Frequency/Duration Dilemma

It is sometimes difficult to determine the appropriate number and frequency of treatment visits. It is common to unintentionally overtreat a patient because the patient's functional goals are not yet met or because symptoms persist longer than anticipated. Yet when looking back over the course of treatment, we can often admit the patient should have been discharged earlier. Continuing to treat the patient those few extra weeks did not accomplish the goals or did not prove to be more beneficial than "letting nature take its course." How do we provide adequate treatment but prevent overtreatment in today's health care environment?

Robin McKenzie states that physical therapists should be "the profession that teaches patients to help themselves."[45] If a patient becomes dependent on passive therapies or gets the impression that using specialized exercise equipment is necessary for full rehabilitation, we have interfered with the patient's ability to help him or herself.

Many of the physical therapist's patients with neuromusculoskeletal problems will need long–term rehabilitation in the form of aggressive exercise, lifestyle training, and education. This is not to say that we must continue treating patient for months and months until the goals of maximal strength, flexibility and fitness are met. The clinician must closely examine any professional involvement with the patient to determine when his or her services are no longer medically necessary. The question we must ask ourselves every day, with every patient is, "Does this patient continue to require the skilled services of a physical therapist?" Defining the desired functional outcome in terms of realistic goals, treatment duration, and prognosis helps us answer this question.

Goals—what goals require the involvement or presence of the clinician? What can be done at home by the patient?

Treatment duration—what is adequate? What is realistic? How long would "nature" have taken?

Prognosis—what is the patient's history? When should we accept that our intervention is no longer necessary or does not benefit the patient?

These three factors must be carefully considered *together* during initial treatment planning. If goals are set without considering realistic duration and the prognosis, the therapist may treat the patient too long and later find out the patient really didn't benefit.

The therapist should try to identify the total anticipated duration of treatment at the time of the initial evaluation. It is certainly acceptable to be wrong because not all facts may be evident, but by estimating the total duration on the first visit, the therapist has set a target that can be modified later with good reason (for example, the prognosis becomes better or worse, or the patient's goals are modified). Estimating the total duration helps the clinician avoid the common trap of seeing the patient in successive 3–4 week blocks of time that quickly add up to several months. In such a case, if the therapist had originally estimated six weeks, a serious look at the feasibility of the goals and prognosis at six weeks of treatment may have prevented overtreatment.

These questions are often asked about the frequency/duration dilemma:

1. Should I continue treating if the functional goals have been accomplished but the patient still has symptoms?

Occasionally, complete pain relief is a legitimate goal. More often, it is either unrealistic or will simply take time and will not progress any faster with the clinician involved. The clinician should consider the patient's history. Is this a chronic problem or one episode in a series of recurring problems? Does the patient have a history of a slow recovery from previous painful conditions? Does the patient have a history of multiple painful conditions for which treatment is frequently sought? A "yes" to any of these questions may be a clue that the symptoms will be difficult to resolve with or without the clinician's intervention. Such a patient should be taught how to enact an independent, long–term pain management program.

2. What should I do when a patient is progressing but not quite enough?

Again, the clinician must consider the original goals, treatment duration, and prognosis. If an original goal is to improve from lifting 30 lb to lifting 70 lb, and the estimated duration is four weeks, the patient must increase 10 lb per week on average. If the patient has only improved to lifting 35 lb on week two, this is not enough progress. Something was miscalculated in the initial evaluation. This is common and certainly acceptable; however, the responsible clinician must reconsider whether the original goals are realistic, the treatments planned are still better than letting nature taking its course, and the prognosis is still reasonably good. If so, continued treatment is acceptable. If not, revisions in the treatment plan should be made without hesitation.

3. What about conditions that require long–term treatment, such as the frozen shoulder or post–surgical ACL reconstructions?

The clinician must make an important distinction: Do such conditions require long–term *treatment* or long–term *monitoring?* The conditions mentioned above may require periodic monitoring and adjustment of the patient's home program for months; however, they may not require frequent visits to the clinic, especially when the patient's progress temporarily plateaus, and the functional status is relatively static. During these static periods, the patient should maintain or slowly progress the home program. Monthly or bimonthly visits are often sufficient. When the patient's functional status changes more rapidly, more frequent visits are justified.

Treatment Strategies

The treatment of any proximal contributing structures should be addressed first. The clinician can determine to what extent problems in these structures affect problems at the more distal joints by analyzing

the results of treatment intervention. For example, if abnormal findings of the lumbar spine are related to hip symptoms, treatment of these abnormal findings should increase function or decrease symptoms at the hip. If treatment of the lumbar spine drastically improves function or symptoms at the hip, the lumbar spine was a significant contributing structure. If the improvement was minimal, the lumbar spine was probably minimally involved. If no improvement was seen, the lumbar spine was either not a contributing structure, or the treatment given was ineffective.

Maximizing patient involvement in treatment is an important strategy. The patient must be taught about weightbearing status, postures, and expected activity levels, including participation in a home exercise program. Compliance must be checked frequently throughout the rehabilitation process. Developing the patient's self–responsibility assures the desired treatment outcome—lasting results!

Common Components of Treatment

While specific treatment programs are based on the patient's problems and goals, there are four components of treatment common to all patients: 1) control symptoms; 2) restore function; 3) modify daily stresses; and 4) prevent recurrence.

Control Symptoms

Patients often come to physical therapy because of pain. They may have decreased range of motion or muscle weakness, but the problem that bothers them the most, and the reason they seek help, is usually pain. However, controlling, decreasing, and eliminating pain and other symptoms are important goals but not usually the primary goal. Physical agents can be used to decrease inflammation, control pain, prevent or reduce swelling, and promote healing. Grade I and II oscillatory joint mobilizations can also be used to control pain. Compression wraps and proper positioning should be used to prevent the formation of dependent edema. After acute injury, immobilization is often necessary to help decrease symptoms. There are a variety of braces and splints for immobilization. Such immobilizers should be gradually reduced and eventually eliminated. Controlling lower extremity symptoms may also entail the use of gait assistive devices. Crutches, walkers, or canes can be used to control weightbearing loads when the patient's symptoms are aggravated by weightbearing activities. Using a cane on the opposite side of the involved limb can reduce the weightbearing load transmitted to the involved hip up to 40%.[6] The patient should be weaned from the assistive device as symptoms resolve and the gait pattern becomes symmetrical.

Modify Daily Stresses

Many clinicians fail to consider the role of modifying daily stresses as a part of a successful treatment program. This often neglected portion of treatment can play a critical role in the patient's response to therapeutic interventions. For example, ultrasound and friction massage applied to a supraspinatus tendon in a patient with supraspinatus tendinitis may seem to have little effect on symptoms if the patient continues to perform overhead reaching and lifting activities at work or is sleeping with arms overhead at night. To be effective, the clinician must work with the patient to find ways to decrease the stresses that may impede progress in rehabilitation.

Beginning with the first visit, the patient should be taught which postures and repeated movements may delay healing. This includes back postures; sleep and work postures; and postures, movements, and activities of the injured extremity. Adaptive devices can be used to facilitate functional use of injured joints and to prevent cumulative trauma. Ergonomic modifications may be necessary at work, in sports, and at home.

Restore Function

Restoring function is the primary goal of any rehabilitation program. Successful rehabilitation aims to improve the patient's functional abilities to allow work, home, and leisure activities without lasting symptom recurrence. Patients must be taught about temporary symptoms that will resolve, for example, post–exercise complaints such as muscle soreness. These temporary symptoms will not interfere with progress in rehabilitation. The patients must also know what symptoms and signs may prevent progress or cause disability, such as chronic effusion, increasing pain frequency or intensity, or loss of joint motion.

Early mobilization after injury is critical to prevent contractures and promote a return to optimal function. The progression from passive to active–assisted to active range of motion should be initiated as soon as possible. Friction massage can be used to decrease symptoms and promote healing of tendinitis or tenosynovitis. Joint mobilization and soft tissue mobilization—that is, myofascial and neural structure mobilization—can be used to restore optimal tissue mobility. Prolonged passive stretching can help restore normal range of motion. Any neural tension problems should be treated to restore optimal neural tissue mobility and decrease symptoms. Functional strengthening exercises should begin as soon as possible. Proprioception exercises and simulation of daily activities can promote functional recovery.

Prevent Recurrence

Preventing recurrence of injuries is a continuous process that begins at the initial visit. The goal is to guide the patient through successful rehabilitation and teach self reliance and self–responsibility. It is closely associated with modifying daily stresses but continues after the patient is discharged from physical therapy. Home activities, work, and recreation should be modified as needed to reduce stress on the injured joints. This may include changing the tools used at work or modifying the way some tasks are performed. Assistive braces and splints can be used to prevent the recurrence of injury and decrease stresses to the joints, as needed.

Treatment can only be effective if it provides lasting results. Recurring symptoms and decreases in function are evidence of ineffective treatment. The clinician should suspect underlying pathology if the patient does not respond favorably to a comprehensive treatment approach.

Post–surgical Treatment Considerations

The clinician should have a thorough knowledge of any surgical procedures and post–surgical precautions. Initiation and progression of treatments should be determined by the structures repaired, the healing constraints of the tissues, and the surgeon's protocol. Post–operative pain, swelling, and stiffness are common. These symptoms usually dissipate in 7–10 days; if they persist they can impede progress in rehabilitation. Prevention of contractures and excessive scar tissue formation is critical to regaining optimal function. Therefore, mobilization should begin as early as possible. Any sling, brace, or splint should be used according to established protocols. Since their continued use can prevent functional muscle development and interfere with mobility, they should be gradually tapered and discontinued. However, some patients may benefit from using a brace on a continuing basis for injury prevention.

Treatment of Acute versus Chronic Conditions

To illustrate how the four components of rehabilitation are used to plan treatment, consider their application to acute and chronic conditions. "Acute" and "chronic" can be clinically useful terms when considering the nature and extent of a patient's signs and symptoms. They provide a way to think about the general treatment components that will direct specific therapeutic interventions for specific problems. They also reflect the nature of the inflammation and repair process discussed before.

Acute disorders are post–traumatic problems that are in the inflammatory phase. Pain is usually felt at rest and can be aggravated by activity. It can be local or diffuse and may be referred into any of the segmentally related areas. Passive and active mobility may be restricted by muscle guarding or pain. Skin temperature may be elevated, and soft tissue or joint edema may be present.

Chronic disorders are problems that are in the remodeling phase. Pain is usually not felt at rest but can be provoked by specific activities. Pain is more likely to be localized. Mobility is usually restricted at or near the end of range, and symptoms are felt during an arc of motion or at end–range.

Treatment of Acute Disorders

The underlying physiological themes in treating acute disorders are:

- *Promote* a progression to a normal tissue healing response

- *Prevent* prolonged inflammation and effusion that may cause muscle inhibition and tissue degradation, which can lead to chronic tissue changes such as muscle

atrophy, adaptive muscle shortening, and arthrofibrosis.

Controlling Symptoms in Acute Disorders

In acute disorders, it can help to use the PRICE acronym to describe initial treatments:

- **Protect** the area using wraps, slings, braces, and gait assistive devices (e.g., crutches or a cane).

- **Rest** the area by avoiding aggravating activities.

- **Ice** the area to decrease pain and muscle spasm and to prevent edema.

- **Compress** the area to prevent and reduce edema.

- **Elevate** the area to prevent and reduce edema.

Physical agents can be used as needed to decrease pain, muscle guarding, and joint or soft–tissue effusion. Concurrently, patients should be encouraged to follow through with taking their medications as prescribed (e.g., non–steroidal anti–inflammatory drugs, muscle relaxants).

Modifying Daily Stresses in Acute Disorders

Methods for controlling aggravating postures, movements, or activities should be addressed. The patient's and the employer's cooperation is essential, so specific instructions should be given to enhance the patient's understanding and compliance. The goal is to modify daily stresses to avoid continued trauma.

Restoring Function in Acute Disorders

Early mobilization of healing tissues can help avoid the deleterious effects of immobilization; however, the inflammatory response should not be prolonged by this intervention. Early passive mobilization performed in a resistance–free range of motion can be used to reduce pain and prevent excessive muscle guarding. Patients should be progressed from passive to active–assisted to active range of motion exercise as soon as tolerated. Strengthening and muscle reeducation can begin with sub–maximal isometric muscle contractions at pain free points in the range of motion. Electrical muscle stimulation can be used to promote muscle reeducation. Functional strengthening and flexibility exercise should be initiated as soon as tolerated. Proprioceptive training should also be initiated within the healing constraints of the problem.

Preventing Recurrence in Acute Disorders

After an acute injury, the patient should be prevented from progressing too rapidly to normal activities. The clinician should specifically guide the return to functional activities. Gradual progression in rehabilitation will set the stage for successful increases in functional activities. Patients should be taught to allow for rest or other symptom relief if problems arise. They must also be able to distinguish between true reinjury and mild symptom provocation.

Treatment of Chronic Disorders

The underlying physiological themes in treating chronic disorders are:

- *Promote* resumption of normal tissue function by reducing mechanical stresses to the tissues; increasing tissue extensibility; increasing neuromuscular strength and control; and increasing the tissues' resistance to stress.

- *Prevent* reinjury, which may lead to abnormal scar tissue formation, excessive tissue hypertrophy, and tissue breakdown.

Controlling Symptoms in Chronic Disorders

Symptom management may be a more appropriate term here. Although the patient may complain of pain, passive treatments should not be used excessively with patients who have chronic disorders. Persistent effusion should be carefully monitored, but symptomatic relief measures should only be applied as needed to encourage progression to an independent exercise program.

Modifying Daily Stresses in Chronic Disorders

The activities or positions that contribute to the patient's problem must be identified and modified to avoid further injury. Protective or assistive devices can be used to allow safe progression to functional activities by controlling stresses.

Examples of using protective devices include the use of braces for knee rehabilitation after surgery; shoe inserts for shock absorption after heel spur excision; and wrist splints to control the effects of cumulative trauma when increasing work time after injury. Patients must be taught to monitor daily stresses and modify positions or activities as needed. The most creative and appropriate treatment regime can be sabotaged by carelessness in daily activities.

Restoring Function in Chronic Disorders

Functional joint movement and positioning requires sufficient capsuloligamentous mobility, adequate myofascial mobility, and sufficient muscle strength to support the muscles' roles as stabilizers, decelerators, or accelerators. Muscles act as shock–attenuators to decrease the joint's share of external loads and play an important role in neuromuscular control of joint stability. Appropriate treatment addresses insufficient capsuloligamentous mobility with specific joint accessory and physiological mobilizations (see Chapter 11, Mobilization Techniques). Poor myofascial mobility could be treated with soft–tissue mobilization and stretching exercises. Muscle strength can be increased through functional strengthening exercises or other resistive training. Coordination exercises and proprioceptive training promote integrated function by helping control movement, position, and functional stability.

Preventing Recurrence in Chronic Disorders

The clinician should guide the progression toward functional activities to ensure the patient does not repeat past injuries. Gradual progression in rehabilitation will set the stage for successful increases in functional activities. Education should be geared toward increasing the patient's ability to identify and modify joint stresses in daily activities and toward increasing patient commitment to independent exercise. Patients should be taught to take rest periods; to use other symptomatic relief measures if problems arise; and to distinguish true reinjury from mild symptom provocation.

Example of Treatment Planning Process

The following clinical example illustrates the treatment planning process.

A 34 year old patient presents in the office of his family physician complaining of right shoulder pain of approximately six weeks' duration. The physician orders an x–ray, which is reported as negative. Rest and a dose of anti–inflammatory medication are prescribed for three weeks. This treatment is ineffective, and physical therapy is prescribed.

The patient complains of right anterior shoulder pain: 1) at work lifting laundry into and out of machines; 2) reaching for the rider's side seat belt in his car; 3) bending his neck toward the left shoulder.

Physical examination provides the following information:

1. limited cervical range of motion in right rotation and right sidebending. Range of motion is about 3/4 normal range

2. right sided cervical muscle stiffness and pain on palpation at the C4–5 joints

3. referred anterior shoulder pain with palpation at C4–5 on the right

4. right anterior shoulder pain and complaints of "tightness" in flexion at 90°

5. tenderness to palpation of the supraspinatus tendon insertion

6. full shoulder range of motion

7. positive impingement sign at the right shoulder

8. negative upper limb tension test (ULTT)

It becomes apparent from the above set of signs and symptoms that this case has more than a single–cause and requires more than a single–treatment.

According to the treatment design steps, the clinician should proceed as follows:

1. Identify the patient's problems.

    - pain in the right shoulder
    - decreased shoulder function at work and in daily activities
    - cervical pain
    - decreased cervical ROM

2. List the treatment goals.

    - reduce right shoulder pain to allow full pain free right shoulder ROM

- improve pain free shoulder function
- reduce cervical pain
- increase cervical ROM to normal range

3. Consider the contributing components of the disorder.

    - Muscles. Anterior shoulder pain is frequently a component of rotator cuff or biceps tendon involvement. The surrounding muscles of the cervical region and anterior chest wall could also refer pain to the shoulder.

    - Joints. The specific joints in the shoulder that could be involved include the glenohumeral, the acromioclavicular, the scapulothoracic, and to a lesser degree the sternoclavicular. These could be directly involved or could refer pain. Furthermore, the right C4–C5 cervical joints could be referring pain to the shoulder.

    - Nerves. The C4-C5 portions of the dura, nerve root sleeve, and brachial plexus could refer pain to the shoulder.

4. Estimate the patient's active role in treatment.

    - During the subjective examination, the patient seemed frustrated with the lack of improvement from the initial treatment of rest and medication. He seemed motivated to participate in rehabilitation, so the clinician estimates good compliance with therapy.

5. Plan realistic and practical guidelines to reduce the contributing stresses.

    - decrease frequency of overhead lifting
    - use left hand to reach for seat belt in car
    - change sleep positions, avoiding putting the arm overhead during sleep
    - review and modify cervical postures

6. Estimate the patient's prognosis.

    - The patient is highly motivated and in relatively good physical condition. His treatment prognosis is excellent.

7. Predict the initial duration treatment

    - The patient's problem is moderately severe

and irritable. It is also fairly chronic at this point. The patient's goals include pain free function in work, which involves lifting laundry, a stressful action for the patient; however, the patient is highly motivated to comply with initial activity restrictions and home exercises. Based on experience with this type of patient, the initial treatment period is estimated to be 3–4 weeks. Monitoring the patient's symptoms, activity level, and home program may require biweekly rechecks for one month.

8. Prioritize treatment interventions.

- It can be clinically valuable to initially treat the spinal components of patients presenting with extremity symptoms. In this case, the patient has cervical stiffness and pain, and the extremity symptoms can be provoked by palpating the cervical joints at C4–5 on the same side as the patient's shoulder complaints. What degree of the patient's right shoulder complaints is caused by the cervical joints? Initial treatment of the spinal component here would help answer this question. If cervical mobilization decreased cervical stiffness and pain but did not affect the shoulder symptoms, then the cervical spine would not seem to be contributing to the shoulder problem; however, cervical mobilization may decrease the shoulder symptoms, and can even lead to increased pain free range of motion of the shoulder.[26]

- Any soft–tissue restrictions should be addressed as well.

- Attention should then turn to the supraspinatus tendons. The examination findings in this case included positive signs for rotator cuff tendon involvement and impingement. These would need to be addressed next along with any joint restrictions found in manual examination. Ultrasound and friction massage could promote healing.

The treatment plan can also be considered in terms of the four components of rehabilitation.

1. *Controlling Symptoms.* Cervical mobilization will be used to decrease cervical and shoulder pain. Ultrasound or another physical agent will be used to control pain at the shoulder.

2. *Modifying Stresses.* The patient should be taught A) to decrease lifting, especially overhead; B) posture and body mechanics principles; C) modification of sleep postures.

3. *Restoring Function.* Cervical and first rib mobilization will be used to increase range of motion. Soft–tissue mobilization to the scalenes or the pectoralis minor muscle can be used if needed. Friction massage and ultrasound will help heal the injured supraspinatus tendon.

4. *Preventing Recurrence.* Throughout the treatment program, the patient will be taught ways to decrease stresses on the neck and shoulder and will also be taught exercises to increase flexibility in the shoulder and cervical spine region.

Reassessment after Treatment Intervention

Application of any therapeutic intervention is not complete without reassessment of the results of treatment. Reassessment validates the treatments given by a clinician by finding out if the treatment works. Reassessments should be both subjective and objective, finding out how the patient feels and any changes in physical signs. Ideally, there will be a correlation between subjective and objective responses to treatment. For example, after mobilization of the shoulder, the patient might report the joint feels less stiff. Physical findings should show increased range of motion at the joint.

Many clinicians use prior experience with successful treatments as a guide for treatment planning. If previous patients with ligament reconstruction responded well to a certain closed kinematic chain exercise, the clinician will likely use the same or similar exercises with future ligament reconstruction patients; however, there is no guarantee that a treatment used in the past will be successful with future patients. Too many variables can affect the result of a given treatment; therefore, it is important to reassess patients frequently to determine if they are responding as desired to treatment. Treatment reassessment helps four ways.[34] First, it helps confirm the examination hypothesis, the clinician's determination of structures that may contribute to the patient's problems. Treatments are based on this hypothesis. If reassessments reveal the patient is responding well to the treatment, the hypothesis is supported. If the patient does not respond to treatments geared toward the hypothesized sources, either the treatments were administered incorrectly, or the patient's problems stem from some other source.

Second, reassessment helps progress treatment. Based on the reassessment, the clinician determines when changing the treatment plan will maximize patient progress. The amounts and types of sign or symptom changes occurring after each treatment help the clinician determine if the treatment is successful.

Third, the reassessment helps confirm clinical patterns. Clinical patterns are consistent sets of signs and symptoms seen with a particular disorder. This includes the way the problem responds to rehabilitation. A clinician recognizes clinical patterns from experience. Reassessments help determine if a patient fits into a particular clinical pattern based on response to treatment.

Finally, reassessments help clinicians develop new clinical patterns. When treatment based on a given clinical pattern is not effective, reassessment ensures that treatment is changed according to the patient's *current* signs and symptoms. The patient's signs, symptoms, and response to treatment no longer fit the clinical pattern originally identified; therefore, this patient's response to treatment serves as the foundation for a new clinical pattern.[34]

Reassessment involves re–evaluating the most significant objective signs and symptoms. These should be reassessed

- during treatments (e.g., between repetitions of a mobilization treatment or between sets of exercises)

- after a treatment

- at subsequent follow–up visits

Frequent reassessments help the clinician monitor the patient's objective signs and symptoms and help validate treatment programs.

TREATMENT OF COMMON NEUROMUSCULOSKELETAL DISORDERS

There are numerous possible sources of extremity pain. Neuromusculoskeletal disorders of the peripheral limbs can be caused by contractile (muscle–tendon unit) or non–contractile (joint, ligament, capsule, bone, and neural) tissues. Spinal disorders can cause neurological signs in the peripheral limbs and may contribute to referred pain felt in the extremities.[10,32,47,64] Adverse mechanical neural tension (AMNT)[6] may be a source of peripheral limb symptoms. Extremity pain can also be caused by visceral or systemic pathology. Many visceral and systemic disorders can refer pain into the joints, muscles, or nerves, so the clinician needs to be familiar with the clinically presenting characteristics of common visceral or systemic pathologies.[2]

Venereal disease, gout, rheumatoid arthritis (RA), and Lyme's disease can cause joint and muscle pain. Angina and myocardial infarctions (MI) may radiate pain to the left shoulder, arm, and neck. Shoulder symptoms can also be related to irritation of the diaphragm, gall bladder, or spleen, which share the same spinal nerve root innervation. The clinician must be able to recognize certain characteristics of visceral and systemic pathology such as involvement in more than one joint, migrating pain, night pain, and, above all, symptoms that are unrelated to and unaltered by movement and position. If the patient's complaint does not present any concrete neuromusculoskeletal findings, or if a patient does not respond in a timely fashion to treatment, these are clues the problem may be something other than a neuromusculoskeletal disorder, and the physician should be consulted before further treatment. In this section, some of the more common types of neuromusculoskeletal injuries are described, and suggestions for treatments are outlined.

MUSCLE DISORDERS

Muscle disorders occur within the contractile unit. The contractile unit consists of the muscle belly, the musculotendinous junction, the tendon, and the tendon's bony attachment. Muscle disorders are characterized by pain with resisted muscle tests and with active movements. Passive movement in the opposite direction may be painful if the muscle is stretched. Palpation may provoke symptoms at specific sites within the muscle.

Adaptive Muscle Changes

Muscles rapidly adapt to length changes caused by joint hypomobility, joint hypermobility, structural changes, or abnormal posture. This is a nonpathological response, but it must be treated.[30]

Treatment

Treatment emphasizing normal physiological function is more effective on adaptive muscle length changes than passive stretching or other passive exercises are.[12] Soft tissue mobilization may help progress the patient toward active exercise. Primary treatment, of course, must be directed toward the cause of the adaptive changes.

Muscle Guarding and Intrinsic Muscle Spasm

Muscle guarding nearly always accompanies pain, regardless of the underlying cause. Muscle guarding can develop wherever pain is felt, even if it is referred. Prolonged muscle guarding leads to a circulatory stasis and metabolite retention. The muscle may begin to spasm, become inflamed (myositis), and develop localized tenderness. Intrinsic muscle spasm adds additional pain and discomfort (Fig 3–5).

Without a thorough examination, it is easy to incriminate muscle guarding and the resulting intrinsic muscle spasm as the primary cause of the patient's problem, but there must be an underlying cause producing the muscle guarding in the first place. It is still often necessary to treat muscle guarding and intrinsic muscle spasm even though it may not be the primary neuromusculoskeletal disorder.

Treatment

Treatment may combine rest, medication, heat or cold, support, massage, electrotherapy, hydrotherapy, and stretching exercises.

Strain (Stress, Pull, Rupture)

Muscle strain is damage to some part of the contractile unit from overuse (chronic strain) or overstress (acute strain). Strains can be graded as mild, moderate, or severe (first, second, and third degree, respectively).[52] A first degree strain may involve a small amount of mechanical injury to the tissue, irritation, and inflammation but no structural damage. In a second degree strain, some portions of the contractile unit are damaged and some degree of functional loss is present, but the entire unit is intact. In a third degree strain, there is loss of function of the muscle, the tendon, or the tendon's attachment due to a complete tear.

The strain will occur at the weakest link of the muscle–tendon unit. Under stress, the muscle may tear, the musculotendinous junction may give way, or the tendon or its bony attachment may be damaged. The patient will also often report a tearing or pulling sensation or, less commonly, a snap.

Resisted muscle tests will cause pain with first and second degree strains. A third degree strain will show loss of strength but may be painless. Passive stretching may also cause localized pain in the case of mild and moderate strains. The involved structures will be tender to palpation. A rupture is often easy to palpate or may be visible as a lump or a depression in the otherwise normal surface anatomy. Rest from movement relieves pain. The patient may report that rest stiffens the involved structures and that movement initially hurts but does help loosen up the stiffness.

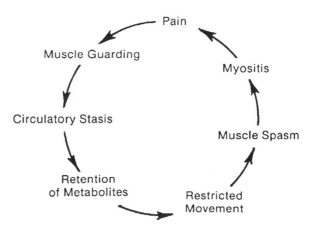

Figure 3–5. The pain-spasm cycle.

Acute strain is the result of a single, violent force applied to the contractile unit that disrupts of some of the fibers of the unit. Muscle or tendon rupture may be complete or may involve just a few fibers. The tendon may be partially avulsed from the bone or be completely torn away.

Chronic strain from overuse fatigues the muscle. This, in turn, may result in muscle spasm, myositis, and ischemia. Overuse may also irritate the musculotendinous junction or tendon, resulting in tendinitis or tenosynovitis. Crepitus may be felt over the involved structure. Although these may seem to be different conditions, they are essentially the same and require the same treatment regime.

Treatment

Treatment of mild and moderate strain consists of rest and protection from further injury. Initially, ice and compression may be indicated, followed by controlled range of motion, functional strengthening, and gradual resumption of activities. Full restoration of mobility and strength should be achieved before the patient is discharged from therapy. Severe strains involving rupture of the muscle, the tendon, or the tendon's insertion may require surgical repair.

Chronic strain treatment consists of rest, local heat or ice, and protection against further strain. These passive treatments should be followed by gradual return to activities and a strengthening program to build up resistance to stress. Cyriax advocates massage when there is muscular involvement and transverse friction massage for tenosynovitis.[14,15] During transverse friction massage, the inner aspect of the tendon sheath is moved repeatedly to and fro across the external aspect of the tendon. With chronic strain, prevention is more important than cure. Treatment should be progressed through gradually increasing activity so the musculotendinous unit can withstand progressively heavier loads.

Contusion (Bruise)

Contusions are caused by a direct blow to the muscle that results in capillary rupture and bleeding, edema formation, and an inflammatory reaction.

Treatment

Treatment consists of limiting bleeding by applying cold and compression and by immobilizing the area and protecting it from further injury. When the bruise begins to resolve, physical agents, rest, protection, and pain free movement can be used to promote healing. Protective padding over the injured area may help decrease the risk of reinjury. Finally, the clinician should be certain full strength and mobility are restored before the patient resumes normal activities.

Muscle Inflammation (Myositis, Tendinitis, Tenosynovitis)

Inflammation of the contractile group occasionally results from sleeping or sitting in a draft, from influenza, or from other systemic diseases. More commonly, inflammation is a natural reaction after strain, contusion, or accompanying intrinsic muscle spasm.

Many of the characteristics of muscle strain and contusion will also be present with muscle inflammation. Nodules and crepitus may be felt over the involved structures, and the muscle fibers may be thick and cord–like. Temperature and color changes may also be present. Patients may report pain and stiffness after rest that eases with activity. Occasionally, calcium deposits will form in the tendon (calcific tendinitis). This is an attempt by nature to heal, and should not alter treatment.

Treatment

Treatment consists of rest and physical agents for symptom control. For myositis, massage can be used to increase tissue mobility; transverse friction massage helps patients with tendinitis and tenosynovitis. Hydrocortisone phonophoresis may be effective, especially with calcific tendinitis.[25] Iontophoresis can also be helpful if the lesion is superficial.[35] Steroid injections are sometimes used to decrease symptoms and promote healing. All use of steroids should be conservative as repeated steroid injections may weaken the tendon and erode the bone.[13,51]

Myositis Ossificans

Myositis ossificans occasionally occurs as a complication of trauma and muscle hematoma. The disorder may appear as a benign growth of bone with a broad base and a sharp extension into the muscle. There may seem to be an involvement of the periosteum rather than the muscle. In this case, the mass is true bone and is firmly attached to the parent bone. In another type of myositis ossificans, there is actually a plaque of bone lying within the muscle. Myositis ossificans can result either from repeated slight injuries or from a single, more severe traumatic event. It may occur in various regions of the body but is most frequent in the thigh, in the upper arm, and around the elbow joint. Myositis ossificans is often evident by palpation before x–rays show the calcified mass.[52] Diagnosis is not difficult once the ossification has matured; however, it is important to recognize the early stages of the condition and prevent the ossification from occurring. If a strain or contusion of the arm or thigh does not resolve promptly, myositis ossificans should be suspected. Myositis ossificans can occur as a complication of strains and contusions, so rehabilitation of these conditions should always occur within the limits of pain. In addition, return to normal activities should not depend on any predetermined treatment duration. Instead, resumption of normal activities should depend on the resolution of symptoms and the return to normal range of motion and strength.

Treatment

The proper care of strains and contusions will prevent most cases of myositis ossificans. The muscle should be rested as soon as ossification is recognized. Ice can be used to decrease pain. Controlled active motion should be permitted only if it is painless. O'Donoghue states that ultrasound, massage, passive stretching, and any activity more vigorous than outlined above is contraindicated.[52] Progressive mobility and strengthening exercises should be carried out well within the limits of pain, at least for the first several months.

Myositis ossificans is a potentially crippling disorder. It is important for clinicians to recognize the early signs of this disease so appropriate treatments can begin.

Contracture

Some clinicians use the terms muscle tightness and muscle contracture interchangeably. In fact, these are two different conditions. Muscle tightness is sometimes seen around joints after immobilization or disuse. The hamstrings, hip flexors, and ankle plantar flexors are commonly involved. In such cases, the problem is either tightening of the tendons or inability to relax the muscle. "Myostatic spasm" describes muscle tightness caused by an inability to fully relax the muscle.[66] Muscle contractures are rare. In contractures, scar tissue is laid down within a muscle. This usually occurs only as a complication of surgery, severe trauma, or disease.

Muscle tightness is reversible with proper physical therapy, but muscle contractures are extremely difficult to overcome. They are often painless but require treatment because they limit function. Progressive contractures involving tendons or fascia are occasionally seen, such as Dupuytren's contracture of the palmar fascia. The etiology of these disorders is often unknown.

Treatment

Treatment consists of stretching exercises and return to functional activities. In more severe cases, massage, physical agents, and more vigorous stretching may be necessary. Ultrasound applied during passive stretch is often an effective treatment for these conditions.

Fibrositis (Fibromyositis)

Fibrositis is synonymous with fibromyositis and myofibrositis. This condition is usually defined as acute or chronic inflammation of the fibrous tissue in the muscle that causes pain and stiffness. Sometimes painful nodules or crepitus are felt, hence the impression that fibrositic nodules or deposits are present. Some fibrositic nodules contain large amounts of metachromatic mucoid substances, mast cells and platelet clots; however, the specific pathological entity of a fibrositic nodule has not been consistently demonstrated, so many authorities refuse to recognize the condition of fibrositis as a true pathological disorder.[66] It is reasonable, therefore, to assume that the nodules and crepitus often attributed to fibrositis are sometimes simply manifestations of inflammation.

Treatment

Regardless of the exact pathological entity, treatment for conditions of this nature should include physical agents to relieve pain, promote healing, improve circulation, and restore function. Local heat or cold, electrotherapy, massage, and stretching exercises are especially effective.

Atrophy

Muscle atrophy is identified by inspection. Weakness from atrophy can also be checked by manual muscle testing (MMT). Circumferential measurements can be used to gauge atrophy, but these measurements alone can be misleading. When a muscle is strengthened, it loses some fat content and may appear leaner, yet when tested will show strength greater than or equal to the uninvolved side. Muscle atrophy can be caused by disuse or by neurological deficit. It is not sufficient to merely recognize muscle atrophy and weakness—it is also necessary to determine why it is present.

Treatment

Treatment should focus on alleviating the cause of the weakness, strengthening exercises, and return to functional activities.

JOINT DISORDERS

For classification purposes, the following structures are considered part of the joint: A) subchondral bone; B) hyaline cartilage; C) menisci; D) synovial lining; E) capsule; F) ligament; and G) bursæ. They are referred to as the noncontractile or "inert" structures.

With joint disorders, both active and passive movements are usually painful or limited in the same direction, with pain at end range. Except in very acute cases, resisted muscle tests are not painful. The patient will often be able to describe the exact mechanism of injury, thus leading the clinician to the exact area of injury. The palpation examination is very important in determining joint involvement because many of the structures can be easily palpated in the extremity joints.

Sprain

A sprain is an injury to the joint capsule or the supporting ligaments resulting from overstress that damages the fibers or their attachments. The joint capsule holds the bone ends together while allowing free movement at the joints. Ligaments reinforce the capsule at points of special stress and prevent abnormal motion of a joint while permitting normal functional motion. The collagen fibers of ligaments are arranged in parallel, which allows very little elasticity; therefore, if a ligament is overstressed, permanent laxity may develop. The collagen fibers of the joint capsule are arranged in an irregular fashion. This arrangement allows a certain degree of play even though the individual collagen fibers are inelastic.

Sprains may be classified as mild, moderate, or severe (first, second, and third degree, respectively). In a mild sprain, some of the fibers have been torn and a small amount of hemorrhaging is present. The ligament is not weakened. In a moderate sprain, a portion of the ligament or capsule is torn, there is a moderate amount of hemorrhaging, and some degree of functional loss is present. In a severe sprain, there is ligamentous or capsular disruption and loss of function due to a complete tear.[49] There is more pronounced hemorrhaging and swelling in the area.

Treatment

Stiffness is inherent in a mild sprain, so treatment is aimed at preventing joint hypomobility and disuse atrophy. Movement and activities are allowed within pain free limits. Physical agents decrease pain and promote healing. Ice, compression bandaging, and elevation help prevent or reduce edema. Gradual and progressive return to normal function is encouraged as the sprain heals.

A moderate sprain must be treated with considerably more precaution to guard against further injury. The capsule or ligaments are already weakened. Even after the joint is "healed"—is pain free—it is still vulnerable to reinjury. If left alone, joint restriction and disuse atrophy may develop. Pain free range of motion and joint mobilization must be integrated into treatment. Physical agents can also be included to relieve symptoms, reduce edema, and promote healing. A ligament requires 6–10 weeks after surgery to heal. A similar time may be necessary after a moderate sprain. It is common for a moderate sprain to be relatively pain free with normal mobility 2–3 weeks after injury, but the injured tissue is still weak. A patient who returns to vigorous physical activity this soon may suffer a second, often more serious, sprain. Many severe sprains in athletics occur under these circumstances.

Sometimes, the severe sprain must be surgically repaired to avoid permanent joint instability. The trend, however, seems to be toward nonsurgical management of many severe sprains. The joint should be splinted or braced in a position that allows optimal healing. This should be followed by controlled motion and a gradual return to functional activities. Proprioception exercises are critical to successful ligament rehabilitation. Restoration of full strength and mobility is the final phase of treatment.

Dislocation

Dislocation is an actual displacement of the opposing surfaces of a joint. In dislocations, some of the joint's ligamentous and capsular structures are stretched or torn. Subluxation is a partial dislocation that may or may not be associated with ligamentous or capsular damage. Either of these conditions may spontaneously reduce, or the bones may lock in the dislocated position. It is also possible to have a chronically dislocating joint without acute ligamentous damage. In this case, the clinician can assume previous damage to the ligaments or capsule.

Treatment

Surgical repair may be considered for acute dislocations with a complete tear of the ligaments. Otherwise, acute dislocation is simply the result of a severe sprain, and it can be treated as such. In the case of chronic dislocation, it is assumed the joint is unstable, and it is treated as such.

Joint Inflammation (Capsulitis, Synovitis, Arthritis)

Joint inflammation, like muscle inflammation, can follow as a natural reaction to injury. It is rarely seen without a history of aggravation or injury. The involved joint may be swollen, red, or warm. As with all joint disorders, movement will hurt, but it is also characteristic for inflammatory disorders to be painful and stiff with rest. Joints that have undergone degenerative changes are more vulnerable to inflammation after overuse or over–stress.

Treatment

Treatment consists of rest, pain free movement and activities, physical agents to promote healing, and restoration of strength and mobility as healing progresses.

Bursitis

A bursa is a sac filled with fluid and situated at places in the tissues at which friction would otherwise develop. Sometimes adventitious bursa develop at sites of friction caused by such abnormalities as pathological bony prominences or protruding metallic inserts. The bursa is highly vascular and has a rich nerve supply.

Bursitis is inflammation of a bursa. It is usually secondary to strains, sprains, or contusions and is often present in cases of tendinitis and myositis. Bursitis is rarely a primary disorder. Calcific deposits (calcific bursitis) occasionally develop as a complication of bursitis. Palpation is often the key to diagnosis. Active and passive range of motion and resisted muscle tests will let the clinician determine if joint or muscle inflammation is present. Bursitis may herald the onset of systemic disease, particularly a collagen disease such as RA or gout. Naturally, unless there is a bursa anatomically in a place from which pain appears to be emanating, the pain cannot be coming from bursitis (Fig 3–6). There are no bursæ located in the back unless they are adventitious. Traumatic bursitis is usually limited to olecranon, ischial, calcaneal, metatarsophalangeal, or intermetatarsal bursæ.[52]

Treatment

Treatment consists of rest, protection from further aggravation, physical agents to promote healing, and restoration of functional activities as healing progresses. Phonophoresis or iontophoresis can also be effective treatments.

Hypomobility (Dysfunction)

Joint hypomobility or dysfunction occurs in two ways: joint impingement and joint contracture.

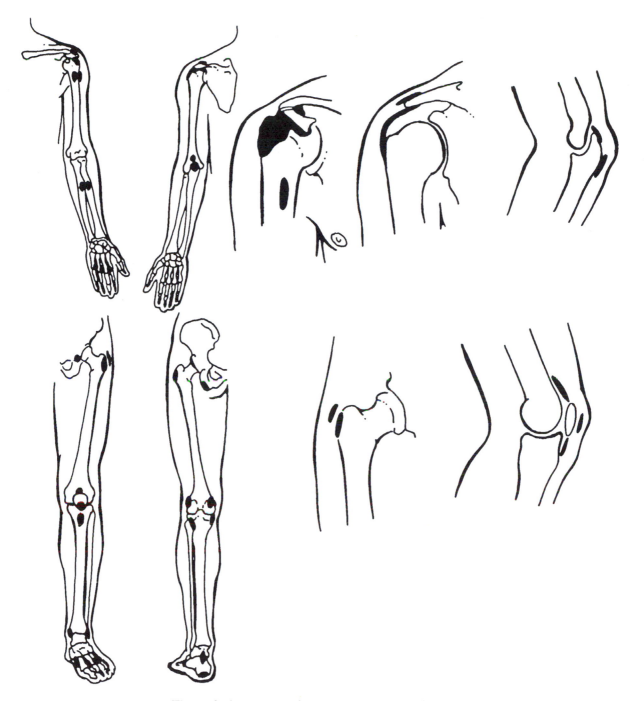

Figure 3–6. Location of bursae throughout the body.

Impingement

The joint seems to lock or be blocked in one particular direction, but may be free to move in other directions. The cause of the blockage is usually a roughened cartilage or a meniscus, a loose body or osteophyte or a nipping of the synovial lining. Joint impingement is most frequently seen in joints that are hypermobile or that show signs of DJD. Although joint impingement or locking happens occasionally in the spine, it rarely happens in the extremity joints. The mechanism of injury is usually a sudden unguarded movement with little or no trauma.

Treatment

Joint manipulation is occasionally indicated as treatment, although the patient will often know how to self–treat the disorder. The patient should be taught to avoid the circumstances that cause the locking. Surgery may be indicated if a torn meniscus or other joint obstruction is the cause of the impingement.

Contracture (Adhesive Capsulitis)

Joint contracture generally involves the entire capsule, although certain parts of the capsule may be more contracted than others due to specific areas of injury and the position of the joint at rest. Joint contracture is usually the result of prolonged immobilization after an injury.

Joint contracture develops when the individual collagen fibers adhere to each other during immobilization. This prevents the play that is normally present between these fibers as the joint moves. This disorder is further complicated when additional collagen is laid down in response to injury and when adhesions are formed. The result is a thickened, tight, constricted capsule.

Ligaments do not become contracted nearly as quickly as the capsule does because the individual collagen fibers are laid down in parallel, and there is normally very little play within the fibers of the ligament. Ligaments do hypertrophy, become thick and stiff, and contribute to joint contracture in cases involving long periods of immobilization.[37]

Active and passive movements will be restricted in a capsular pattern, and resisted muscle tests will be painless.[14,37] Muscle atrophy and weakness may be present. The joint capsule will often be tender to palpation. The patient's chief complaint will often be stiffness and restriction of movement rather than pain. Although joint contracture will not show up on x–ray initially, prolonged joint hypomobility may lead to joint degeneration, which will eventually be evident with x–rays.

Treatment

Treatment consists of joint mobilization and stretching techniques. Heat, especially ultrasound, is useful before mobilization. Ultrasound produces a deep heating effect precisely at the joint structures (muscle–bone interface) increasing the extensibility of these tissues. Hold–relax stretching exercises and functional active exercises are also indicated due to the adaptive muscle shortening often present after prolonged immobilization. Joint contracture can be prevented in most cases by properly managing acute sprains, strains, and inflammations and by using fracture management techniques that allow some joint movement early in the healing process.

Hypermobility

Joint hypermobility involves laxity of the joint capsule or ligaments and is commonly associated with congenital defects or severe trauma. Patients with joint hypermobility often complain of pain after vigorous activity. They often cannot maintain any joint position for more than a few minutes without pain. The patient will often describe a "slipping" or "popping" in the joint with certain movements. This slipping or popping can be repeated over and over. Chronic dislocation may be a complaint in severe cases. Occasional, inconsistent popping is usually meaningless. Joint hypermobility may lead to early joint degeneration because of increased wear and tear and abnormal biomechanical stresses to which the joint is subjected.

Treatment

Joint hypermobility should be treated with muscle strengthening or, in extreme cases, support such as bracing or splinting. Strengthening the rotator cuff and scapulothoracic muscles is especially effective if the glenohumeral joint is unstable.

Degenerative Joint Disease (Osteoarthritis–DJD)

Degenerative joint disease (DJD) is characterized by loss of articular cartilage; subchondral bony sclerosis; cartilage and bone proliferation at the joint margins with subsequent osteophyte formation; and capsular thickening with synovial inflammation.

In severe, advanced stages of this disorder, pain is present with all movement, especially with activities that cause approximation of the joint surfaces such as lifting a heavy weight (upper extremity) or weightbearing (lower extremity). This is because the protective articular cartilage is worn away, and bone is moving on bone. In other stages, DJD itself is usually symptom free. The pain associated with mild to moderate DJD is more likely to be caused by contracture than DJD itself: the clinician can easily distinguish between the two by determining whether joint approximation or joint movement increases the patient's pain. Patients with DJD are more vulnerable to joint sprain and inflammation because only a slight amount of overstress or overuse is often enough to aggravate the symptoms.

There are many theories about the cause of DJD. Although there is evidence of genetic, metabolic, and endocrine factors, three principle causes are commonly seen:

1. Joints that are hypomobile are susceptible to DJD. The hyaline cartilage is avascular and receives its nutrition through the synovial fluid. Normal movement is vital to this exchange. Laboratory experiments have shown that a joint that is immobilized will soon begin to show signs of DJD.[44,45]

2. Joint hypermobility will lead to DJD because of abnormal biomechanical stresses. Clinical experience shows that joints that are unstable or hypermobile due to old injury, repeated overstress, or congenital defects will often develop DJD.

3. Wear and tear plays an important role in development of DJD. A joint subjected to abnormal biomechanical stresses or repeated injuries will often show signs of joint degeneration.

Treatment

Since mild to moderate DJD is usually symptom free, treatment is directed toward correcting or supporting abnormal biomechanical stresses; mobilizing hypomobility; and managing the joint sprains or inflammations, which are often the true causes of the patient's complaint. An example of abnormal biomechanical stress is uneven leg length. The patient is likely to stand more on the short leg, thus increasing the weightbearing stress on that leg. The patient is also apt to develop genu recurvatum of the short leg due to abnormal hyperextension at toe–off.[63] The spine will develop a compensatory scoliosis with increased facet weightbearing and decreased facet joint mobility on the concave side. Any of these factors could cause early DJD in the involved joints. These severe consequences of leg length discrepancy are particularly unfortunate since

the condition can be easily corrected with a shoe lift. There are many other examples of abnormal biomechanical stresses that can precipitate DJD, such as pes planus, pronated foot, genu valgus, genu varus, and depression of the metatarsal arch. Joint hypermobility or instability can also cause abnormal stress.

If joint hypomobility is present with DJD, the clinician should try mobilization. If successful, restoration of normal joint mobility may interrupt the degenerative process. In severe DJD, any attempt to increase the mobility or activity may result in increased pain or inflammation. In such cases, correcting abnormal biomechanical stresses may still be feasible, as may support with braces, foot orthoses, splints, and other assistive and labor saving devices.

Osteochondritis Dissecans

Osteochondritis dissecans is the separation of a fragment of articular cartilage from the underlying matrix. It occurs most frequently at the knee and elbow. Some believe the disorder results from spontaneous ischemic necrosis due to circulatory insufficiency, while others believe it is due to repeated trauma. The latter seems more probable.[59] Osteochondritis dissecans is easily identifiable on x–ray.

Treatment

Treatment varies from no treatment, except for protection from further trauma, to surgical excision. The clinician must be aware of this disorder. Failure to improve with appropriate physical therapy management may indicate osteochondritis dissecans, and it again points out the need for x–ray examination in cases involving trauma, repeated or unusual stresses, or conditions that do not respond in a timely way to physical therapy management.

NERVE DISORDERS

Although positive neurological signs and symptoms are often found in the extremities, they are usually due to pathology in the brain or spinal cord or to spinal nerve root impingement. Central nervous system dysfunction is not within the scope of this text; treatment of spinal nerve root impingement is discussed in *Evaluation, Treatment and Prevention of*

Musculoskeletal Disorders, Volume I—The Spine. Only the neurological disorders directly associated with pathology in the extremities are dealt with here.

Nerve Contusion

The peripheral nerves most often contused are the axillary nerve at the shoulder, the radial nerve in the radial groove of the humerus, the ulnar nerve at the elbow, and the peroneal nerve behind the fibular head.

The injury is usually from a direct blow on the nerve, causing pain and numbness. The condition may be transient or there may be persistent aching along the distribution of the nerve because of swelling and congestion within the nerve and nerve sheath. In isolated cases, there may be paralysis of the muscles supplied by the nerve.[52]

Treatment

Treatment should include measures to protect from overuse and further contusion. Cold compresses initially, followed by local heat or hydrotherapy on the second or third day, can be used to promote healing. Recovery is almost always complete and fairly rapid.[52] Muscle strengthening and re–education may be necessary in cases of prolonged paralysis.

Nerve Stretch

Another type of nerve injury is caused by overstretch. Examples include overstretching the common peroneal nerve after lateral collateral ligament (LCL) ruptures at the knee or overstretching the median nerve after elbow dislocation. The symptoms will vary with the severity of the injury. If there is a complete avulsion there will be immediate and complete loss of function; if the nerve is stretched but not torn, there will be hemorrhage and shock to the fibers and perhaps subsequent scarring around the nerve, in which case function will return more slowly and less completely.[52]

Treatment

Most cases will recover gradually. Physical therapy to maintain joint function, prevent deformity during complete paralysis, and regain muscle strength as the nerve function returns is important. Surgical

exploration and repair is sometimes necessary, but should be approached conservatively.[52]

Peripheral Nerve Entrapment

Peripheral nerve entrapment can cause pain, numbness, and muscle atrophy in the structures supplied by the entrapped nerve. Peripheral nerve entrapment symptoms follow the specific nerve distribution rather than a dermatome pattern, which is characteristic of spinal nerve root entrapment. The patient with peripheral nerve entrapment will often have normal muscle stretch reflexes. Night pain may be a symptom, especially if the nerve is subjected to postural stresses.

Peripheral nerves can be entrapped at many areas. Some of these sites include soft tissue tunnels, such as the Arcade of Froshe (see Chapter 5, <u>The Elbow</u>), or bony tunnels like the ulnar groove. Peripheral nerves are also subject to mechanical irritation such as friction and stretch or intermittent compression as a result of non–functional postures, movements, or repetitive stresses. Peripheral nerve entrapment may be as obvious as signs or symptoms in the corresponding distribution of the affected nerve. Subtle symptoms may be present before the presentation of objective signs in the early stages of peripheral nerve entrapment. There are several excellent references concerning the diagnosis, classification, and treatment of these injuries.[39,16,57,48,7]

Treatment

Conservative measures such as soft–tissue mobilization or stretching exercises may help mobilize an entrapped nerve. Patients should be taught methods to eliminate the stresses that aggravate the problem. Neural mobilization can be used if the patient shows positive neural tension signs. Surgical release or nerve transposition is occasionally necessary if conservative treatment fails.

BONE DISORDERS

Bone disorders are characterized by pain at rest that is aggravated by activity. Symptoms provoked by percussion on examination or by unusual joint crepitus after injury indicate a fracture. The patient presenting with a fracture and without an acute injury may have an underlying metabolic pathology (e.g., metastatic cancer).

Fracture

Any case involving trauma should be x–rayed to see if a fracture is present. Although fracture diagnosis is done primarily with x–rays, certain signs and symptoms should cause the clinician to suspect fracture. These include pain in locations unusual for a sprain or strain; a deep aching pain at rest; and grinding or grating sensations with movement. Since fractures are occasionally missed with x–ray, the clinician should be aware of these signs and symptoms and seek further radiological examination if the patient's symptoms persist beyond a normal expected treatment time.

Treatment

Fractures require medical management. Clinicians may be involved in preserving and restoring mobility and strength as the fracture heals.

Stress Fracture

Stress fractures are usually seen in people who have a rather rapid increase in their level of physical activity. The term "march fracture" was coined to describe the fracture of the metatarsal shaft that is caused, not by acute injury, but by repeated stress. Military recruits, athletes starting quickly into a new activity, runners who have increased their mileage rapidly, or anyone who has gone from a sitting occupation to one that requires standing and walking are susceptible to stress fractures.

This disorder is particularly deceptive since there is no history of traumatic injury. Early x–rays are negative, yet the symptoms persist. X–rays confirm the diagnosis only if they show new bone formation at the site of insult. These circumstances often occur without an actual fracture line ever appearing across the bone. A bone scan is a useful diagnostic procedure. It will be "hot" within 24 hours of symptom onset.[8,54]

While stress fractures are common in the foot, they can occur almost anywhere, especially in the lower extremities and pelvis. Patients will not have a history of specific trauma but will be tender over the bone. Stress fracture pain is felt as a deep aching that often persists even at rest. A vibrating tuning fork placed over a suspected fracture site will produce pain.

Treatment

Once the diagnosis is confirmed, the patient should be protected from further stress until the lesion is solidly healed, followed by gradual resumption of activities. Early detection permits prompt treatment and prevents progression of the pathology. Addressing the causes is an important part of preventing further injury.

SUMMARY

The body's response to trauma and the deleterious effects of immobilization have been outlined. A procedure for planning treatments was described. Effective treatment includes consideration of all potential sources of neuromusculoskeletal problems. Four components of rehabilitation common to all patients were identified and their relationship to the treatment planning process was described. Finally, common neuromusculoskeletal pathologies and their treatments were discussed.

REFERENCES

1. Binkley JM, Peat M: The Effect of Immobilization on the Ultrastructure and Mechanical Properties of the MCL of Rats. Clin Orthop Rel Res 203:301-308, 1986.

2. Boissonnault W, Janos S: Screening For Medical Disease: Physical Therapy Assessment and Treatment Principles. In Examination in Physical Therapy Practice: Screening For Medical Disease. Churchill-Livingstone, New York NY 1991.

3. Booth F, Kelso J: Effect of Hindlimb Immobilization on Contractile and Histochemical Properties of Skeletal Muscle. Pflugers Arch 342:231-238, 1973.

4. Booth F: Physiologic and Biochemical Effects of Immobilization on Muscle. Clin Orthop Rel Res 219:15-20.

5. Bourdeaux B, Hutchinson W: Etiology of Traumatic Osteoporosis. JBJS 35:479, 1953.

6. Brand RA, Crownshield RD: The Effect of Cane

Use on Hip Contact Force. Clin Orthop and Rel Res 147:181, 1980.

7. Butler D: <u>Mobilisation of the Nervous System</u>. Churchill-Livingstone, Edinburgh 1991.

8. Cahill BR: Stress Fracture of the Proximal Tibial Epiphysis: A Case Report. Am J Sports Med 5: 186-187, 1977.

9. Candolin T, Videman T: Surface Changes in the Articular Cartilage of Rabbit Knee during Immobilization: A Scanning Electron Microscopic Study of Experimental Osteoarthritis. Acta Pathol Microbiol Immunol Scand 88:291, 1980.

10. Cloward R: Cervical Discography: A Contribution to the Etiology and Mechanism of Neck, Shoulder and Arm Pain. Annals of Surgery 150(6) 1052-1064, 1959.

11. Cooper R: Alternatives During Immobilization and Regeneration of Skeletal Muscle in Cats. JBJS 54:919, 1972.

12. Cummings G: <u>Proceedings of the Ninth Annual Dogwood Conference</u>. Dogwood Institute, Alpharetta GA 1984.

13. Cyriax J, Coldham M: Treatment By Management, Manipulation, and Injection. In <u>Textbook of Orthopaedic Medicine</u>. Volume 2, 11th ed. Bailliere-Tindall, London England 1984.

14. Cyriax J: Diagnosis of Soft Tissue Lesions. In <u>Textbook of Orthopædic Medicine</u>, Vol 1, 8th edition. Bailliere-Tindall, London 1982.

15. Cyriax J: Treatment by Manipulation. Massage and Injection. In <u>Textbook of Orthopaedic Medicine</u>, Vol 2, 10th edition. Bailliere-Tindall, London 1980.

16. Dawson DM, Hallet M, Millender LH: <u>Entrapment Neuropathies</u>. Little-Brown, Boston MA 1983.

17. DeAndrade J, Grant C and Dixon A: Joint Distension and Reflex Inhibition in the Knee. JBJS 47:313-322, 1965.

18. Dickinson A, Bennett K: Therapeutic Exercise. Clin Sports Med 4:417-429, 1985.

19. Donaldson C, et al: Effect of Prolonged Bed Rest on Bone Mineral. Metabolism 19:1071, 1970.

20. Donatelli R, Owens-Burkhardt: Effects of Immobilization on the Extensibility of Periarticular Connective Tissue. JOSPT 3: 67-72, 1981.

21. Fleisch H, Russeu, Simpson B, and Muhlbauer R: Prevention by a Diphophonate of Immobilization Osteoporosis in Rats. Nature 223:221, 1969.

22. Gamble JG, Edwards CC, Max SR: Enzymatic Adaptation in Ligaments during Immobilization. AMJ Sports Med 12:221-228, 1984.

23. Garrett G: Effects of Injury on Muscle and the Patellofemoral Joint. Advances on the Knee and Shoulder. Cincinnati Sports Medicine and Deaconess Hospital, Cincinnati OH 1989. Symposium.

24. Geiser M, Trueta J: Muscle Action, Bone Rarefaction, and Bone Formation. JBJS 40:282.

25. Griffin J, et al: Patients Treated with Ultrasound Driven Hydrocortisone and with Ultrasound Alone. Physical Therapy 47: (594-601, 1967.

26. Groom D: The Neck and Shoulder: Does Treatment of Spinal Structures Speed Recovery from Shoulder Dysfunction? Lincoln School of Health Sciences, La Trobe University, Victoria, Australia 1988. Unpublished thesis.

27. Hardt A: Early Metabolic Responses of Bone to Immobilization. JBJS 54:119, 1972.

28. Harrelson GL: Shoulder Rehabilitation. In <u>Physical Rehabilitation of the Injured Athlete</u>. JR Andrews and GL Harrelson, ed. WB Saunders, Philadelphia PA 1991.

29. Howell D: Osteoarthritis-Etiology and Pathogenesis. In <u>American Academy of Orthopædic Surgeons: Symposium on Osteo-Arthritis</u>. CV Mosby Co, St. Louis MO 1976. Seminar manual.

30. Janda JV: On the Concept of Postural Muscles and Posture in Man. Aust J Physiother 29:83-85, 1983.

31. Janda V: Muscles, Central Nervous Motor Regulation And Back Problems. In The Neurological Mechanisms in Manipulative Therapy. IM Korr, ed. Plenum Press, New York NY1978.

32. Jayson M and Barks J: Structural Changes in the Intervertebral Disc. Annuls Rheum Dis 32:10-15, 1973.

33. Jayson M, Dixon A: Intra-articular Pressure in Rheumatoid Arthritis of the Knee III: Pressure Changes During Joint Use. Annuls Rheum Dis 29:401-406, 1970.

34. Jones M, Butler D: Clinical Reasoning. In <u>Mobilisation of the Nervous System</u>. D Butler, ed. Churchill-Livingstone, Melbourne Australia 1991.

35. Kapandji I: <u>The Physiology of the Joints</u>, 5th ed. Churchill-Livingstone, New York NY 1982.

36. Kennedy J, et al: Nerve Supply of the Human Knee and Its Functional Importance. Am J Sports Med 10:329-335, 1982.

37. Kessler R, Hertling D: The Hip-Common Lesions. In <u>Management of Common Musculoskeletal Disorders-Physical Therapy Principles and Methods</u>, 2nd ed. JB Lippincott, Philadelphia PA 1992.

38. Kirkaldy-Willis WH: The Pathology And Pathogenesis Of Low Back Pain. In <u>Managing Low Back Pain</u>, 2nd edition. W Kirkaldy-Willis, ed. Churchill Livingstone, New York NY 1988.

39. Kopell H and Thompson W: <u>Peripheral Entrapment Neuropathies</u>. Krieger, Huntington NY 1975.

40. Lindboe C, Platou C: Effects of Immobilization of Short Duration on Muscle Fiber Size. Clinical Physiology 4:183, 1984.

41. MacDougall J, Elder G, Sale D, et al: Effects of Strength Training and Immobilization on Human Muscle Fibers. European Journal of Applied Physiology 43:25, 1980.

42. MacDougall J, et al: Biomechanical Adaptation of Human Skeletal Muscle to Heavy Resistance Training and Immobilization. Journal of Applied Physiology 43:700-703, 1977.

43. Max S: Disuse Atrophy of Skeletal Muscle: Loss of Functional Activity of Mitochondria. Bio Chem Bio Phys Res Commun 46:1384-1398.

44. McFadden J: Smoking May Be Significant Risk Factor in Failed Back Surgery. Back Pain Monitor 4:41-52, Apr 1986.

45. McKenzie R: The Lumbar Spine. Spinal Publications, Waikanae New Zealand 1981.

46. Minaire P, et al: Quantitative Histological Data on Disuse Osteoporosis. Calcif Tissue Res 17:57, 1974.

47. Mooney V and Robertson J: The Facet Syndrome. Clin Orthop and Rel Res 115:149-156, Mar/Apr 1976.

48. Nerve Compression Syndromes. RM Szabo, ed. Slack, Thorofare 1989.

49. Noyes FR, Grood ES, et al: Clinical Biomechanics of the Knee: Ligament Restraints and Functional Stability. AAOS Symposium on the Athlete's Knee. CV Mosby, St Louis MO 1981.

50. Noyes RR, Mangine RE, Barber S: Biomechanics of Ligament Failure: An Analysis of Immobilization, Exercise, and Reconditioning Effects in Primates. JBJS 56:1406.

51. Noyes, F: Advances in the Understanding of Knee Ligament Injury, Repair and Rehabilitation. Medicine and Science in Sports and Exercise 16:427-443, 1984.

52. O'Donoghue DF: Treatment of Injuries to Athlete, 2nd ed. WB Saunders, Philadelphia PA 1970.

53. Rifenberick D, Max S: Substrate Utilization by Disused Rat Skeletal Muscles. American Journal of Physiology 226:295-297.

54. Roy S, Irving R: Sports Medicine: Prevention, Evaluation, Management, and Rehabilitation. Prentice Hall, Englewood Cliffs NJ 1983.

55. Salter R, Field P: The Effects of Continuous Compression on Living Articular Cartilage. JBJS 42:31-49, 1960.

56. Stoke M, Young A: A Contribution of Reflex Inhibition to Arthrogenic Muscle Weakness. Clinical Science 67:7, 1984.

57. Sunderland S: Nerves and Nerve Injuries. Churchill-Livingstone, Edinburgh 1978.

58. Trias A: Effects of Persistent Pressure on Articular. JBJS 43:376-386, 1961.

59. Turck S: Orthopædics. 2nd edition. Lippincott, Philadelphia PA 1967.

60. Uhthoff H, Jaworski Z: Bone Loss in Response to Long-Term Immobilization. JBJS 60:420, 1978.

61. Videman T: Connective Tissue and Immobilization. Clin Orthop Rel Res 221:26-32, 1987.

62. Videman T: Experimental Osteoarthritis in the Rabbit. Comparison of Different Periods of Repeated Immobilization. Acta Orthop Scand 53:339, 1982.

63. Walker H and Schreck R: Relationship of Hyperextended Gait Pattern to Chondromalacia Patellæ. Phys Ther 55: 259-262, 1975.

64. Wyke B: The Neurological Basis of Thoracic Spinal Pain. Rheumatology and Physical Medicine 10:356-367, 1970.

65. Young A, Stokes M and Iles J: Effects of Joint Pathology on Muscle. Clin Orthop 219:21-27, 1987.

66. Zohn D and Mennell J: Musculoskeletal Pain: Diagnosis and Physical Treatment. Little-Brown, Boston MA 1976.

SECTION 2
The Upper Quarter

CHAPTER 4
THE SHOULDER

INTRODUCTION

Shoulder problems can be a challenge to the clinician. Effective function of this highly mobile joint complex requires movement across four joint structures. This requires coordinated neuromuscular control of several muscular force couples while maintaining the integrity of the neurovascular structures that exit the neck and thorax. The balance between force couple interactions determines the health of the shoulder—its ability to assume postures and perform a wide range of daily activities while resisting the physical stresses of those postures and activities. Shoulder symptoms can originate from the cervical spine and thoracic cage; the viscera; or the shoulder complex itself.[2,4] A thorough medical examination will rule out or confirm serious pathologies. Effective shoulder management must include all the related neuromusculoskeletal structures considered in an appropriate functional manner.

FUNCTIONAL ANATOMY

Osseous and Capsuloligamentous Components

The sternoclavicular, acromioclavicular, and glenohumeral joints are the true joints of the shoulder complex, while the scapulothoracic joint is a functional joint.[42] The bony structure of the joints is shown in Figure 4–1, and the ligamentous support of the joints is shown in Figure 4–2.

Sternoclavicular Joint

The sternoclavicular joint is a saddle–shaped synovial joint between the medial end of the clavicle, the sternal manubrium, and the first costal cartilage. This joint forms the only bone–to–bone attachment of the arm to the trunk. Its stability is supplemented by an intra–articular disc which blends with the capsuloligamentous tissues. When the shoulder moves into elevation or depression, the clavicle moves on the disc and cushions forces from the arm.[5,19] In cases of trauma to the clavicle and its joints, the acromioclavicular joint and the clavicle are most likely to be injured; however, there may be concurrent injury to the sternoclavicular joint.

Acromioclavicular Joint

The acromioclavicular joint is a plane synovial joint between the acromion process of the scapula and the lateral end of the clavicle. It augments the range of motion at the glenohumeral joint and is stabilized by a weak capsule that is fortified by several ligaments. Many people have an acromioclavicular intra–articular disc that increases the stability at this joint.[5] The coracoacromial ligament blends with the trapezius and deltoid muscle attachments to form a roof over the humeral head that helps prevent upward displacement of the humeral head. Since the coracoacromial ligament covers the supraspinatus muscle, it can be involved in shoulder impingement syndrome. The coracoclavicular ligament is composed of the trapezoid ligament anterolaterally and the conoid ligament posteromedially. This ligament is the primary suspensory ligament that

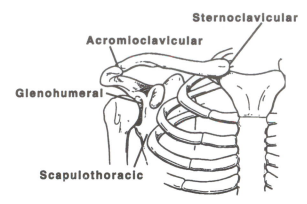

Figure 4–1. Joints of the shoulder.

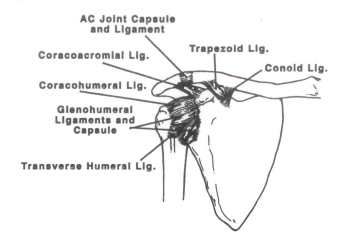

Figure 4–2. Shoulder ligaments (anterior view).

prevents separation of the scapula from the clavicle.[5] The acromioclavicular ligament lies over the superior aspect of the acromioclavicular joint, reinforcing the joint's capsule. Injury to the ligament structures—a "separated shoulder"—can render the acromioclavicular joint unstable and contribute to pain and dysfunction at the shoulder complex.

Glenohumeral Joint

The glenohumeral joint is a multiaxial ball–and–socket joint between the head of the humerus and the glenoid cavity of the scapula. It is a highly mobile joint with little inherent stability. Stabilization of the humeral head in the glenoid fossa is accomplished through both static and dynamic mechanisms.[48] *Circle stability* is provided by opposing structures on each side of the joint.[48] At the glenohumeral joint, the anterior and posterior joint capsule provides circle stability. Some additional support is provided by the glenoid labrum, a fibrocartilaginous rim that slightly deepens the glenoid cavity and makes the joint surfaces more congruent. The long head of the biceps

muscle that arises from the supraglenoid tubercle is continuous with the labrum. It helps prevent upward displacement of the humeral head.[47]

The ligamentous support of the glenohumeral joint is provided by three ligaments. Each ligament is actually a thickened area of the joint capsule. The ligaments are the superior glenohumeral ligament (SGHL); the middle glenohumeral ligament (MGHL); and the inferior glenohumeral ligament (IGHL) (Fig 4–3). These three ligaments act as static restraints to prevent excessive translation of the humeral head on the glenoid. The ligaments and their functions are listed in Table 4–1.[12]

The tendons of the rotator cuff muscles provide additional joint stability through their insertions on the joint capsule (Fig 4–4).[5,47] When the rotator cuff muscles are relaxed, the humeral head rests in the upper portion of the glenoid cavity. Contraction of the rotator cuff muscles pulls the humeral head down into the lower and wider portion of the glenoid cavity, allowing full overhead elevation of the arm. If the

Table 4–1. Glenohumeral Ligaments and their Functions

Structures	Function
SGHL and IGHL (both bands)	Prevent inferior displacement
SGHL, MGHL and IGHL (anterior band)	Prevent anterior displacement
IGHL (posterior band)	Prevent posterior displacement
SGHL, MGHL and IGHL (anterior band)	Limit external rotation
IGHL (posterior band)	Limit internal rotation

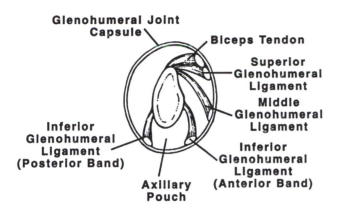

Figure 4–3. Glenohumeral ligaments blend with the joint capsule (adapted from O'Brien, et al[31]).

static stability of the glenohumeral joint is compromised, asynchronous muscle firing may ensue and cause subacromial impingement.

In summary, the four joints of the shoulder must work together to raise the arm overhead. Only 120° of elevation (flexion or abduction) occur at the glenohumeral joint. An additional 60° of elevation occur with scapular rotation.[47] The clavicle elevates ≈35–45° at the sternoclavicular joint during the first 90° of shoulder abduction.[36] In addition to elevation of the clavicle, 45–50° of backward rotation occur at the acromial end of the clavicle to allow full scapular rotation.[19] Although most authors agree that the overall ratio of scapular to humeral motion is 1:2, this can vary throughout the range of elevation of the arm.[19,33,42] The term *scapulo–humeral rhythm*[11] describes the integrated motion of all shoulder complex segments needed to fully elevate the arm.[19,33,42] Table 4–2 summarizes the movements and range of motion at the shoulder.

Scapulothoracic Joint

The scapulothoracic joint is not a true joint. It actually consists of the body of the scapula and the myofascial structures covering the posterior chest wall. The scapulothoracic joint functions as an integral part of the shoulder complex and is critical to providing dynamic stability and full range of motion for the shoulder complex.[35]

Neuromuscular Components

Muscular Structures

The shoulder complex is composed of three bony segments that function together as a kinematic chain.[2] The muscles of the shoulder complex act in combination to produce motion. Precise timing of these muscle contractions is essential for normal movement. There are three mechanisms that integrate the function of the shoulder complex prime movers: muscular force couples, the rotator cuff, and the scapular stabilizers. The posterior muscles of the shoulder are shown in Figure 4–5.

Muscular Force Couples

A force couple is formed by two equal but opposite forces that rotate a part around its axis of motion. There are several force couples critical to shoulder complex dynamics. During shoulder elevation, the deltoid and the rotator cuff muscles form a force couple that balances the upward pull of the deltoid with the downward pull of the rotator cuff. This centers the humeral head in the glenoid fossa and allows smooth movement (Fig 4–6). Injury to the rotator cuff mechanism can contribute to pain and dysfunction in the shoulder complex because of this critical role in fine tuning the position of the humerus.

The trapezius and serratus anterior muscles form a force couple that upwardly rotates the scapula during arm elevation (Fig 4–7). During the initial elevation, the upper trapezius and the upper portion of the serratus are most active, with some contribution from the levator scapulæ muscle. After 90° of elevation, the lower trapezius and lower serratus complete the motion. The lower trapezius is more

Table 4–2. Movements and Range of Motion at the Shoulder

Flexion	160-180°
Extension	50-60°
Abduction	170-180°
Adduction	50-75°
Internal rotation	60-100°
External rotation	80-90°

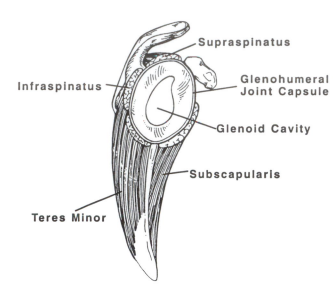

Figure 4–4. Tendons of the rotator cuff insert into the glenohumeral joint capsule (lateral view).

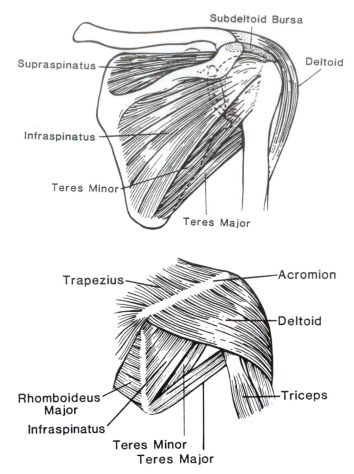

Figure 4–5. The posterior muscles of the shoulder

active in abduction of the shoulder, and the lower serratus is more active in flexion.[34,42]

Similarly, the rhomboids; teres major; levator scapulæ; pectoralis minor; and latissimus dorsi form a force couple that downwardly rotates the scapula during purposeful shoulder extension, as seen in functional motions such as chopping wood or performing pull–ups.

Rotator Cuff Mechanism

In addition to its role in the force couples previously discussed, the rotator cuff also increases the stability of the glenohumeral joint via the tendinous insertion of the muscles into the joint capsule.[12] When these muscles contract, tension is produced within the capsule, centering the humeral head in the fossa by ligament tension.[9,48] This provides dynamic circle stability of the glenohumeral joint.

Scapular Stabilization

The muscles that attach to the scapula control its rotation and position, and ultimately determine the positions available to the humerus. As already discussed, the serratus anterior and trapezius muscles control upward rotation of the scapula during

shoulder flexion and abduction. The rhomboids; levator scapulæ; teres major; pectoralis minor; and latissimus dorsi muscles downwardly rotate the scapula when lowering the arm to the side. The upward rotators work eccentrically to control scapular rotation during this movement. The serratus anterior and pectoralis minor perform scapular protraction. The rhomboids; levator scapulæ; and the middle and lower trapezius retract the scapula. The pectoralis minor can depress and upwardly tilt the scapula; thus, many muscles function as a group to dynamically stabilize the shoulder complex. Poor scapular stability can be caused by altered neuromuscular control after a shoulder injury and can contribute to further shoulder pain and dysfunction.

In summary, the neuromuscular structures play an important role in functional stability of the shoulder complex. Understanding these roles will help the clinician determine how these structures contribute to shoulder problems. Table 4–3 provides

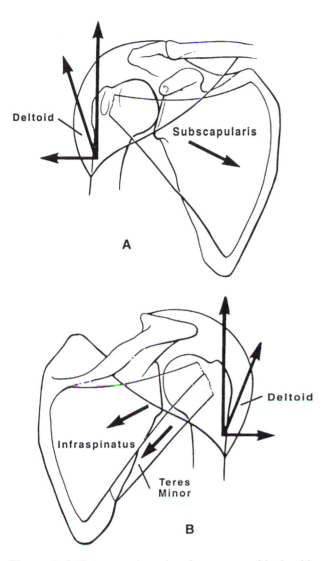

Figure 4–6. Force couple action that occurs with shoulder elevation. As the deltoid lifts the humerus, the rotator cuff pulls the head of the humerus inferiorly in the glenoid fossa. A) anterior view; B) posterior view.

a summary of the shoulder muscles with their actions and their peripheral and segmental nerve innervations.

Neurovascular Structures

The shoulder complex is particularly vulnerable to neurovascular compromise due to its intimate anatomical relationship with the brachial plexus and upper extremity vascular supply.[43]

Neural Structures

Cervical nerve roots merge to form the trunks, divisions, and cords of the brachial plexus. The

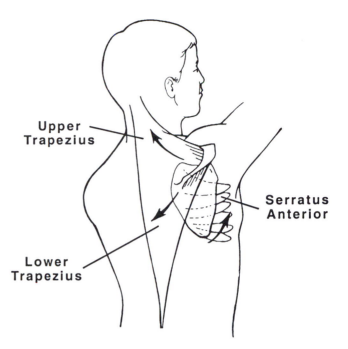

Figure 4–7. Force couple action that occurs with shoulder elevation. The action of the lower trapezius pulling inferomedially opposes the anterolateral force of the upper trapezius and serratus anterior. These opposing forces center the humeral head in the glenoid fossa.

plexus can be compromised at several sites between the neck and the shoulder (Fig 4–8).[29] As the cervical nerve roots merge to form the brachial plexus, they pass between the anterior and middle scalene muscles. Two nerves of clinical significance branch off before the trunks of the plexus form. The long thoracic nerve forms from branches of cervical roots from C5, C6, and C7. This nerve innervates the serratus anterior muscle. Injury to the long thoracic nerve adversely affects scapular stability and causes "scapular winging" (Fig 4–9). The dorsal scapular nerve, which innervates the levator scapulæ and rhomboids, is formed from branches of cervical roots C5 and C6. Injury to this nerve can affect scapular retraction and downward rotation.

The upper, middle, and lower trunks of the brachial plexus form as they pass over the first rib. The C8 and T1 nerve roots pass on either side of the head of the first rib (Fig 4–10). First rib dysfunction can affect the nerve trunks, and cause a variety of symptoms.

The suprascapular nerve arises from the upper trunk of the plexus, originating from the C4, C5, and

Table 4-3. Muscles of the Shoulder: Actions, Peripheral Nerve Supplies, and Nerve Roots

Muscles	Actions	Peripheral Nerve Supply	Spinal Segment
Anconeus	Elbow extension	Radial	C7, C8, (T1)
Biceps (when strong contraction required)	Forward flexion	Musculocutaneous	C5, C6, C7 (lateral cord)
Biceps Brachii	Elbow flexion	Musculocutaneous	C5, C6
Brachialis	Elbow flexion	Musculocutaneous	C5, C6, (C7)
Brachioradialis	Elbow flexion	Radial	C5, C6, (C7)
Coracobrachialis	Forward flexion	Musculocutaneous	C5, C6, C7 (lateral cord)
Deltoid	Abduction	Axillary	C5, C6 (posterior cord)
Deltoid (anterior fibers)	Forward flexion/ horizontal adduction/ internal rotation	Axillary	C5, C6 (posterior cord)
Deltoid (posterior fibers)	Extension/horizontal abduction/external rotation	Axillary	C5, C6 (posterior cord)
Flexor carpi ulnaris	Elbow flexion	Ulnar	C7, C8
Infraspinatus	Horizontal abduction/ abduction/external rotation	Suprascapular	C5, C6 (brachial plexus trunk)
Latissimus Dorsi	Extension/adduction/ internal rotation/ depression of scapula/ protraction (forward movement) of scapula	Thoracodorsal	C6, C7, C8 (posterior cord)
Levator scapulæ	Elevation of scapula/ medial (downward) rotation of inferior angle of scapula	C3, C4 nerve roots Dorsal scapular	C3, C4 C5
Long head of biceps (if arm externally rotated first, trick movement)	Abduction	Musculocutaneous	C5, C6, C7 (lateral cord)
Pectoralis major	Horizontal adduction/ adduction/internal rotation/ depression of scapula/ protraction (forward movement) of scapula	Lateral pectoral	C5, C6 (lateral cord)
Pectoralis major (clavicular fibers)	Forward flexion	Lateral pectoral	C5, C6 (lateral cord)
Pectoralis major (sternocostal fibers)	Extension	Lateral pectoral Medial pectoral	C5, C6 (lateral cord) C8, T1 (medial cord)
Pectoralis minor	Depression of scapula/ protraction (forward movement) of scapular retraction (backward movement) of scapula	Medial pectoral	C8, T1 (medial cord)
Pronator teres	Elbow flexion	Median	C6, C7

Table 4–3 (continued).   Muscles of the Shoulder: Actions, Peripheral Nerve Supplies, and Nerve Roots

Muscles	Actions	Peripheral Nerve Supply	Spinal Segment
Rhomboid major	Elevation of scapula/ retraction (backward movement) of scapula/ medial (downward) rotation of inferior angle of scapula	Dorsal scapular	(C4), C5
Rhomboid minor	Elevation of scapula/ retraction (backward movement) of scapula/ medial (downward) rotation of inferior angle of scapula	Dorsal scapular	(C4), C5
Serratus anterior	Depression of scapula/ lateral (upward) rotation of inferior angle/protraction (forward movement) of scapula	Long thoracic	C5, C6, (C7)
Subscapularis	Abduction/adduction	Subscapular	C5, C6 (posterior cord)
Subscapularis (when arm is by side)	Internal rotation	Subscapular	C5, C6 (posterior cord)
Supraspinatus	Abduction	Suprascapular	C5, C6 (brachial plexus trunk)
Teres major	Extension/horizontal abduction/adduction/ internal rotation	Subscapular	C5, C6 (posterior cord)
Teres minor	Extension/horizontal abduction/abduction/ external rotation	Axillary	C5, C6 (posterior cord); C5, C6 (brachial plexus trunk)
Trapezius	Retraction (backward movement) of scapula	Accessory	Cranial nerve XI
Trapezius (lower fibers)	Depression of scapula	Accessory C3, C4 nerve roots	Cranial nerve XI
Trapezius (upper and fibers)	Lateral (upward) rotation of inferior angle of scapula	Accessory C3, C4 nerve roots	Cranial nerve XI C3, C4
Trapezius (upper fibers)	Elevation of scapula	Accessory C3, C4 nerve roots	Cranial nerve XI
Triceps	Elbow extension	Radial	C6, C7, C8
Triceps (long head)	Extension	Radial	C5, C6, C7, C8, T1 (posterior cord)

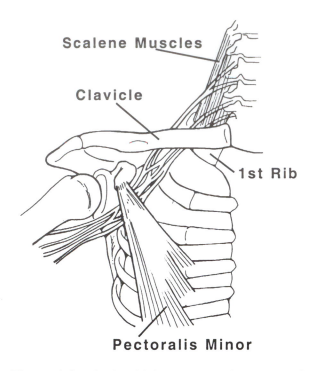

Figure 4–8. The brachial plexus can be compromised between the scalene muscles; between the clavicle and the first rib; and under the insertion of the pectoralis minor.

C6 nerve roots. This nerve passes beneath the trapezius through the suprascapular notch to innervate the supraspinatus and infraspinatus muscles. The suprascapular nerve can be impinged at this notch by the overlying superior transverse scapular ligament (Fig 4–11), causing pain and affecting abduction and external rotation at the shoulder.

The trunks of the brachial plexus divide into the anterior and posterior divisions just beneath the clavicle. The lateral, posterior, and middle cords of the plexus are formed beneath the pectoralis minor muscle (Fig 4–8). Postural dysfunction or traumatic injuries can cause impingement of the plexus beneath the clavicle or the pectoralis minor. The median, ulnar, radial, axillary, and musculocutaneous nerves form from the cords of the plexus as they pass under the pectoralis minor muscle.

Vascular Structures

In the shoulder region, the vascular structures closely follow the path of the neural structures. The subclavian and axillary arteries are commonly compromised. They can be compressed between A) the scalenus anticus and medius; B) the clavicle and

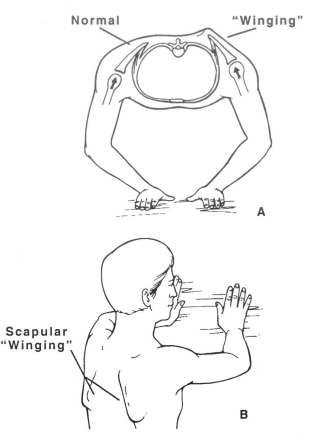

Figure 4–9. Scapular winging can be caused by injury to the long thoracic nerve.

the first rib (or a cervical rib); or C) the pectoralis minor muscle and the ribs (Fig 4–12). The resulting symptoms can seem to be neurological. Signs and symptoms of this vascular compression have been traditionally grouped under the diagnosis Thoracic Outlet Syndrome (TOS) (see the "Common Clinical Conditions" section of this chapter). Compression of the posterior humeral circumflex artery (with or without the axillary nerve) is less frequent, but can occur in the quadrilateral space (Fig 4–13).[6]

EVALUATION

Subjective Examination

The subjective examination should proceed as outlined in Chapter 2, Principles of Extremity Evaluation. The patient's main complaints give the clinician valuable clues about the current problems and help plan the objective examination. Any recent trauma should be documented, especially if the static stability of the shoulder could be compromised. Chronic problems can be clarified by identifying

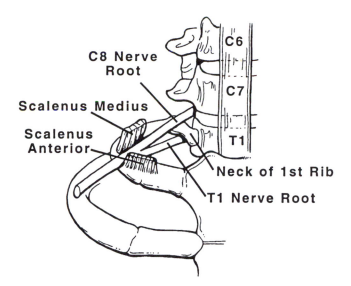

Figure 4–10. The C8 and T1 nerve roots pass on either side of 1st rib (right shoulder, anterior view).

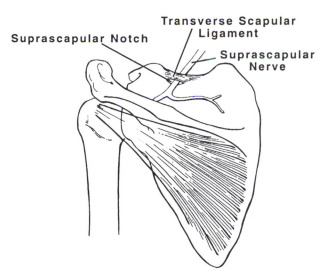

Figure 4–11. The suprascapular nerve can become entrapped at suprascapular notch (left shoulder, posterior view).

contributing factors, including cumulative trauma caused by repetitive shoulder motions.

The general medical history should be noted, especially any previous injuries or surgeries to the shoulder complex or cervical spine. Shoulder pain can have many sources including the myocardium and viscera (diaphragm, gall bladder, liver, kidney, and lung); therefore, current or past problems with these systems should be carefully noted. The results of any diagnostic or laboratory tests should be noted. Advances in the use of MRI to diagnose shoulder complaints and pathology make it a useful tool, especially for looking at rotator cuff problems, labrum injuries, or other sub–acromial pathology. The results of standard radiographs should be

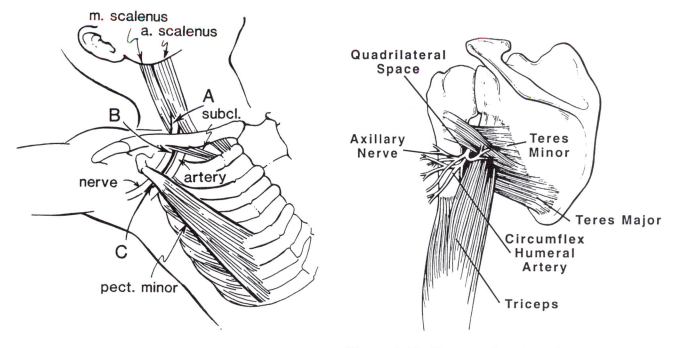

Figure 4–12. Thoracic outlet syndrome sites: A) scalene-first rib syndrome; B) costoclavicular syndrome; and C) pectoralis minor or hyperabduction syndrome.

Figure 4–13. The posterior circumflex artery can be compressed in the quadrilateral space (left shoulder, posterior view. Adapted from Baker, et al[1]).

obtained to identify any degenerative changes or evidence of calcified tendons or other recent or previous instability at the shoulder joints.

Planning the Objective Examination

Based on the subjective clues, the clinician must make decisions about which tests to perform during the objective examination. There is no need to perform every shoulder test on every patient complaining of shoulder problems. Excessive testing can provoke the patient's symptoms and may lead to an inaccurate picture of the patient's condition; therefore, before beginning the objective examination, it helps to plan which tests to perform based on the severity, irritability and nature (SIN) of the problem. If the shoulder problem is severe, the patient will have difficulty maintaining a position, so the mobility examination should be limited to pain free points in the range. Shoulder problems that are provoked easily but don't settle down easily are considered irritable. For patients with irritable conditions, the number of motions tested should be limited to avoid exacerbating symptoms. Sometimes the nature of the problem limits the objective examination. For example, an acute or unhealed fracture of the humeral head would prevent a full shoulder examination. Recent acute trauma to the shoulder, such as a acromioclavicular sprain, glenohumeral dislocation, or rotator cuff tear may limit the examination due to the severity of the complaints, the irritability of the symptoms, and the nature of the problems. In such cases, only the most essential tests should be performed during the initial evaluation. At this point, treatment should be geared toward controlling symptoms. Further evaluation can be conducted as the condition resolves.

The Cervical Component of Shoulder Disorders

The cervical spine and shoulder have an intimate anatomical, biomechanical, and neural relationship that is complex and not yet fully understood.[17] Shoulder disorders can be caused by shoulder pathology, spinal structures, or both.

Stimulation of the anterolateral portion of cervical discs can refer pain to the medial border of the ipsilateral scapula.[10] These sites of interscapular pain are referred to as "Cloward's Areas" (Fig 4–14).

Irritation of the posterolateral disc refers pain to the scapula and the posterior shoulder region.[10] Cervical disc pathology can irritate neuromeningeal structures and refer pain to the shoulder.[17] Injecting 6% saline solution into the interspinous muscles between C3 and T2 spinal segments produces characteristic patterns of pain referral into the shoulder and upper limb.[14]

Diagnostic blocks of the medial branch of the dorsal ramus and facet joints at the C5–C6 spinal segments temporarily gave complete relief to patients with neck and shoulder pain.[3] Several studies have shown that passive mobilization of the cervical spine can improve shoulder mobility and decrease shoulder pain.[18,22,45] These studies all strongly suggest that the clinician should be prepared to examine the cervical spine in any patient with shoulder complaints.

Cervical Examination Considerations

The challenge, then, is for the clinician to differentiate sites of symptom complaints from their potential sources. Even vague subjective complaints of neck and upper back stiffness or pain should be followed up in the examination. The contribution of cervical complaints may only be a small part of the clinical picture, but they should not be overlooked.

The quadrant test identifies cervical components of shoulder complaints (see Chapter 2, Principles of Extremity Evaluation). If the quadrant test does not provoke shoulder symptoms, but there are signs of decreased cervical joint mobility on the same side as the shoulder complaints, the cervical spine should be examined further but not necessarily immediately. If the quadrant test is negative, the cervical spine can be ruled out for the time being but should be reassessed at a later visit if the patient does not progress as expected. A quadrant test that provokes shoulder symptoms warrants a more extensive examination of the cervical spine.

Cervical spine palpation or mobilization often reproduces shoulder complaints and implicates neck involvement fairly clearly. Shoulder mobility should be reassessed after any cervical palpation or mobilization to find any changes in mobility or symptom response in the shoulder complex. Differentiating between cervical and shoulder components can be difficult but should be a routine

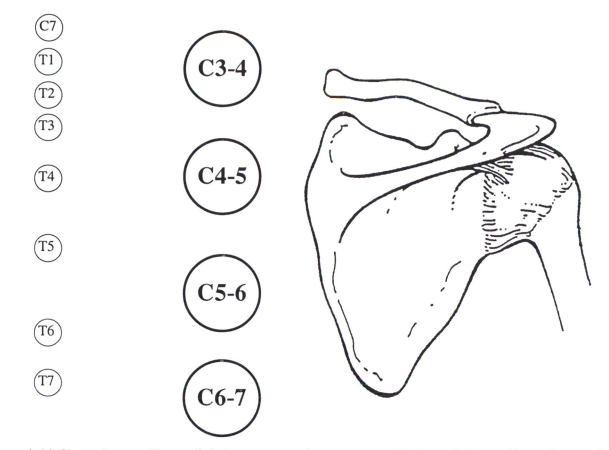

Figure 4–14. Cloward's areas. The small circles represent spinous processes. The large circles are Cloward's areas. Pain in these general areas corresponds to possible disc pathology at the level indicated inside the large circles.

part of the examination. Simple maneuvers such as adding contralateral cervical side–bending to any active motion of the shoulder at points of symptom response can give valuable information about the role of the cervical spine. If shoulder symptoms are increased with cervical sidebending, further evaluation of the cervical spine is indicated.

Objective Examination

Structural

Structural observation begins when the patient enters the clinic. The position and the way the patient carries the arms when walking, disrobing, and getting on the examination table should be noted. This will give the clinician an initial idea about potential functional restriction, pain, or weakness in the upper quarter. The status of the entire upper limb is often reflected in the vasomotor changes observed in the forearm and hand (shiny skin, edema, etc.).

The patient's overall posture should be noted since the position of the head, neck, and upper back will influence the posture of the shoulder complex. Postural malalignments can affect the available range of motion and compromise the neurovascular structures as they exit the neck and thorax. The level and contour of the shoulders and the clavicles and the position and symmetry of the scapulæ should be noted. A high riding clavicle can indicate problems at the acromioclavicular joint. Deformities along the clavicle may be the sites of old fractures. Any muscle atrophy should be noted and compared to the opposite limb. Many people, especially athletes, exhibit hypertrophy and lower shoulder position on the dominant limb.[41]

Some specific structural deviations may be observed. A patient with a recent biceps tendon rupture may present with the biceps muscle "balled up," with bruising and ecchymosis over the injury. Scapular winging can be caused by serratus anterior weakness. Finally, the skin should be inspected and any discoloration, scars, incisions, or swelling should be noted.

Mobility

Physiological Mobility

Physiological mobility refers to the movement of the shoulder in standard planar movements and functional combined movements.

Active Mobility

Active shoulder motions that can be tested include:

- elevation of the arm in three positions: flexion, abduction, and in the plane of the scapula (approximately midway between flexion and abduction. This motion is called "scaption." [Fig 4–15])

- extension

- horizontal adduction

- internal and external rotation (checked with arms at sides, in the neutral position, and in 90° of abduction)

- combined extension, internal rotation, and adduction (commonly called "hand behind the back")

- combined external rotation and abduction

- elevation, depression, protraction, and retraction of the shoulder girdle

It can be valuable to assess both limbs simultaneously to compare motion symmetry, scapulohumeral rhythm, and dynamic scapular stability. Scapular control should be observed during active elevation of the shoulder (abduction, flexion, and scaption) (Fig 4–16). Observing the patient perform the following specific sequence of active movements can help:

1. flexion to 90°

2. horizontal abduction with scapular retraction

3. external rotation

4. abduction

5. adduction (arms to side)

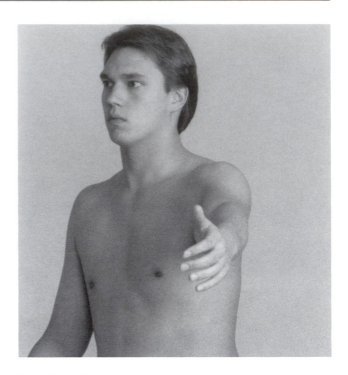

Figure 4–15. Scaption—elevation of the arm in the plane of the scapula.

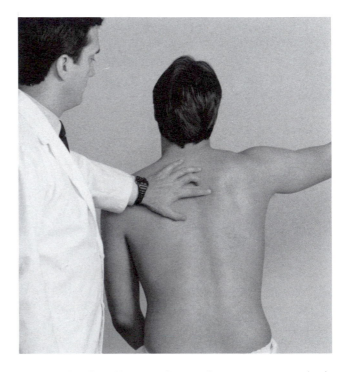

Figure 4–16. When testing active movements it is important to observe scapular stability while the patient raises and lowers the arm.

This sequence of movements lets the clinician observe dynamic scapular stability in concentric and eccentric contractions. Common findings during active mobility testing include a painful arc during elevation, suggestive of subacromial impingement and rotator cuff tear; or poor scapulohumeral rhythm, suggestive of adhesive capsulitis (Fig 4–17). Active mobility can be tested in standing or sitting.

Passive Mobility

Passive mobility testing assesses the integrity of the non–contractile components of the shoulder. Passive mobility should be examined in any active motion that was not within normal limits of motion or where the clinician was unable to test the end–feel. The limb is taken through the available range, with overpressure applied at end range. The following should be noted: the range of motion; the symptom response; the end–feel; and the pattern of motion restriction, if any. The affected extremity should be compared to the contralateral extremity and to normal. The pattern of motion restriction can be considered capsular or non–capsular. The overall capsular pattern of the shoulder complex is *greatest limitation in external rotation, followed by abduction, then flexion and internal rotation*. The normal end–

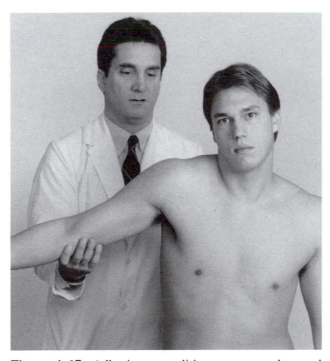

Figure 4–17. Adhesive capsulitis can cause abnormal glenohumeral rhythm.

feel of the shoulder complex is a tissue stretch, or "capsular" end–feel.

The symptom response to passive motion can reveal the stage of the problem (see Chapter 2, Principles of Extremity Evaluation). Testing can include any of the active motions and can be performed with the patient supine or prone (Fig 4–18).

Accessory Mobility

Accessory joint mobility refers to component motions and joint play (see Chapter 2, Principles of Extremity Evaluation). Accessory mobility should be assessed for each movement in which the physiological range of motion was limited or abnormal in some way. Joint play movements of the shoulder are usually examined with the patient supine, but can be checked with the patient prone or sidelying (see Chapter 11, Mobilization Techniques). The specific joint play movements of the glenohumeral joint that should be examined include: anterior glide; posterior glide; inferior glide; caudal distraction; and lateral distraction. These can be combined and tested in various positions of physiological motion to identify specific barriers of restriction to movement. Joint play movements of the sternoclavicular, acromioclavicular, and scapulothoracic joints should also be tested. The clinician should compare the findings to the contralateral limb and to normal. These findings include the available range; the end–feel; any crepitus noted; and any symptoms provoked. The results should be consistent with the findings of the physiological mobility examination. For example, when a patient presents with active and passive motion limitation in the capsular pattern, the clinician will usually find that the coinciding joint play movements of anterior and inferior glide will also be restricted.

Strength

Specific manual muscle testing (MMT) assesses the status of the contractile elements of the shoulder complex. These tests are performed in the mid range of motion to avoid stress on the non–contractile structures. The patient is told to gradually increase effort to a voluntary maximum contraction. This helps avoid substitution of synergistic muscles. The

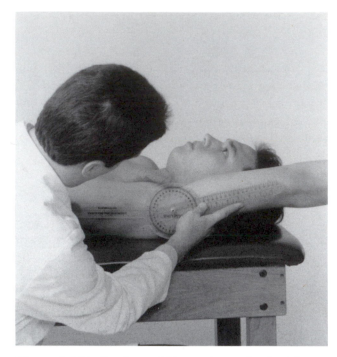

Figure 4–18A. Passive mobility testing at the shoulder: flexion.

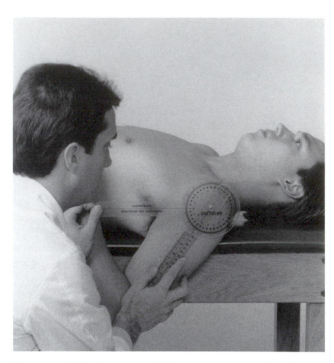

Figure 4–18B. Passive mobility testing at the shoulder: extension.

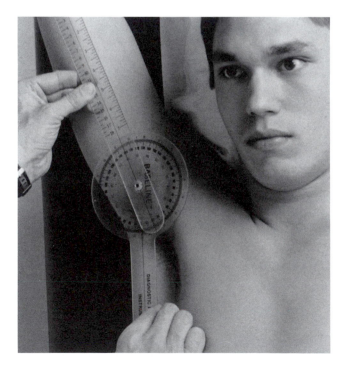

Figure 4–18C. Passive mobility testing at the shoulder: abduction.

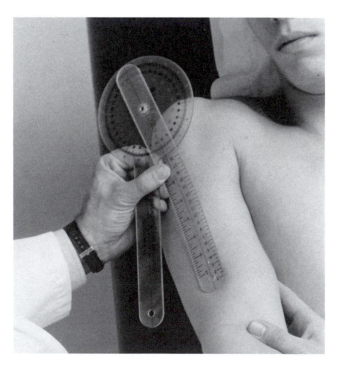

Figure 4–18D. Passive mobility testing at the shoulder: adduction.

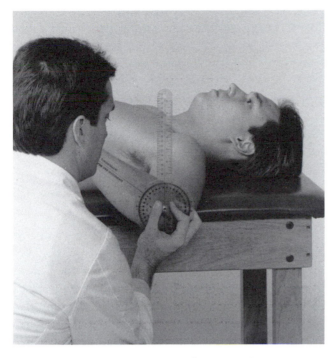

Figure 4–18E. Passive mobility testing at the shoulder: internal rotation.

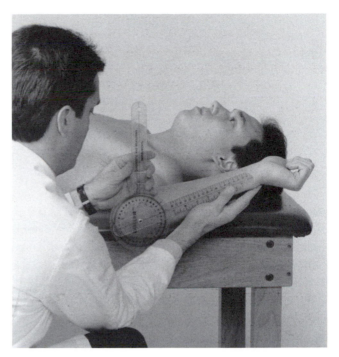

Figure 4–18F. Passive mobility testing at the shoulder: external rotation.

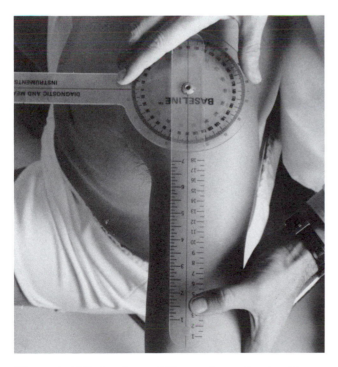

Figure 4–18G. Passive mobility testing at the shoulder: horizontal abduction.

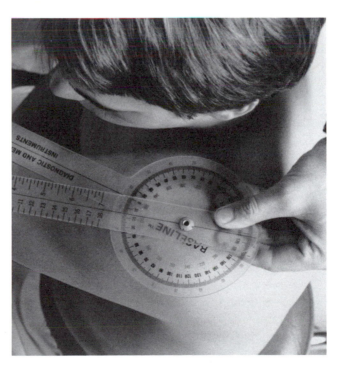

Figure 4–18H. Passive mobility testing at the shoulder: horizontal adduction.

clinician resists the tests isometrically. The muscle strength should be graded and any symptom response noted. Any muscle acting on the shoulder complex should be tested, including the biceps and triceps brachii. Cyriax's four patterns of response (see Chapter 2, Principles of Extremity Evaluation) can help with the assessment and the treatment plan.

Some authors suggest "functional strength testing."[32] Functional strength testing can include sitting push–ups, shoulder shrugs, and lifting loads (0–5lb) in a number of functional planes (e.g., flexion, abduction, and scaption).[32] Bilateral comparison for symmetry should be noted since research suggests strength norms vary by age, gender, and activity.[30] Although functional strength testing has merit, it has not been extensively researched and is not a widely practiced procedure.

Neurological

The neurological examination should be carried out as outlined in Chapter 2, Principles of Extremity Evaluation. Indications for neurological testing include paresthesia, anesthesia, weakness, or other complaints that make the clinician suspect neurological involvement. The neurological examination includes testing motor function, light touch sensation, and deep tendon reflexes (DTR's). Motor function is assessed in the cervical myotomes per the upper quarter screening examination (see Chapter 2, Principles of Extremity Evaluation). Light touch sensation should be tested in the upper limb including the C4–T1 dermatomes and the regional cutaneous nerve fields (see Fig 2–12 on pages 24 and 25). The relevant DTR's include the biceps (C5–C6), brachioradialis (C6–C7), and triceps (C7–C8). Unilateral and bilateral comparison for symmetry should be noted. Research suggests that proprioception should also be assessed because position sense is impaired after anterior dislocation of the glenohumeral joint.[44]

There are many tissue interfaces that can subject the neural tissues to adverse mechanical stresses in the neck and shoulder. These include the intervertebral foramen as the nerves exit the spinal canal; the scalene muscles (where the brachial plexus runs between the anterior and middle portions); the first rib (where the lower trunks of the brachial plexus lie); the pectoralis minor (under which pass the three

cords of the brachial plexus); the superior–medial brachium (where the median and ulnar nerves lie); and the radial groove of the humerus (where the radial nerve lies). Trauma to these areas can affect neural tissue mobility. Patients with such trauma can have limited shoulder mobility secondary to pain complaints. The ULTT should be performed on any patient with shoulder complaints where a neural tension disorder may contribute (see Chapter 2, Principles of Extremity Evaluation.

Palpation

Palpation examination should proceed as discussed in Chapter 2, Principles of Extremity Evaluation. The process should be consistent with layered palpation, gradually moving from surface tissues to deeper tissues as tolerated. Unilateral and bilateral comparison for symmetry should be noted. The skin, bones, joints, muscles, tendons, and bursæ of the shoulder complex should be examined:[5,26]

Anterior (Fig 4–19)

- sternoclavicular joint
- clavicle
- acromioclavicular joint
- scalene muscles
- coracoid process of the scapula
- bicipital groove and biceps tendon
- rotator cuff insertions (especially the supraspinatus tendon)
- muscles of the axilla (subscapularis, latissimus dorsi, pectoralis major, pectoralis minor)

Posterior (Fig 4–20)

- acromioclavicular joint
- infraspinatus muscle–tendon junction
- supraspinatus muscle–tendon junction
- spine of the scapula
- scapular borders
- triceps tendon origin
- trapezius muscle
- levator scapulæ

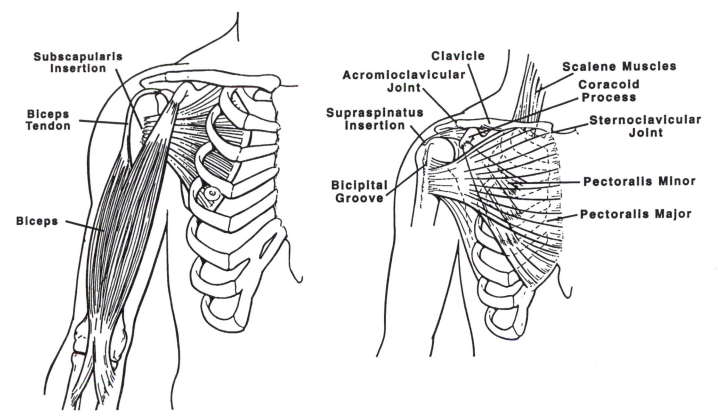

Figure 4–19. Structures to palpate at the shoulder: anterior surface. Infraspinatus and teres minor not shown.

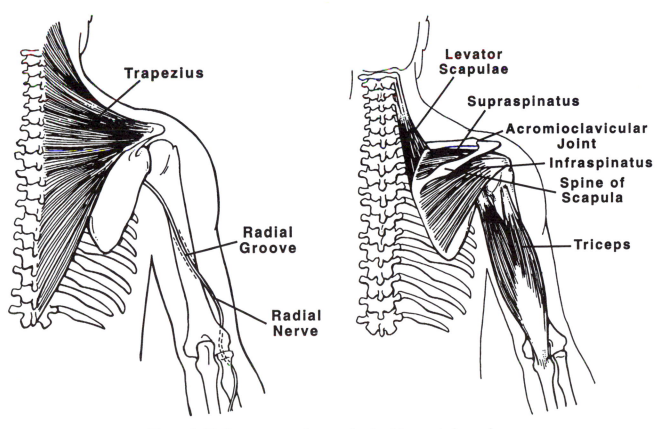

Figure 4–20. Structures to palpate at the shoulder: posterior surface.

• radial nerve (at the radial groove)

Other structures that should be palpated include the anterior chest wall (ribs and muscles); scalene muscles; first rib; brachial plexus; cervical and thoracic spinal segments; and the radial groove of the humerus. It is important to correlate the palpation findings with the rest of the objective examination.

Special Tests

Special tests help the clinician identify the specific structures that contribute to the patient's problems. There are three types of special tests at the shoulder: neurovascular, musculotendinous, and joint/ligamentous. The special tests for the shoulder are summarized in Table 4–4.

Neurovascular Tests

Thoracic outlet syndrome (TOS) was usually considered a compromise of the vascular structures exiting the thorax, but recent research has challenged this. The brachial plexus can also be compromised, and some authors suggest that over 90% of TOS cases are actually neurological in origin.[46] TOS can involve compression or stretching of the subclavian artery, subclavian vein, or the brachial plexus as they pass through the thoracic outlet; therefore, the ULTT should be performed (see Chapter 2, Principles of Extremity Evaluation) in addition to the traditional vascular tests for TOS. These vascular tests require assessment of the pulse response and symptom complaints in varying positions of the cervical spine and upper limb. The positions used for testing can compromise the vascular structures at three interfaces: anterior and middle scalenes; first rib and clavicle; and pectoralis minor and ribs.

Adson's Test

Adson's Test helps determine if the neurovascular bundle is being compressed as it passes between the scalenus anticus and medius. In some people, the bundle passes through the muscle mass rather than between the two muscles. There is no consensus on the exact method for performing Adson's Test. The goal of the test is to place the neurovascular bundle and scaleni on maximum stretch. The test described here combines elements from several authors.[7,19,21,27]

The clinician should palpate the patient's radial pulse at the wrist as the patient takes a deep breath and holds it. The patient's arm is abducted and extended, and the patient extends and rotates the cervical spine toward the arm being tested (Fig 4–21). The test is positive if the radial pulse is markedly decreased or obliterated and the patient's symptoms are reproduced. The test is repeated with cervical extension and rotation away from the arm being tested.

Costoclavicular (Military Bracing) Test

The costoclavicular test checks for compression of the neurovascular bundle as it passes between the clavicle and first rib by approximating the two structures. Again, the clinician palpates the radial pulse at the wrist. The patient is asked to assume an exaggerated military position by drawing the scapulæ backward and downward (Fig 4–22). The test is positive if the radial pulse is markedly decreased or obliterated and the patient's symptoms are reproduced.

Hyperabduction Test

The hyperabduction test helps determine if the neurovascular bundle is being compressed between the pectoralis minor muscle and the ribs. The clinician palpates the radial pulse at the wrist while abducting the shoulder as far as possible (Fig 4–23). The clinician should concentrate on performing true abduction (without flexion).[23] The test is positive if the radial pulse is markedly decreased or obliterated and the patient's symptoms are reproduced.

Roo's Test (EAST)

This test identifies general compression of the neurovascular bundle. Named for Dr. David Roo, this test is also called the Elevated Arm Stress Test (EAST). The patient holds the position of bilateral full shoulder external rotation and abduction to 90° for three minutes while repeatedly opening and closing the fists (Fig 4–24). After completing the test, the clinician quickly looks for objective changes and the patient's subjective response. The test is positive if the patient has increased pallor, cyanosis, swelling, vein distention, tingling, numbness, or pain. The clinician should compare the affected limb to the unaffected limb.

Table 4–4. Special Tests for the Shoulder

Test Type	Test Name	Purpose
Neurological	Adson's Test	Compression of neurovascular bundle between anterior and middle scalenes
	Costoclavicular (military bracing)	Compression of neurovascular bundle between the 1st rib and the clavicle
	Hyperabduction	Compression of neurovascular bundle between pectoralis minor and the ribs
	Roo's Test (EAST Test)	Thoracic outlet syndrome
Musculotendinous	Neer's Test	Subacromial impingement
	Hawkin's Test	Subacromial impingement
	Active Impingement	Subacromial impingement
	Drop Arm Test	Integrity of rotator cuff
	Speed's Test	Bicepital tendonitis
	Gilchrist's Sign	Bicepital tendonitis
	Lippman's Test	Bicepital tendonitis
	Ludington's Test	Biceps tendon rupture
Joint/Ligamentous	Anterior Apprehension Test	Anterior instability
	Rockwood Test	Anterior instability
	Relocation Test	Anterior instability
	Anterior Drawer Test	Anterior instability
	Rowe Test	Anterior instability
	Fulcrum Test	Anterior instability
	Clunk Test	Tear of glenoid labrum
	Posterior Apprehension Test	Posterior instability
	Posterior Drawer Test	Posterior instability
	Jerk Test	Posterior instability
	Norwood Stress Test	Posterior instability
	Push-Pull Test	Posterior instability
	Sulcus Sign	Inferior instability
	Feagin Test	Inferior instability
	Rowe Test for Multidimensional Instability	Multidirectional instability
	Lateral Scapular Glide	Scapulothoracic instability
	Acromioclavicular Instability	Acromioclavicular instability

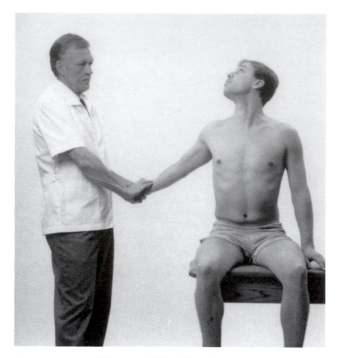

Figure 4–21. Adson's test.

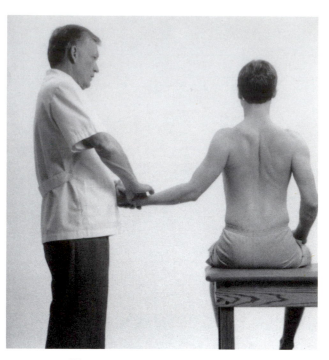

Figure 4–22. Costoclavicular test.

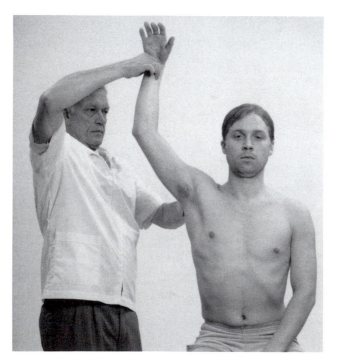

Figure 4–23. Hyperabduction test.

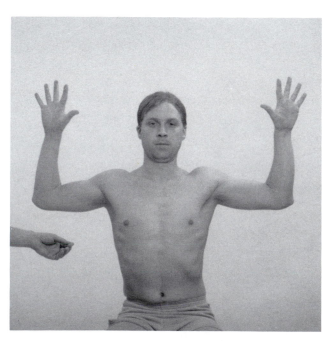

Figure 4–24. Roo's (EAST) test.

Musculotendinous Tests

Impingement Tests

Subacromial impingement is a common clinical condition. Impingement and instability can be part of a pathology continuum rather than two separate entities;[35] therefore, any findings in this section should be correlated with any findings of instability. There are two types of tests for subacromial impingement: passive and active.

Neer's Test

Neer's Test is a passive impingement test. With the patient sitting or standing, the arm is brought into full flexion with overpressure (Fig 4–25). This test is positive for impingement if it produces pain.

Hawkin's Test

Hawkin's Test is a passive test for subacromial impingement. The patient sits or stands with the arm in ≈90° of shoulder elevation in the scapular plane (scaption). The clinician applies forcible overpressure into full internal rotation of the arm (Fig 4–26).[20] The test is positive if pain is produced by the test position.

Active Impingement Tests

There are two active tests for impingement. The first is simply active flexion and active abduction of the arm. A painful arc of motion during active motion indicates possible impingement.

The second active test for impingement is active scaption. This test, called the "empty can" test, assesses the integrity of the supraspinatus muscle (Fig 4–27). The test is positive if pain is produced or the patient's symptoms are provoked.

Drop Arm Test

The drop arm test is a traditional test used to assess the integrity of the rotator cuff. The patient is asked to abduct the arm to 90°, then lower it slowly (Fig 4–28). The test is positive if the patient is unable to control the movement of the arm or if the test provokes extreme pain, indicating a tear in the rotator cuff.

Biceps Tendon Tests

Speed's Test

This test identifies bicipital tendinitis. The clinician palpates the biceps tendon while resisting

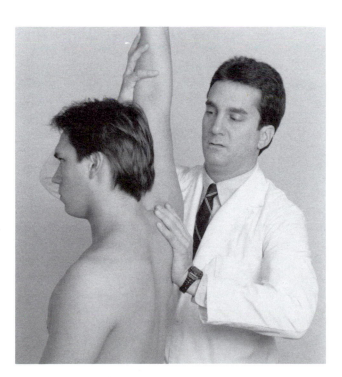

Figure 4–25. Neer's test.

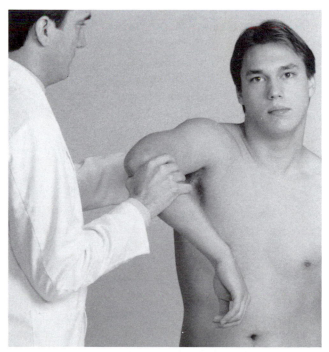

Figure 4–26. Hawkin's test.

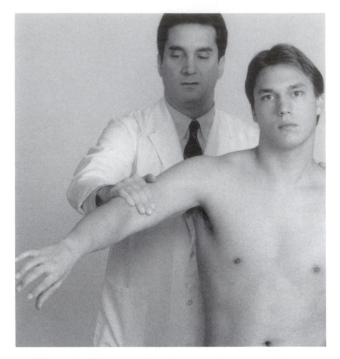

Figure 4–27. Active impingement (empty can) test.

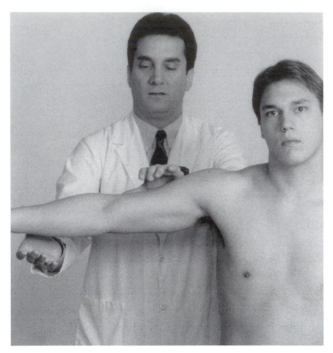

Figure 4–28. Drop Arm test.

shoulder flexion (with the patient's elbow extended and forearm supinated) (Fig 4–29). This test is performed at 90° (causing impingement) or in extension (causing stretch). A positive sign is increased pain at the biceps tendon.

Gilchrist's Sign

This test identifies bicipital tendinitis. The patient is asked to lower the arm to the side from full abduction with external rotation while holding a 5 lb weight (Fig 4–30). The test is positive if the test position causes pain or an audible snapping of the biceps tendon in the groove.

Joint and Ligamentous Tests

Ligamentous tests assess the stability of the joints. The tests for glenohumeral instability can be grouped as anterior, posterior, and inferior instability. The clinician may find multidirectional instability. These tests can be performed in a variety of positions based on patient comfort and relaxation, the patient's complaints, and the clinician's needs (patient size, clinician's skill level, etc.). As a group, these tests are provocative, so careful manual handling is required. The tests for instability are positive if there is apprehension, muscle guarding, or excessive joint

play movement. Symptom response and joint noise (crepitus) may accompany these findings.

Anterior Glenohumeral Instability Tests

Anterior Apprehension Test (Crank Test)

This test identifies anterior glenohumeral instability. The clinician fully externally rotates the shoulder while applying an anterior force in varying positions of abduction. The traditional test is performed at 90° of abduction (Fig 4–31). A positive test is any sign of anxiety in the patient's face, indicating apprehension of subluxation.

Rockwood Test

In the Rockwood Test (a modification of the crank test), the clinician fully externally rotates the arm and applies an anterior force with the arm at the side and at 45°, 90°, and 120° of abduction (Fig 4–32).[38] Patients usually have the most severe symptoms at 90° of abduction.

Relocation Test

Occasionally the clinician may need to relocate the humeral head during testing. The relocation test can ensure correct alignment has been attained.

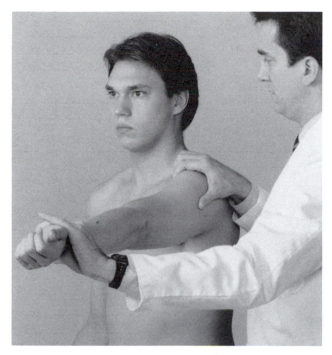

Figure 4–29A. Speed's test performed in flexion.

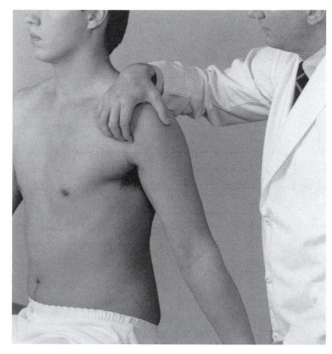

Figure 4–29B. Speed's test performed in extension.

The clinician externally rotates the arm at 90° abduction with the patient supine). If the patient becomes apprehensive, a posterior stress is applied to relocate the proximal humerus (Fig 4–33). The test is positive if the apprehension signs are eliminated and there is an increase in pain free (and apprehension–free) external rotation range.

Anterior Drawer Test

This test assesses anterior instability. The patient is supine with the arm in a relaxed position. The clinician stabilizes the scapula with one hand while pulling the humeral head anteriorly (Fig 4–34). The test is positive if the patient shows apprehension, guarding, or pain.

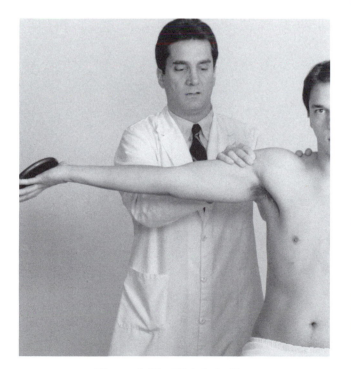

Figure 4–30. Gilchrist's Sign.

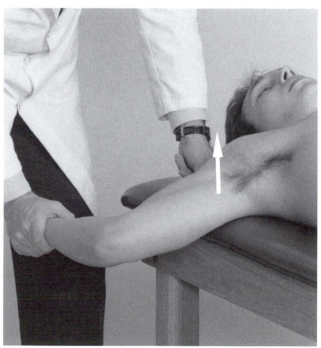

Figure 4–31. Anterior apprehension (crank) test.

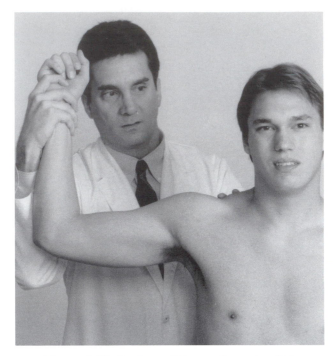

Figure 4–32. Rockwood Test performed at 90°.

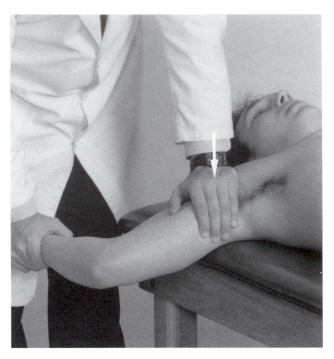

Figure 4–33. Relocation test.

Rowe Test

The Rowe Test identifies anterior instability. The patient is supine with the hand behind the head. The clinician places a closed fist under the proximal humeral head and presses the humerus into horizontal abduction (Fig 4–35). A positive test is pain, apprehension, or muscle guarding.

Fulcrum Test

The fulcrum test assesses anterior instability. The patient is supine with the arm at 90° abduction and the clinician's hand under the proximal humeral head. The clinician externally rotates and horizontally abducts the arm (Fig 4–36). The test is positive if the patient has pain, apprehension, or muscle guarding.

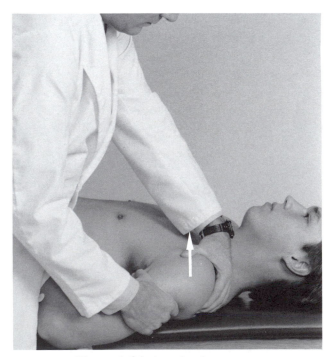

Figure 4–34. Anterior drawer test.

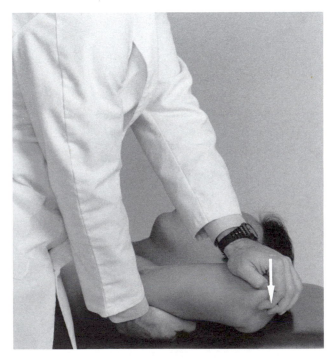

Figure 4–35. Rowe test.

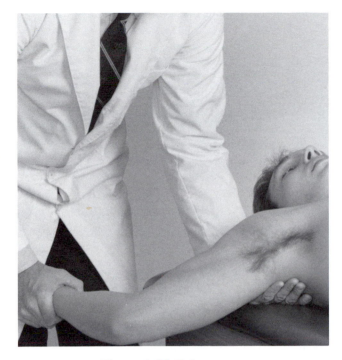

Figure 4–36. Fulcrum test.

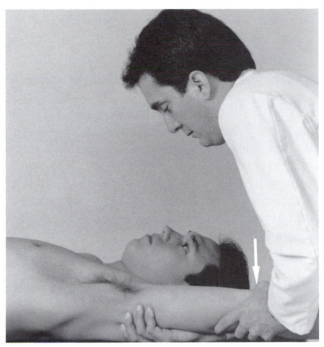

Figure 4–37. Clunk test.

Clunk Test

The clunk test assesses anterior instability. The clinician positions the patient in supine with full shoulder abduction, supporting the proximal humerus posteriorly. Overpressure is applied, then repeated with external rotation of the humerus (Fig 4–37). The test is positive if it provokes a "clunk" or grinding sensation, consistent with a tear of the glenoid labrum. This test can also show anterior instability if the patient exhibits apprehension on testing.

There are other options for testing for anterior instability,[15,24,37] and any joint play test for anterior glide could be used (see Chapter 11, Mobilization Techniques).

Posterior Glenohumeral Instability Tests

Posterior Apprehension Test

This test identifies posterior instability. The clinician applies a posterior force on the humeral head through the elbow with the patient's arm flexed to 90° and internally rotated (Fig 4–38). The test is positive if the patient shows apprehension, guarding, or pain.

Posterior Drawer Test

The posterior drawer test identifies posterior instability. With the patient supine, the clinician applies a posterior force on the humeral head while

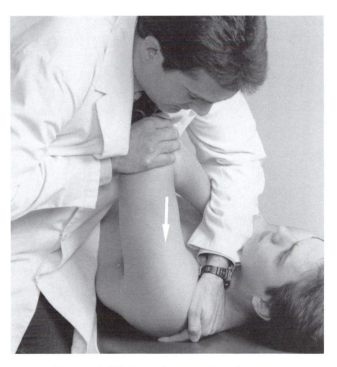

Figure 4–38. Posterior apprehension test.

stabilizing the scapula (Fig 4–39). The test is positive if the patient shows apprehension, guarding, or pain.

Jerk Test

The jerk test is another test for posterior instability. The patient's arm is posteriorly loaded through the long axis of the humerus while the shoulder is internally rotated and flexed to 90°. The clinician stabilizes the trunk, and horizontally adducts the arm across the body (Fig 4–40). The test is positive if a "jerk" occurs as the humeral head subluxes posteriorly. As the arm is brought back to the start position, a relocation "jerk" can occur as the humeral head realigns in the glenoid fossa.

Push–Pull Test

Another test for posterior instability is the push–pull test. The patient is supine with the arm in 90° of abduction and slight horizontal adduction and the elbow flexed to 90°. The clinician pushes the head of the humerus posteriorly with one hand and pulls the wrist anteriorly toward the ceiling with the other (Fig 4–41). The test is positive when there is greater than 50% posterior translation of the humeral head.

The other options for testing posterior instability include any joint play test for posterior glide (see Chapter 11, Mobilization Techniques).

Inferior Glenohumeral Instability Tests

Sulcus Sign

A positive sulcus sign indicates inferior instability. The patient sits or stands with the shoulder fully relaxed. The clinician pulls distally on the arm, distracting the arm inferiorly (Fig 4–42). The test is positive if there is an increased space between the tip of the acromion process and the humeral head when compared with the opposite side.

Feagin Test

The Feagin Test assesses inferior instability. The clinician applies an inferior force on the patient's proximal humerus with the arm abducted to 90° (Fig 4–43). The test is positive if it provokes pain, apprehension, or muscle guarding.

Other options for testing for inferior instability include any joint play test for inferior glide (see Chapter 11, Mobilization Techniques).

Multidirectional Glenohumeral Instability Tests

Rowe Multidirectional Instability Test

A patient with inferior instability often also has signs of multidirectional instability. This test is

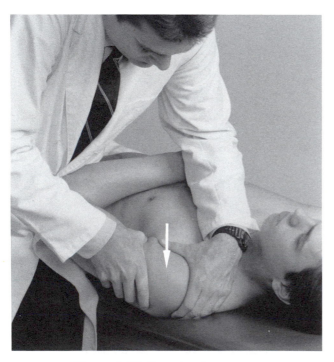

Figure 4–39. Posterior drawer test.

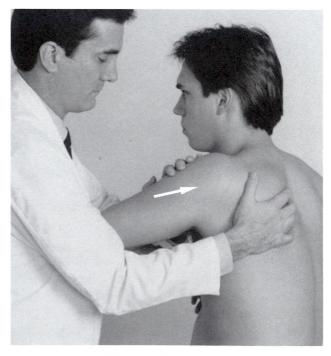

Figure 4–40. Jerk test.

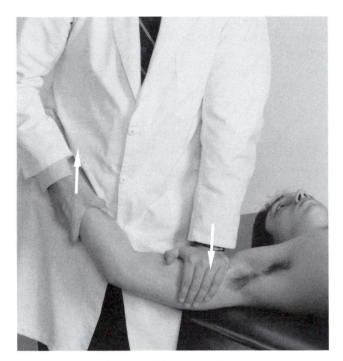

Figure 4–41. Push-Pull test.

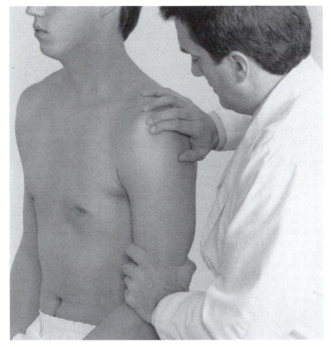

Figure 4–42. Sulcus sign.

performed with the patient leaning over and the involved arm relaxed at ≈45° of elevation. The clinician applies and maintains distal distraction while pushing the proximal head anteriorly, then posteriorly, and finally inferiorly (Fig 4–44). The test is positive if there is excessive mobility when compared to the uninvolved limb. Apprehension, muscle guarding, or pain are also positive signs.

Multidirectional instability can also be assessed by combining joint play movements of the shoulder and assessing the responses (see Chapter 11, Mobilization Techniques).

Other Instability Tests

Lateral Scapular Glide Test

The lateral scapular glide test assesses the stability of the scapulothoracic joint. The distance between the spinous process of T7 and the inferior angle of the scapula is measured in five different shoulder positions: 0° abduction (arm at side), 45° abduction, 90° abduction with full internal rotation, 120° abduction, and 150° abduction (Fig 4–45). The test is positive (scapula is unstable) if there is a difference >1 cm from one side to the other.

Acromioclavicular Instability Tests

In many cases, laxity of the acromioclavicular joint can be easily observed on structural examination. The patient actively depresses the

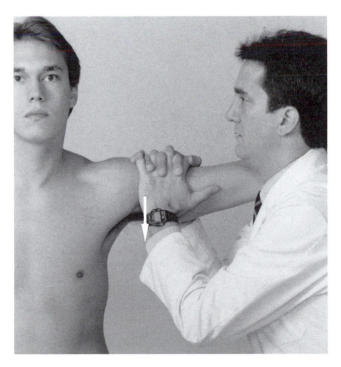

Figure 4–43. Feagin test.

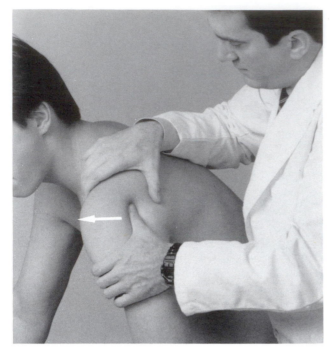

Figure 4–44A. Rowe Multidirectional Instability Test: anterior.

shoulder girdle while the clinician palpates the joint line between the clavicle and the acromion process of the scapula. If unable to perform active shoulder depression, the patient can hold a 10–15 lb weight and relax the shoulder girdle while the clinician palpates

the joint. These tests are positive if there is increased "step–off" between the clavicle and acromion process. Any joint play movement of the acromioclavicular joint can also be used to test for instability (see Chapter 11, <u>Mobilization Techniques</u>).

Objective Examination Summary

Shoulder pain can be caused by many factors. The four joints of the shoulder complex; the musculotendinous units; the cervical joints and soft tissues; and the mechanical interfaces of the nerves as they exit the neck and thorax are the areas most commonly involved. Systematically analyzing the examination results will help the clinician determine if joints, muscles, or nerves are the cause of the patient's problem. Other sources of shoulder complaints include the viscera, chest wall, and the elbow. Re–evaluation should include reconsideration of any of the potential contributing areas, especially if the patient is not benefiting from treatment.

At the conclusion of the evaluation, the clinician determines what problems the patient has and develops a problem list to be used to set goals and plan treatment.

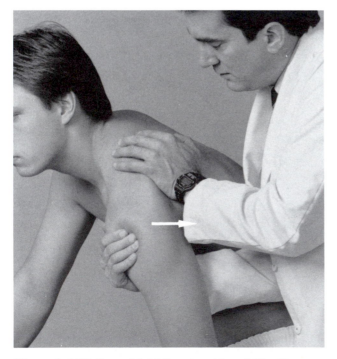

Figure 4–44B. Rowe Multidirectional Instability Test: posterior.

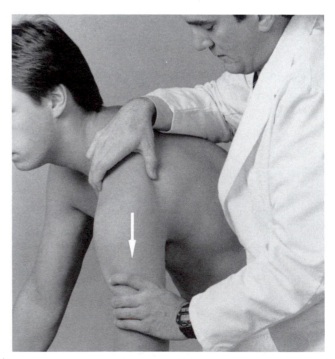

Figure 4–44C. Rowe Multidirectional Instability Test: inferior.

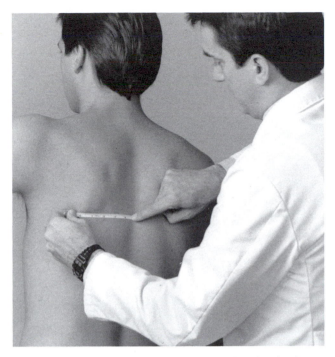

Figure 4–45. Lateral scapular glide test. Testing is shown at 90° abduction.

TREATMENT STRATEGIES

The contribution of the cervical spine; the four joints of the shoulder complex; the rotator cuff and scapula stabilizers; and the neural tension components are the four areas considered for treatment of most shoulder disorders. Any cervical components should be treated first. After cervical treatment, the patient should be reassessed to see if there are any changes in shoulder mobility or symptoms. The remaining components of the problem should be treated next.

Throughout the rehabilitation program, the patient should be taught about the effects of postures and repetitive movements on shoulder problems. Proper posture also helps prevent compromise of the neurovascular structures exiting the neck and thorax. A kyphotic thoracic posture causes a protracted scapular position with internal rotation of the humerus. This posture prevents full glenohumeral motion, and can cause subacromial impingement. Scapular stabilization exercises are often an important part of a shoulder rehabilitation program. These exercises should be started as soon as possible to provide proximal stability of the shoulder complex.

General treatment strategies are discussed in Chapter 3, Pathology and Treatment Principles. See *Evaluation, Treatment and Prevention of Musculoskeletal Disorders*, Volume I, Chapter 5, Treatment of the Spine by Diagnosis, and Volume I, Chapter 6, Treatment of the Spine by Problem, for treatment techniques for the cervical spine. See Chapter 11, Mobilization Techniques, and Chapter 12, Exercise, of this book for sections relating to mobilization techniques, stretching, strengthening, and proprioceptive exercises for the shoulder complex.

COMMON CLINICAL CONDITIONS

Glenohumeral Instability

The glenohumeral joint is anatomically predisposed to instability secondary to the small and shallow glenoid cavity that articulates with the larger humeral head. There are three common types of instability found at the glenohumeral joint. They are: *anterior, posterior,* and *multidirectional* instability. *Anterior* instability is the most common type and is often associated with glenoid labrum tears. *Posterior* instability is less common and can be easily missed on examination due to a less dramatic presentation than anterior instability. *Multidirectional* instability occurs in patients with generalized ligament laxity[49] and chronic instability. Most patients who have inferior instability also have anterior and posterior (multidirectional) instability. This problem can be caused by acute dislocation or subluxation; recurrent dislocation or subluxation; or cumulative microtrauma (gradual attenuation of tissues). The direction of the instability and its correlation to symptoms and functional complaints can only be established by careful examination. Instability can be part of an injury continuum that results in rotator cuff problems.[35] Glenoid labrum tears can also result from glenohumeral joint instability.

History

In many cases, the instability is caused by acute trauma, frequently a fall onto an outstretched arm. Anterior instability can occur when the arm is in an externally rotated position during a fall or when an excessive force is applied to the arm while it is externally rotated and elevated. Posterior instability can occur when the arm is internally rotated during a fall. It can also arise from violent muscle contractions that occur during an epileptic seizure or an electrical shock. Multidirectional instability is usually found in patients with a history of prolonged anterior or posterior instability or in patients with a generalized joint laxity. All three types of instability can occur gradually by repeated microtrauma during daily activities. The biomechanical positions that may correlate with the gradual attenuation of the tissues should be identified. For example, patients with anterior instability may work (or play) in positions in which the arm is externally rotated, elevated, and horizontally abducted. Patients with posterior instability may frequently be in postures of shoulder internal rotation, elevation, and horizontally adduction. Direct trauma to the anterior or posterior shoulder can also cause acute instability. Patients with subtle instabilities may not have a history of acute trauma but may present with other injuries or complaints.

Signs/Symptoms

Patients with shoulder instability may complain of apprehension with shoulder movements. Shoulder pain during and after activity is a common complaint. The patient with an acute or recurrent instability will complain of the shoulder "going out." They may also complain of an intermittent feeling of loss of power, referred to as the "dead arm syndrome." This can be caused by a stretch on the surrounding neurovascular structures. The objective examination should include tests for instability (see the "Special Tests" section of this chapter). Positive signs of instability are apprehension, pain, muscle guarding, and excessive joint play. It is important to avoid dislocating the joint during examination to limit tissue injury. Increased joint play findings should be compared to the uninvolved shoulder. Crepitus during the examination can indicate labral injury, bony lesions, or other pathology. The patient may show concurrent signs and symptoms consistent with secondary rotator cuff involvement.

Diagnostics

Radiographs are often not necessary, but they can help diagnose acute dislocations of the glenohumeral joint (Fig 4–46). Anterior instability is consistent with the Hills–Sachs finding on radiograph. Hills–Sachs is a bony lesion on the posterior humeral head from the

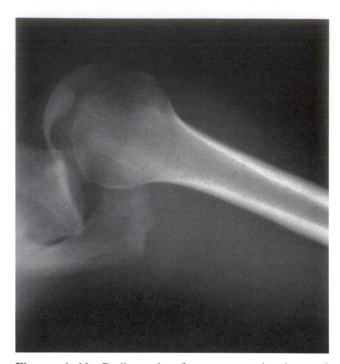

Figure 4–46. Radiograph of an acute glenohumeral dislocation.

trauma of anterior dislocation or subluxation. On radiograph, patients with posterior instability may have the Reverse Hills–Sach finding (Fig 4–47), a bony lesion on the anterior humeral head from the trauma of a posterior dislocation or subluxation. MRI

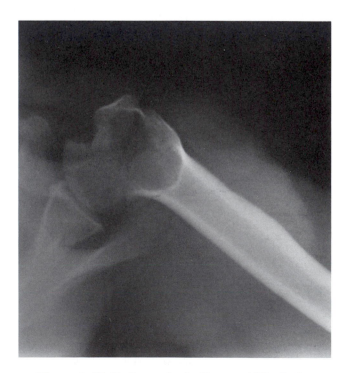

Figure 4–47. Radiograph of a Reverse Hills-Sachs.

can provide information about pathology related to the glenoid labrum and rotator cuff.

Problem List

Patients with acute instability can have the following problems:

1. Severe pain

2. Inability to use the shoulder in functional activities

3. Transient neurovascular symptoms

4. Moderate to severe apprehension of dislocation

5. Temporary disability in daily activities.

Patients with chronic instabilities can have the following problems:

1. Recurrent shoulder pain with activity

2. Recurrent subluxations with certain movements, positions, and activities

3. Decreased tolerance of certain activities

4. Progressive episodes of reinjury with increased pain and disability.

Treatment

Treatment of the acute dislocation should progress through three phases: protective, mobility, and strengthening. In the protective phase, the patient is immobilized for three days to six weeks, depending on the specific injury. Physical agents can decrease pain and swelling during this time.

In the mobility phase, the patient may continue to use a sling, but it should be removed for passive mobility exercises several times each day. Postural scapular stabilization exercise should be started as soon as tolerated. Active exercises should be added gradually, avoiding positions that reproduce pain, apprehension, and instability.

The strengthening phase usually begins 4–6 weeks after an acute injury but can be started sooner if there are no symptoms or instability signs. Resistive exercises should be functional and specifically attend to the muscle groups responsible for preventing

further instability (the posterior rotator cuff and shoulder horizontal adductors and abductors for anterior instability; the posterior rotator cuff and shoulder horizontal abductors for posterior instability). Scapular stabilization and proprioception exercises should be progressed as tolerated. The patient should be taught which activities, movements, or positions to avoid to keep the joint out of positions that may compromise stability.

Recurrent instability treatment should emphasize strengthening the scapular stabilizers and rotator cuff muscles and balancing the strength of internal and external rotators. Identifying biomechanical instability factors is critical. Correcting those factors involves educating patients and possibly changing their technique in sports or at work. Many patients with instabilities also have rotator cuff problems, and concurrent treatment of these problems is essential for optimal rehabilitation. Proprioceptive activities are important in preventing injury recurrence and improving kinesthetic sense.[13,44]

When conservative care fails, surgery may be necessary. There are many possible surgical procedures to try to "correct" instability. Post–operative rehabilitation should progress in a fashion similar to the acute dislocation; however, the clinician should work closely with the surgeon to carry out a rehabilitation program consistent with the specific procedure performed.

Acromioclavicular Sprain

Injury to this joint is commonly called the "separated shoulder." There are three grades of sprains to the acromioclavicular joint. Grade I sprains are characterized by mild damage to the supporting ligaments without any displacement. Grade II sprains involve rupture of the acromioclavicular ligaments and a sprain of the coracoclavicular ligaments. Usually there is displacement between the clavicular and acromial articular surfaces that is easily palpated on examination. Grade III sprains are characterized by rupture of both the acromioclavicular and coracoclavicular ligaments. There is obvious displacement between the clavicle and acromion that is easily observed on examination.

History

There are three common injuries to the acromioclavicular joint. They are: A) a fall on the tip of the shoulder that depresses the acromion inferiorly; B) a fall on an outstretched arm that transfers the forces superiorly on the acromion; and C) repetitive overhead activities. The clinician should identify these factors and any others that may cause injury to the acromioclavicular joint.

Signs/Symptoms

The patient may complain of pain on moving the arm overhead or across the body into horizontal adduction; these movements compress the acromioclavicular joint. Active shoulder depression may recreate instability and cause pain. Patients often complain of pain when trying to sleep on the injured shoulder. The joint should be tested for instability as outlined in the "Special Test" section of this chapter. There may be crepitus when palpating the joint during mobility testing. Grade II and III sprains should be easily detected by a palpable step–off of the high–riding clavicle, which will be displaced superiorly. The clinician should also inspect and examine the sternoclavicular joint, which is often involved when the acromioclavicular joint is injured.

Diagnostics

Radiographs of Grade I injuries of the acromioclavicular joint will not show displacement with stress views (stress views are taken with the patient's arm at the side holding a weight. The weight inferiorly displaces the acromion on the clavicle.). Radiographs of patients with chronic complaints at this joint may show degenerative changes and sometimes osteolysis of the joint. Grade II and III sprains will show displacement of the joint on stress views (Fig 4–48).

Problem List

Patients with acromioclavicular sprains may present with the following problems:

1. Pain with reaching across the body

2. Pain with overhead activities

3. Complaints of crepitus or grinding with active movement

4. Pain when lying on the involved shoulder

5. Decreased tolerance to certain activities

Treatment

Grades I and II sprains of this joint are treated conservatively; Grade III treatment is controversial. Some physicians recommend surgery for Grade III sprains. Others favor conservative care. For any grade of sprain, physical agents can decrease symptoms and inflammation. A short period of immobilization can help Grade II sprains. Mobility exercises can be started as soon as tolerated for Grades I and II injuries. Resistive exercises should be started when pain free normal range of motion has been restored. The scapular stabilizers should be included in the strengthening program. The clinician should carefully avoid extremes of range, especially in horizontal adduction. Extremes will stress the joint and provoke symptoms or compromise stability.

If treated conservatively, Grade III sprains may require 4–6 weeks of immobilization. Passive mobility exercises can be progressed gradually,

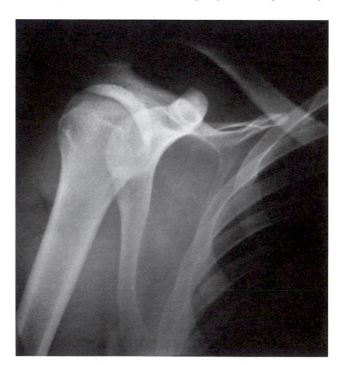

Figure 4–48. Stress view radiograph of an acromioclavicular sprain.

respecting the healing constraints. Scapular stabilization exercises should be initiated as the range of motion increases, with resistive exercises added as tolerated. Initially these exercises should be performed with the arm elevated no greater than 90°, avoiding horizontal adduction and active depression of the shoulder. Post–operative treatment of the surgically repaired or reconstructed acromioclavicular joint should progress as the conservative management of the Grade III sprain, with modifications as needed according to the procedure performed. Close follow–up with the surgeon promotes optimal rehabilitation.

Rotator Cuff Injury

The usual nature of onset and progression differs for older and younger patients. The patient younger than 35 years of age typically injures the cuff with microtrauma from overuse. The microtraumas result in instability, and recurrent instability leads to subacromial impingement, which may eventually cause a rotator cuff tear. The typical rotator cuff patient over age 35 develops problems from underuse and progressively worsens. Underuse results in decreased vascularity and decreased neuromuscular function. These problems can lead to functional instability. Instability leads to spur formation, which can compromise the subacromial space and cause chronic impingement and bursitis. Eventually, degenerative rotator cuff tears occur, and even the biceps tendon may rupture. Asynchronous firing of the scapular stabilizers and rotator cuff muscles can occur after an initial injury, causing dynamic instability and increasing the problems. The clinician can use this continuum to explain the mechanisms of rotator cuff injury and to guide rehabilitation.

Of course, not all patients will exactly fit these profiles—especially those who suffer acute trauma and subsequent injury. Patients' conditions can also be classed as primary or secondary impingement. *Primary impingement* is caused by mechanical crowding of the subacromial space. This can be caused by a tight posterior capsule or weak humeral head depressors (rotator cuff muscles).[8] Repetitive trauma can cause spur formation or thickening of the subacromial bursa and the rotator cuff, leading to even further crowding. *Secondary impingement* is caused by glenohumeral instability or scapulothoracic

instability, causing a relative crowding of the subacromial space and subsequent transient impingement.[35] This classification scheme can help explain the problem to the patient and help design the treatment program.[35]

History

Patients may report a history of repetitively reaching or lifting overhead. Acute flare ups are possible after unaccustomed activities. Acute injury can occur with a fall on an outstretched arm or on the shoulder directly.

Signs/Symptoms

Common complaints include pain with overhead reaching or lifting. Daily aggravating factors include getting dressed and pain when sleeping on the shoulder or with the arm overhead. There may be complaints of weakness with pain. Severe weakness with minimal pain may indicate a rotator cuff tear. Objective examination will be consistent with signs of impingement (see the "Special Tests" section of this chapter). The subacromial bursa and the rotator cuff tendons may be tender to palpation. Joint play testing may reveal posterior capsule tightness. There may be signs of weakness, and specific muscle testing should be performed to identify the involved muscle–tendon structures. When testing strength, the clinician should differentiate between true muscle weakness and "give–way" weakness because of pain. Substitution patterns, especially of the shoulder elevators, may be present in the patient with a rotator cuff tear. The glenohumeral joint may show signs of instability, and the scapular stabilizers may be weak.

Diagnostics

Radiographs of the shoulder can offer insight into rotator cuff problems. Calcific tendons and spur formation can be easily identified and potentially correlated with the symptoms and functional complaints. Degenerative rotator cuff tears will be consistent with radiographic findings of a superiorly migrated humeral head due to lack of adequate humeral head depression (Fig 4–49). MRI has replaced the arthrogram to identify rotator cuff tears. Even minor changes of fibrotic tendon thickening and local edema can be picked up by MRI.

Problem List

Patients with rotator cuff problems may show any of the following clinical problems:

1. Pain when sleeping on the involved shoulder

2. Pain with reaching, lifting, or getting dressed

3. Pain after lifting or throwing

4. Grinding and clicking in the shoulder joint

5. Progressive symptoms of anterior shoulder pain with activity

Treatment

Although symptomatic relief measures can decrease pain and inflammation, treatment of rotator cuff problems will not succeed unless the underlying causes are identified. These include poor scapular stabilization, tight posterior capsule, limited subacromial space, weak rotator cuff muscles, acromioclavicular involvement, and glenohumeral instability.[35] Conservative management includes treating these causes rather than only treating the symptoms. Joint mobilization and self stretching exercises can decrease capsular tightness. Specific exercises to strengthen the rotator cuff muscles should be carried out in a pain free range. Dynamic elastic band or tubing with very light freeweights can be used with low loads and high repetitions. Specific exercises to strengthen the scapular stabilizers and provide proximal stability should be included in the treatment. Proprioceptive exercises should be included to augment dynamic scapular and rotator cuff stability and static glenohumeral stability. Teaching patients to change or eliminate the predisposing mechanical stresses is important.

Subacromial decompression or debridement is sometimes needed to relieve pressure on the rotator cuff tendons. Post–operative rehabilitation usually progresses rapidly. Mobility and strengthening exercises can be initiated after a 1–2 week immobilization phase. Restoring full pain free motion is critical to the success of the resistive exercise phase. The patient with rotator cuff repair will require a longer immobilization phase (using a sling or splint) of up to 6 weeks. After this immobilization period, the goal is to regain full passive range of motion as soon as possible without violating the healing constraints or increasing the symptoms. Resistive exercises for the rotator cuff should not start until the tissues heal at about 6 weeks; however, scapular stabilization can be initiated as soon as tolerated. The clinician should work closely with the surgeon to understand the surgical procedure and to provide appropriate treatment and follow–up.

Adhesive Capsulitis

This common clinical problem is often called the "frozen" shoulder. This condition typically presents as a general capsular tightening of the glenohumeral joint. In most cases the problem is idiopathic—no apparent cause is known. Women are affected more than men and middle aged to older people more often than younger ones. Many clinicians consider adhesive capsulitis to be self limiting, resolving ≈12 months after onset; however, clinical experience shows that with an appropriate treatment regime, many patients improve satisfactorily in 3–5 months.

History

Patients may have a history of trauma before onset of their complaints, but in most cases there is a

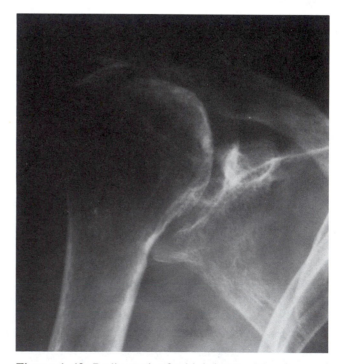

Figure 4–49. Radiograph of a high humeral head caused by a rotator cuff degeneration.

gradual onset with no known precipitating factors. We have found that many patients presenting with a "frozen" shoulder have a history of similar complaints on the opposite shoulder. The restricted mobility has begun to interfere with daily activities and sleep by the time the patients arrive at the clinic.

Signs/Symptoms

Patients usually complain of lateral upper arm pain at rest that increases in severity with attempts to move the shoulder. They often have difficulty getting to sleep because of problems finding a comfortable position. They may awaken with pain if they roll onto the shoulder. Problems in daily activities include fixing hair, fastening a bra, reaching into the back pocket of pants, and putting on shirts and coats. The findings on objective examination include a marked limitation of glenohumeral motion actively and passively in the capsular pattern: *external rotation limited more than abduction, which is limited more than flexion and internal rotation.* Extension, as in the functional hand–behind–the–back maneuver, may also be greatly reduced. In acute cases the patient presents with pain and muscle guarding at the end of passive range. Patients with chronic conditions may have range of motion limited by tightness, with pain on overpressure. Resistive muscle testing may provoke pain in the acute phase, but this should resolve as the range of motion improves. There may be concurrent signs of rotator cuff tear, which would show up as weakness on MMT. With decreased range of motion, the movement of neural structures in the shoulder region can become restricted. It is common to find a positive ULTT, especially in the patient whose pain prevents improvements in range of motion.

Diagnostics

There are no routine diagnostic tests for adhesive capsulitis. Standard radiographs may show some degenerative changes at the glenohumeral joint; however, recent clinical research has used the arthrogram to identify a decreased capsular filling consistent with a tight capsule. Experimental saline solution injections into the subscapularis bursal sac inferiorly (hydrodilation) have shown promising results with marked increases in range of motion of the shoulder immediately after the procedure.[16]

Problem List

Patients with adhesive capsulitis may present with any of the following problems:

1. Decreased functional use of the arm during daily activities

2. Inability to reach the hand behind the back

3. Shoulder pain with lifting or with reaching, especially overhead

4. Marked decrease in shoulder range of motion

5. Shoulder muscle weakness

Treatment

Initial treatment in the acute stage can include physical agents to decrease pain and muscle guarding. Grades I and II oscillatory mobilizations can be used to relieve symptoms, beginning with inferior glides. It is useful to begin passive range of motion exercises in the pain free and resistance–free range before starting the patient on a home program. Scapular stabilization exercises should be started as soon as tolerated. These exercises will promote normal scapulo–humeral posture in preparation for any resistive exercise program that may be indicated.

When the patient's condition allows, capsular tightness can be treated with more aggressive joint mobilization. Grade III oscillations can be used initially since the patient can usually tolerate them. The patient may experience some pain with these treatments, so the clinician should carefully avoid provoking muscle guarding. Muscle guarding will inhibit progress. Eventually, Grade IV oscillations or Grade III sustained mobilizations should be used to stretch the tight capsule. Again, the patient may have some pain with treatment, but these grades of mobilizations should be used as long as the pain resolves quickly after the treatment. It is important to prevent symptoms from building up and lasting. The treatments may occasionally result in pain that persists for an extended period (greater than two hours after treatment) or come on several hours after the treatment has been completed. In such cases, the intensity of the treatment should be decreased to avoid increasing symptoms and losing range of motion. Inferior and anterior mobilizations are usually performed; however, the clinician should mobilize into any joint play directions found to be limited on examination. Deep heating agents can help joint mobilizations. Accessory mobilizations should be combined with a passive physiological stretch to provide the most effective gains in mobility. Patients can be taught self–mobilization to supplement treatments (see Chapter 11, Mobilization Techniques).

The time required to treat frozen shoulders can be extensive. Aggressive home exercise, close follow–up, and critical reassessment promote lasting results. Any gains in range of motion or function should be positively reinforced, as this problem can take 3–5 months (or more) to resolve.

Thoracic Outlet Syndrome

Thoracic outlet syndrome (TOS) is a collection of signs and symptoms attributed to compression of the neurovascular bundle, including the brachial plexus and the subclavian and axillary arteries. "Thoracic inlet" has been used to describe problems with the subclavian vein. Recent authors have proposed that over 90% of TOS patients have a neurological basis for their complaints.[46] This contradicts traditional thinking and testing for a vascular origin of the problems.

There are three anatomical sites that can be involved in TOS (Fig 4–12). The first is the point at which the brachial plexus and subclavian artery are compressed as they pass over the first rib between the anterior and middle scalene muscles (scalene/first–rib syndrome). The second is the point at which the axillary artery and brachial plexus are compressed between the clavicle and first rib (costoclavicular syndrome). The final point of compression is at the coracoid process between the pectoralis minor muscle and the ribs (pectoralis minor syndrome or hyperabduction syndrome). The patient must be examined carefully to differentiate complaints and to plan appropriate treatment.

History

Gradual onset of symptoms is common. Symptoms are usually reported in the distal limb at the hand and fingers and often occur at night or in the morning. There is usually no history of acute trauma. Some patients assume prolonged postures that may be related to the onset of symptoms or perform repetitive motions that provoke the symptoms.

Signs/Symptoms

TOS patients commonly complain their hands and fingers "fall asleep." Aggravating factors include staying in prolonged kyphotic postures and working or sleeping with the arms overhead for prolonged periods. Sleeping with arms overhead can also increase pain due to the prolonged stretch on the neurovascular bundle. Reaching with the arms overhead or behind the body in horizontal abduction may also aggravate the complaints.

With arterial compression, the patient will report pain and fatigue during activity that goes away with rest. Symptoms will often start distally and proceed proximally. In later stages, cold sensitivity may be present. Any signs of emboli, such as cyanosis in one or more fingers, are serious and require immediate medical attention.[23] When arterial compression is present, positive objective findings may include any of the following: A positive Adson's test, costoclavicular test, hyperabduction test, or Roo's Test (EAST).

Venous compression may lead to edema, skin tightness, cyanosis, pain, and fatigue. Venous distention may be seen in the extremity after activity. When possible, the therapist should try to reproduce the position or activity that causes the symptoms. Other possible causes of peripheral vascular symptoms should be ruled out before a definitive diagnosis is made. The edema should decrease after a change in the aggravating position. The edema that does not diminish may be a sign of venous thrombosis. The patient should be referred to a physician for further evaluation.

Nerve compression causes various symptoms including pain, tingling. or numbness. Symptoms usually follow the nerve trunk. Ulnar nerve symptoms are more common than median nerve symptoms.[23] Night pain is common.[23,28]

Diagnosis for brachial plexus compression in the thoracic outlet is primarily done through ruling out other pathology in the cervical spine and upper extremities that could cause similar symptoms.[23] Objectively, if Adson's Test, the costoclavicular test, the hyperabduction test, or Roo's Test reproduces neurological symptoms, and if other pathology is ruled out, TOS is a likely cause of the patient's neurological symptoms. The neural tension tests for the upper limb discussed in Chapter 2, Principles of Extremity Evaluation, are important as well.

The ULTT with a median or ulnar nerve bias may be positive. The standard neurological examination is usually negative.

Diagnostics

Radiographs of the cervical and thoracic spines may show a cervical rib, an anatomic anomaly that can put stress on the neurovascular bundle. An MRI may show structural changes at the site of neurovascular compromise, but this test is usually not necessary. Arteriograms and venograms can also aid diagnosis. Venous compression is diagnosed objectively through plethysmography.

Problem List

Patients with thoracic outlet syndrome can have the following clinical problems:

1. Pins and needles (falling asleep) sensations in the upper extremity

2. Complaints of fatigue with use of arms and hands for overhead reaching activities

3. Pain with upper extremity stretching

4. Functional limitations due to pain and paresthesias

5. Sleep postures aggravating the condition

Treatment

Due to the intimate relationship between the neurovascular structures and the shoulder girdle, posture correction is critical. Work, leisure activities, and sleep postures should be modified as needed to decrease pressure on the structures. Scapular stabilization exercises will help promote an upright posture. Physical agents can be used to help soft tissue mobilization and to help stretch the scalenes,

pectoralis minor, or other involved soft tissues. Related neural tension findings should be addressed (see Chapter 11, Mobilization Techniques). Mobilization of the first rib and clavicle may be necessary. Specific instructions will help the patient use improved postures, avoid repetitive movements, and perform self stretches. Without patient compliance in these areas, only temporary improvement may occur.

The patient must be taught early on that TOS may take several weeks or months to resolve. Careful, consistent attention to the patient's home exercise program is necessary for long term resolution.

In some cases, surgical resection of a cervical rib or other surgical release techniques can be successful; however, successful surgical management must include patient education and exercise to prevent factors such as poor posture, repetitive activities, and poor ergonomic conditions from causing the patient's symptoms to recur.

SUMMARY

The evaluation, treatment, and prevention of shoulder problems has been presented. Patients with shoulder complaints are commonly referred to physical therapy and present a formidable challenge to any clinician. Management of patients with shoulder complaints is complicated because the shoulder is a common site of symptom referral from visceral sources and the cervical spine. Poor posture in the cervical and shoulder region can lead to shoulder pain, dysfunction, and neurovascular compromise. Proper upright posture is necessary for normal shoulder function across its four joint structures. Optimal shoulder function requires synchronous muscle balance between the scapular stabilizers and the rotator cuff. Effective shoulder problem management must include all related neuromusculoskeletal structures.

Please refer to Chapter 11, Mobilization Techniques; Chapter 12, Exercise; and Chapter 13, Prevention of Extremity Injuries for expanded information on mobilization techniques, stretching and resistive exercises, and prevention of problems with the shoulder complex.

REFERENCES

1. Baker CL, Liu SH, Blackburn TA: Neurovascular Syndromes of the Shoulder. In Rehabilitation of the Athletic Shoulder. KE Wilk, ed. Churchill-Livingstone, New York NY 1993.

2. Bernhardt D: Evaluation of the Shoulder Complex. In Post-graduate Studies in Sports Physical Therapy. Forum Medicum, Berryville VA 1991.

3. Bogduk N, Marsland A: On the Concept of Third Occipital Headache. Journal of Neurology, Neurosurgery, Psychiatry 49: 775-780, 1986

4. Boissonnault W, Janos S: Screening For Medical Disease: Physical Therapy Assessment and Treatment Principles. In Examination in Physical Therapy Practice: Screening For Medical Disease. Churchill-Livingstone, New York NY 1991.

5. Booher J, and Thipodeau G: Athletic Injury Assessment. Times Mirror/Mosby College Publishers, New York NY 1989.

6. Cahill BR, Palmer RE: Quadrilateral Space Syndrome. Journal of Hand Surgery 8(1):65-69, 1983.

7. Cailliet R: Neck and Arm Pain. FA Davis, Philadelphia PA 1964.

8. Cain PR, et al: Anterior Instability of the GH Joint: A Dynamic Model. American Journal of Sports Medicine 15:144-148, 1987.

9. Cleland J: On the Actions of Muscles Passing Over One Joint. Journal of Anatomical Physiology 1:85-93, 1966.

10. Cloward R: Cervical Discography: A Contribution to the Etiology and Mechanism of Neck, Shoulder and Arm Pain. Annals of Surgery 150(6) 1052-1064, 1959.

11. Codman E: The Shoulder. Thomas Todd, Boston MA 1934.

12. Culham E, Peat M: Functional Anatomy of the Shoulder Complex. JOSPT 18(1):342-350, 1993.

13. Davies G, Dickoff-Hoffman S: Neuromuscular Testing and Rehabilitation of the Shoulder Complex. JOSPT 18(2):449-458, 1993.

14. Feinstein B, Langton J, et al: Experiments on Pain Referred from Deep Somatic Tissues. JBJS 36A:981-997, 1954.

15. Gerber C, Ganz R: Clinical Assessment of Instability of the Shoulder. JBJS 66B:551-556, 1984.

16. Groom D: The Neck and Shoulder: Does Treatment of Spinal Structures Speed Recovery from Shoulder Dysfunction? Lincoln School of Health Sciences, La Trobe University, Victoria, Australia 1988. Unpublished thesis.

17. Groom D: Cervical Spine and Shoulder Seminar, Minneapolis MN 1993. Personal Communication.

18. Groom D: Cervical Spine and Shoulder. Seminar presented in Minneapolis MN 1993.

19. Halbach J and Tank R: The Shoulder. In Orthopedic and Sports Physical Therapy, Vol 2. J Gould and G Davies, ed. CV Mosby, St Louis MO 1985.

20. Hawkins R, Kennedy J: Impingement Syndrome in Athletics. Am J Sports Med 8:151-163, 1980.

21. Hoppenfeld S: Physical Examination of the Spine and Extremities. Appleton-Century-Crofts, Norwalk CT 1976.

22. Hunkin K: The Neck and Shoulder: Can Treatment of the Cervical Spine Relieve Shoulder Pain and Disability? School of Physiotherapy: South Australia Institute of Technology, 1978. Unpublished thesis.

23. Koontz C: "Thoracic Outlet Syndrome, Diagnosis and Management." In Orthopedic Physical Therapy Forum series. AREN, Pittsburgh, PA 1987. Videotape.

24. Leffert RD and Gumley G: The Relationship Between Dead Arm Syndrome and Thoracic Outlet Syndrome. Clin Orthop and Rel Res 223:20-31, 1987.

25. Ludington N: Rupture of the Long Head of the Biceps Flexor Cubiti Muscle. Annals of Surgery 77:358-363, 1923.

26. Magee D: Orthopedic Physical Assessment. WB Saunders, Philadelphia PA 1992.

27. Mennell J: Back Pain. Little-Brown, Boston MA 1964.

28. Mennell J: Differential Diagnosis of Visceral From Somatic Back Pain. Joul of Occ Med 8:477-80, Sept 1966.

29. Mosley LH, et al: Cumulative Trauma Disorders and Compression Neuropathies of the Upper Extremities. In Occupational Hand and Upper Extremity Injuries. M Kasdan, ed. Hanley & Belfus, Philadelphia PA 1991.

30. Murray M, Gore D, Gardner G, et al: Shoulder Motion and Muscle Strength of Normal Men and Women in Two Age Groups. Clin Orthop 192:268-273, 1985.

31. O'Brien SJ, Neves MC, Arnoczky SP, et al: The Anatome and Histology of the Inferior Glenohumeral Ligament Complex of the Shoulder. Am J Sports Med 18(5): 449-456, 1990.

32. Palmer M, Epler M: Clinical Assessment Procedures in Physical Therapy. JB Lippincott, Philadelphia PA 1990.

33. Perry J: Biomechanics of the Shoulder. In The Shoulder. C. Rowe, ed. Churchill-Livingstone, New York NY 1988.

34. Perry J: Muscle Control of the Shoulder. In The Shoulder. C. Rowe, ed. Churchill-Livingstone, New York NY 1988.

35. Pink M, Jobe F: Shoulder Injuries in Athletes. Orthopaedics 11(96): 39-47, 1985.

36. Poppen N, Walker P: Normal and Abnormal Motion of the Shoulder. JBJS 58:195-201, 1976.

37. Protzmanv R: Anterior Instability of the Shoulder. JBJS 62A:909-918, 1980.

38. Rockwood C: Subluxations and Dislocations About the Shoulder. In Fractures in Adults-1. C Rockwood and D Green, ed. JB Lippincott, Philadelphia PA 1984.

39. Rowe C: Dislocations of the Shoulder. In The Shoulder. C Rowe, ed. Churchill-Livingstone, Edinburgh 1988.

40. Saha SK: Mechanics of Elevation of the Glenohumeral Joint. Acta Orthop Scand 44:668-678, 1973.

41. Savoie F: Evaluation of the Shoulder: Examination of the Throwing Athlete. Joul Miss State Med Assoc 66:1866-1877, 1989.

42. Schenkman M, Rugo de Cartaya V: Kinesiology of the Shoulder Complex. JOSPT 8:438-450, 1987.

43. Sillman JF, Dean MT: Neurovascular Injuries to The Shoulder Complex. JOSPT 18(1): 442-448, 1993.

44. Smith R, Brunoli J: Shoulder Kinesthesia After Glenohumeral Joint Dislocation. Physical Therapy 69:23-29, 1992.

45. Terry P: Comparable Spinal Signs in Patients with Known Shoulder Pathology. Lincoln School of Health Sciences, La Trobe University, Victoria, Australia 1991. Unpublished thesis.

46. Toby EB and Koman LA: Thoracic Outlet Compression Syndrome. In Nerve Compression Syndromes. RM Szabo, ed. Slack, Thorofare, London 1989.

47. Wadsworth C: Manual Examination and Treatment of the Spine and Extremities. Williams and Wilkins, Baltimore MD 1988.

48. Wilk K, Arrigo C: Current Concepts in the Rehabilitation of the Athletic Shoulder. JOSPT 18(1):365-378, 1993.

49. Zarins B, Rowe C: Current Concepts in the Diagnosis and Treatment of Shoulder Instability in Athletes. Med Sci Sports Exerc 16(5):444-448, 1984.

CHAPTER 5

THE ELBOW

INTRODUCTION

The elbow is composed of three joints and four groups of muscles that synergistically control its motion. There are several two–joint muscles that attach around the elbow and influence its function. It is also the origin of the muscles that control the wrist and hand, and is the gateway for neurovascular structures as they enter the forearm.

The elbow is commonly injured from repetitive trauma at work or during sport activities but can also be acutely injured in a fall or by a direct blow. Symptoms felt at the elbow may be referred from the cervical spine, shoulder, and forearm. Evaluation, treatment, and prevention of elbow problems should include these related structures in an integrated management program.

FUNCTIONAL ANATOMY

Osseous and Capsuloligamentous Components

The elbow is a compound synovial joint composed of three joints: the ulnohumeral, radiohumeral, and superior radioulnar. Since the capsule and joint spaces are continuous for all three joints, injury to one joint will affect the other two. The

middle radioulnar joint should also be considered when examining the elbow. Figure 5–1 shows the bony and ligamentous structures of the elbow.

Ulnohumeral Joint

The ulnohumeral joint is a uniaxial hinge joint formed between the trochlear notch of the ulna and the trochlea of the humerus. The distal humerus and proximal ulna are offset 45° anteriorly to allow full range of motion without the ulna impinging on the humerus (Fig 5–2). The trochlea of the humerus is asymmetrical. Its axis of motion points superolateral to inferomedial. This causes an angulation of the elbow called the "carrying angle." When the arm is at the side, the carrying angle is 10–15° in men and 20–25° in women (Fig 5–3).[29] The asymmetry of the trochlea allows the amount of joint play needed for full range of motion. The joint gaps medially in full extension, laterally in full flexion, and glides side–to–side in supination and pronation. The ulna rotates internally 5° in early elbow flexion and externally 5° at end range of flexion.[7,43] The ulnohumeral joint is stabilized medially by the ulnar collateral ligament.

Radiohumeral Joint

The radiohumeral joint is a uniaxial hinge joint between the head of the radius and the capitulum of the humerus. The radial collateral ligament provides lateral stability to the joint. Trauma to the radiohumeral joint may interfere with elbow flexion and extension.

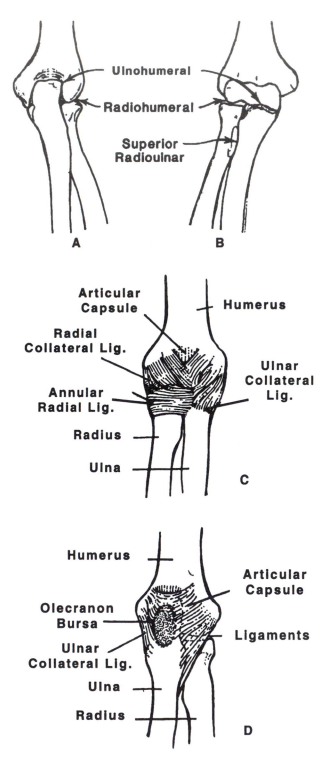

Figure 5-1. Joints, bones, and ligaments of the elbow (right elbow; A&D, posterior view; B&C, anterior view).

Superior Radioulnar Joint

The superior radioulnar joint is a uniaxial pivot joint between the proximal head of the radius and the medial portion of the proximal ulna. The spherical head of the radius allows the rotation needed for forearm supination and pronation. The joint is stabilized by the annular ligament that surrounds the head of the radius. Injury to this joint may limit the ability to control the position of the hand.

Middle Radioulnar Joint

The middle radioulnar joint is formed by the interosseous membrane and the oblique cord running perpendicular to each other between the ulna and the radius. The interosseous membrane stabilizes the elbow by resisting proximal displacement of the radius on the ulna during pushing movements. The oblique cord resists distal displacement of the radius during pulling movements (Fig 5-4).

In summary, the ulnohumeral, radiohumeral, superior radioulnar, and middle radioulnar joints

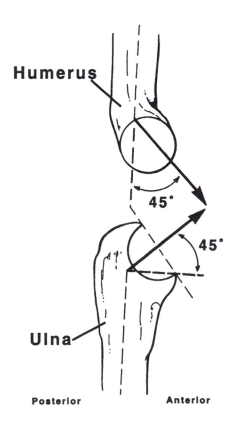

Figure 5-2. The relationship between the humerus and the ulna (side view).

contribute to the movement and stability of the elbow. Table 5–1 summarizes the movements and ranges of motion at the elbow.

Neuromuscular Components

Muscular Structures

Eight muscles exert the major forces to flex and extend the elbow and to supinate and pronate the forearm. Each of these movements will be discussed as isolated and coordinated movements in the open and closed kinematic chain. While the muscles that flex and extend the wrist have their origin at the elbow and may cause symptoms at this joint, these muscles will be discussed in Chapter 6, The Wrist and Hand. The muscles that act on the elbow are shown in Figure 5–5.

Flexor Function

The brachialis, biceps brachii, and brachioradialis muscles are the major elbow flexors. The pronator teres and flexor carpi ulnaris can also contribute to flexion. The brachialis is the "workhorse" of elbow flexion: it helps when the forearm is in pronation or supination and when the shoulder is flexed or extended.[3] The biceps brachii helps elbow flexion when lifting loads >2lb.[3] The brachioradialis flexes the elbow, and it stabilizes supination and pronation during strong resistance.

Extensor Function

The triceps brachii and anconeus muscles are the elbow extensors. The medial triceps appears to be the most active, the long head the least active, and the lateral triceps the strongest.[16] The anconeus helps

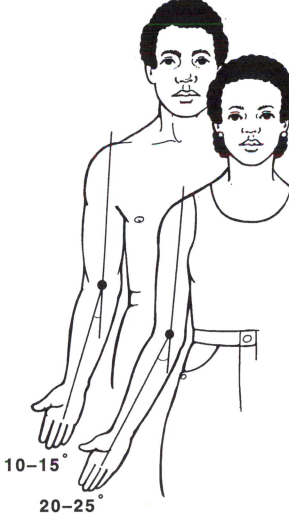

10–15°

20–25°

Figure 5–3. The carry angle of the elbow.

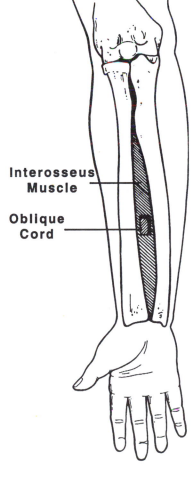

Interosseus Muscle

Oblique Cord

Figure 5–4. The right middle radioulnar joint.

Table 5–1. Movements and Range of Motion at the Elbow

Flexion	140-150°
Extension	0-15°
Supination	90°
Pronation	80-90°

with extension and helps stabilize in pronation and supination.[2] The pectoralis major and anterior deltoid muscles can facilitate elbow extension in a closed kinematic chain (e.g., during push–ups or when pushing heavy objects).

Supination and Pronation

The supinator muscle probably acts alone to supinate the forearm under low loads and when performing slow movements; however, when the elbow is flexed to 90°, the biceps brachii performs supination four times more effectively than the supinator muscle.[18]

The pronator quadratus is the prime mover of pronation under low loads. The pronator teres is most active when performing pronation and stabilizing elbow flexion.[18] The flexor carpi radialis may also help pronate. The anconeus and brachioradialis muscles stabilize supination and pronation.[2,3]

Integrated Function

The elbow must work with other joints for most functional activities. This requires coordination between muscle antagonists. When pulling objects toward the body, the biceps brachii flex the elbow while the shoulder extends. The triceps aid this motion by controlling elbow flexion and helping shoulder extension. When pushing, the triceps extend the elbow while the biceps control elbow extension and help with shoulder flexion. When turning doorknobs or screwdrivers clockwise, the biceps supinate the forearm while the flexion action of the biceps is countered by the triceps. When using a fork, the biceps provide supination and flexion to bring the fork to the mouth, and contract eccentrically to control putting the fork down (pronation and extension).

These examples illustrate the importance of considering the integrated muscle functions when managing elbow problems. The muscles, their actions, and their segmental and peripheral nerve innervations are shown in Table 5–2.

Neural Structures

Four nerves have critical roles as they traverse the elbow: the ulnar, the median, the musculocutaneous, and the radial. The path of the nerves will be discussed in relation to the anatomical tissues that can cause mechanical nerve irritation or entrapment.

Ulnar Nerve

The ulnar nerve originates from the C8–T1 nerve roots and descends into the upper extremity from the medial cord of the brachial plexus. It passes in an anterior–posterior direction in the upper arm through the Arcade of Struthers, ≈8 cm proximal to the medial epicondyle.[14] This "arcade" is a fascial bridge between the medial head of the triceps and the medial intermuscular septum.[30] The ulnar nerve then passes behind the medial epicondyle and through the cubital tunnel—the most common site of ulnar nerve trauma. The cubital tunnel is the area between the ulnar collateral ligament and the arcuate ligament (the tendon expansion of the flexor carpi ulnaris muscle). As the elbow flexes, the nerve becomes taut[6] and is compressed by ligamentous tightening.[15] The ligamentous structure that forms the "roof" over the cubital tunnel is the cubital tunnel retinaculum.[22] This retinaculum is absent in up to 10% of the population, predisposing the nerve to subluxation over the medial epicondyle.[34] The ulnar nerve sends small branches to the joint capsule and then enters the forearm by passing between the two heads of the flexor carpi ulnaris. The three areas that can mechanically irritate the ulnar nerve around the elbow are 1) the Arcade of Struthers; 2) the cubital tunnel; and 3) the area between the two heads of the flexor carpi ulnaris (Fig 5–6).

Median Nerve

The median nerve originates from the C5–T1 nerve roots and descends into the upper extremity from branches of the medial and lateral cords of the brachial plexus. The nerve passes anteromedially in the upper arm beneath the brachial fascia and over the

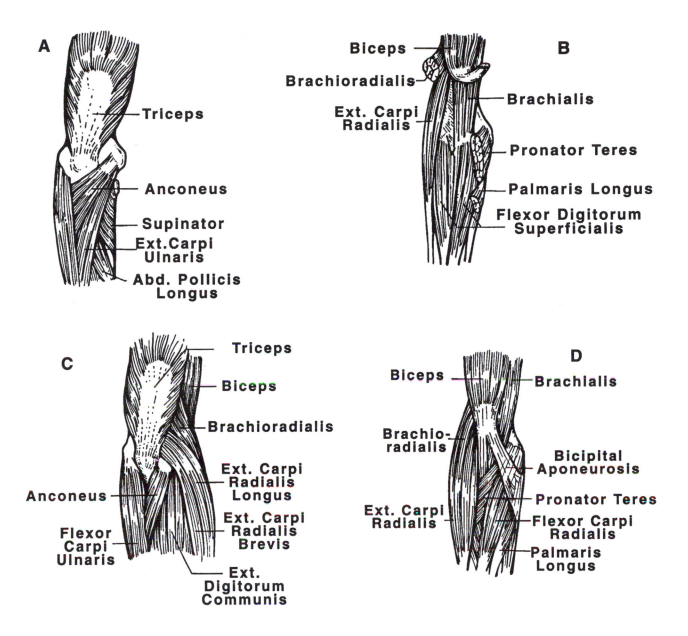

Figure 5–5. Muscles of the elbow (right elbow; A&C, posterior view; B&D, anterior view).

Table 5–2. Muscles of the Elbow: Actions, Peripheral and Segmental Innervations

Muscles	Actions	Peripheral Nerve Supply	Spinal Segment
Anconeus	Extension	Radial	C7, C8 (T1)
Biceps brachii	Flexion/supination	Musculocutaneous	C5, C6
Brachialis	Flexion	Musculocutaneous	C5, C6 (C7)
Brachioradialis	Flexion	Radial	C5, C6 (C7)
Flexor carpi radialis	Pronation	Median	C6, C7
Flexor carpi ulnaris	Flexion	Ulnar	C7, C8
Pronator quadratus	Pronation	Median (anterior interosseus)	C8 (T1)
Pronator teres	Flexion/pronation	Median	C6, C7
Supinator	Supination	Radial (posterior interosseus)	C5, C6
Triceps brachii	Extension	Radial	C6, C7, C8

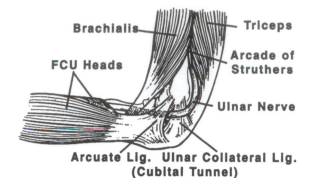

Figure 5-6. Ulnar nerve pathway and potential entrapment sites at the Arcade of Struthers, cubital tunnel and flexor carpi ulnaris heads (right elbow; medial view).

brachialis muscle. At the elbow, it continues near the medial aspect of the antecubital fossa, medial to the biceps tendon and the brachial artery. When present, an anomalous structure called the Ligament of Struthers can cause mechanical entrapment of the median nerve proximal to the antecubital fossa. The Ligament of Struthers is found in ≈1% of the population.[32] The median nerve continues distally, passing under the bicipital aponeurosis and between the two heads of the pronator teres muscle. The anterior interosseus branch of the median nerve descends along the anterior aspect of the interosseus membrane, arising inferior to the border of the pronator teres. The three areas that could compromise the median nerve are 1) the Ligament of Struthers (if present); 2) the bicipital aponeurosis; and 3) the two heads of the pronator teres (Fig 5-7).

Musculocutaneous Nerve

The musculocutaneous nerve originates from the C5-7 nerve roots, coming off the lateral cord of the brachial plexus. The nerve passes between the biceps brachii and the brachialis muscles to pierce the brachial fascia lateral to the biceps tendon. The nerve can be mechanically irritated or entrapped between the biceps tendon and the brachial fascia and as the nerve passes through the brachial fascia (Fig 5-8).[4]

Radial Nerve

The radial nerve originates from the C6-C8 nerve roots (with fibers from C5 and T1 in some people) and descends into the arm from the posterior cord of the brachial plexus. The nerve then passes laterally in the upper arm through the radial groove of the humerus. It continues distally to pierce the lateral intermuscular septum, then passes anteriorly to the lateral epicondyle behind the brachialis and brachioradialis muscles. The radial nerve divides into the posterior interosseus and superficial radial nerve branches at the antecubital space distal to the radiohumeral joint. The superficial branch courses under the brachioradialis muscle and over the top of the supinator and pronator muscles. The posterior interosseus branch passes around the posterolateral radius and then between the two heads of the supinator muscle. In some cases, the radial nerve has a fibrous attachment to the radial head. It sometimes

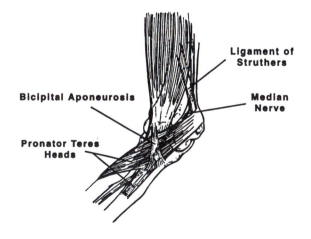

Figure 5-7. Median nerve pathway and potential entrapment sites at the Ligament of Struthers, bicipital aponeurosis, and pronator teres (right elbow; medial view).

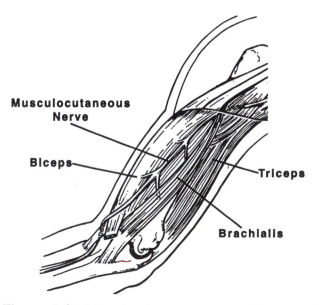

Figure 5-8. Musculocutaneous nerve pathway and potential entrapment sites at the biceps tendon and brachial fascia (right elbow; medial view).

passes under a fibrous arch called the radial tunnel, or Arcade of Froshe.[6] This arcade lies proximal to the supinator muscle and is present in ≈30% of the population.[32]

The three areas that could compromise the radial nerve by mechanical irritation or entrapment are 1) the radial groove; 2) the radial head; and 3) the supinator muscle (alone or via the radial tunnel) (Fig 5–9).

EVALUATION

Subjective Examination

The subjective examination should proceed as outlined in Chapter 2, Principles of Extremity Evaluation. The patient's main complaints provide valuable clues about current problems and will help the clinician plan the objective examination. In acute trauma, the mechanism of injury should be noted. Did the patient fall directly on the elbow? Was there a fall on an outstretched arm that may have caused a hyperextension injury? A patient complaining of elbow pain who is unable to supinate may have a dislocated radial head. This condition is sometimes seen in children whose parents have pulled on their arm. If the injury is subacute or chronic, questions should focus on factors that aggravate the symptoms. Many elbow problems are the result of repetitive activities that cause cumulative trauma. Overuse of the hand and wrist can result in elbow symptoms such as medial or lateral epicondylitis. Careful questioning about the specific demands of work and leisure activities will help functional assessment of elbow problems.

The patterns of the patient's complaints will further guide the objective examination. Paresthesias in the hand or forearm can be caused by irritation of nerves at the elbow. For example, ulnar nerve problems may result from leaning on the elbows, or from sleeping with the elbows in full flexion. Complaints of sensory changes or muscle weakness indicate the need for neurological testing.

Planning the Objective Examination

The objective examination of the elbow should be based on the information gained from the subjective examination. Excessive provocation of the problem can lead to an inaccurate picture of the patient's condition; therefore, it helps to plan which tests to perform based upon the severity, irritability and nature (SIN) of the problem before beginning the objective examination. If the patient is unable to maintain certain positions, the condition is relatively severe and these positions should not be stressed on the initial evaluation. For example, it is a good idea to avoid applying overpressure into extension for a

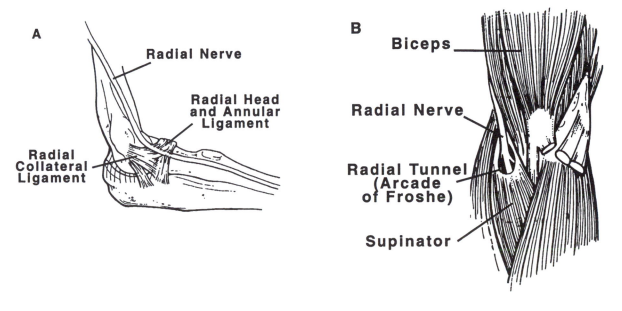

Figure 5–9. Radial nerve pathway and potential entrapment at radial head and supinator muscle. Not shown is its potential entrapment at the radial groove (right elbow; A, lateral view; B, anterior view).

patient with an acute hyperextension injury. If symptoms are easily provoked, the condition is irritable and the number of motions tested should be limited initially. The objective examination may also be limited by the nature of the patient's complaints. If a patient has acute inflammation, overpressures and palpation should be minimized.

Objective Examination

The objective examination should proceed as outlined in Chapter 2, Principles of Extremity Evaluation. Evaluation of the cervical spine, shoulder, wrist, and hand should be included if these areas are suspected contributors to the patient's problem. The quadrant test (see "Clearing Tests" in Chapter 2, Principles of Extremity Evaluation) will rule out the cervical spine as the source of complaints. Elbow symptoms easily provoked by neck movements or positions warrant a complete examination of the cervical spine. The shoulder should be checked if the patient complains of pain radiating from the shoulder to the elbow with movements of the arm. The wrist and hand should be screened in any patient complaining of elbow

problems. Refer to "Clearing Tests" in Chapter 2, Principles of Extremity Evaluation, for specific techniques to clear the shoulder, wrist, and hand.

Structural Observation

Symmetrical observation of bilateral upper limbs is performed with the arms exposed. Visual observation should begin as the patient enters the office. The clinician should observe how the patient uses the elbow while undressing and moving about, then have the patient stand in the anatomical position and note the carrying angle (Fig 5–3). Some patients may exhibit a carrying angle deformity from a prior fracture, called a "gunstock deformity." Swelling is commonly located at the posterolateral and anteromedial elbow. This differs from swelling present from an olecranon bursitis that is well encapsulated at the posterior olecranon (Fig 5–10). Soft tissue symmetry should be assessed. It is common to find the dominant forearm muscles better developed than on the non–dominant side, especially in athletes and laborers. Any soft tissue or bony deformities, discolorations, or scars should be inspected. Finally, the clinician should note the

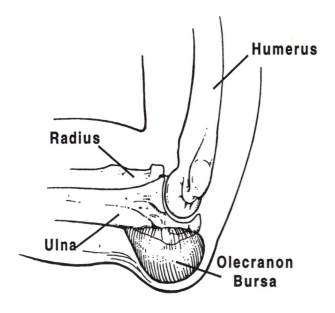

Figure 5–10. Enlarged olecranon bursa (right elbow; medial view).

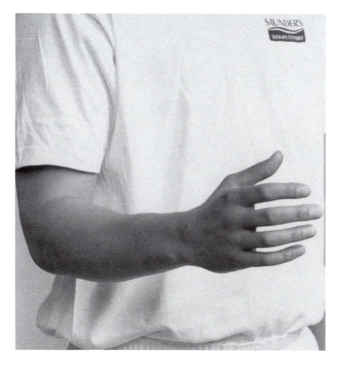

Figure 5–11. The functional position of the arm.

patient's ability to maintain the functional position (90° flexion with the forearm positioned midway between supination and pronation) (Fig 5–11).[16]

Mobility

Physiological Mobility

Physiological mobility is the movement of joints in planar movements and in combined functional movements. Active and passive physiological mobility should be assessed.

Active Mobility

Active mobility assesses the patient's willingness and ability to move the elbow. The motions that can be included in active mobility testing at the elbow are flexion, extension, supination, pronation, flexion with supination, flexion with pronation, extension with supination, and extension with pronation. Overpressure is applied at the end of the available active range of motion. The important findings to note include: available active range of motion; the symptom response to motion; any crepitus felt or heard; and the response to overpressure. The clinician should note if overpressure reproduced the patient's symptoms or increased the available range of motion. Tests can be performed with the patient standing, sitting, or supine.

Active mobility can be limited by connective tissue tightness, pain, swelling, edema, or weakness. Common findings after immobilization include limitations in supination–pronation, most notably at the end ranges of flexion and extension. Some authors have shown that most daily activities can be performed in less–than–normal ranges, so the patient's functional complaints frequently may not represent the limitations demonstrated by the objective findings.[37]

Passive Mobility

Passive mobility testing assesses the integrity of non–contractile tissues. Passive testing is indicated for each motion that shows limitations or reproduces symptoms during active testing. When moving the joint passively, the clinician should note the range available, symptom response, end–feel, and the pattern of motion restriction. Comparisons should be made to the contralateral extremity and to normal.

The pattern of motion restriction may be capsular or non–capsular. The capsular pattern at the elbow is *flexion limited more than extension* and *equal limitation of supination and pronation.*

The symptom response to passive motion can reveal the stage of the problem (see Chapter 2, Principles of Extremity Evaluation). Passive testing can be performed with the patient standing, sitting, or supine. Figure 5–12 shows passive mobility testing for elbow flexion and extension and forearm supination and pronation.

Accessory Mobility

Accessory mobility refers to component motions and joint play (see Chapter 2, Principles of Extremity Evaluation). It can be assessed with the patient in any position, but testing is usually easiest with the patient supine. The specific accessory motions to be tested include distraction, medial glide, and lateral glide at the ulnohumeral joint; anterior and posterior glide, rotation, and proximal and distal glides at the superior radioulnar joint; and anterior and posterior glide at the radiohumeral joint (see Chapter 11, Mobilization Techniques). The distal radioulnar joint should also be tested for accessory mobility, particularly if the patient shows limitation or symptoms with supination or pronation. The findings should be compared to the contralateral limb and to normal accessory mobility for that joint. When testing accessory motion, the clinician must note the amount of movement allowed, the quality of the movement, the end–feel, any crepitus, and any symptom provocation. The findings should be correlated with findings from the tests of physiological mobility. In particular, it is important to note whether passive physiological mobility limitations are caused by decreased accessory mobility. For example, a limitation in supination can be caused by a limitation in anterior glide at the superior radioulnar joint (see Chapter 11, Mobilization Techniques).

Strength

Resisted muscle testing assesses the contractile tissues. Specific manual muscle tests (MMT) are performed in the mid–range of motion to avoid stress on the non–contractile structures. The patient is told to gradually increase effort to a voluntary maximum contraction. This avoids substitution of synergistic

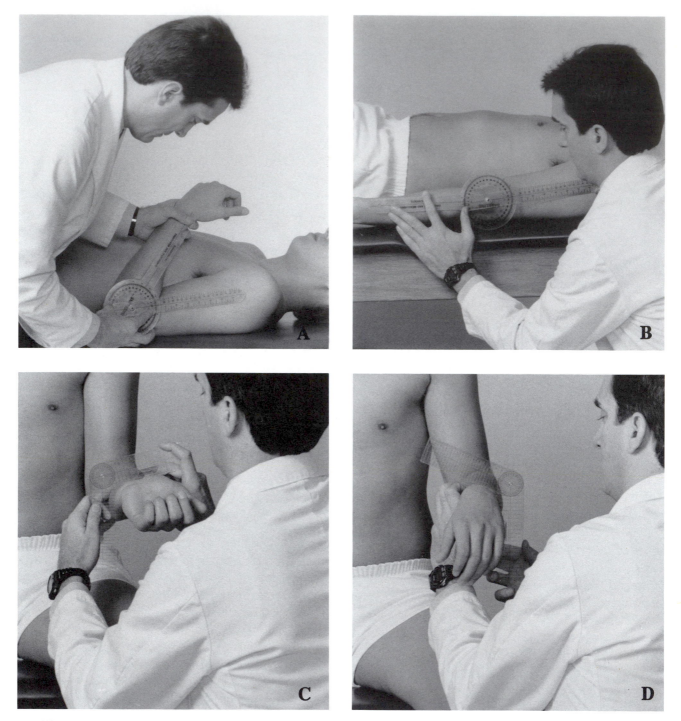

Figure 5–12. Passive mobility testing at the elbow. A) Elbow flexion; B) elbow extension; C) forearm supination; D) forearm pronation.

muscles. The clinician resists the attempt with an isometric contraction. The muscle strength should be graded and any symptom responses noted. Cyriax's four patterns of response help interpret the results of resisted tests (see Chapter 2, <u>Principles of Extremity Evaluation</u>). Any muscle acting on, acting across, or influencing the elbow should be included in muscle

strength testing. This includes the muscles of the wrist and hand that have their origins around the elbow. Grip testing with a dynamometer is also appropriate for patients with elbow complaints (Fig 5–13).

Some clinicians advocate functional strength testing of the elbow since the length of the forearm

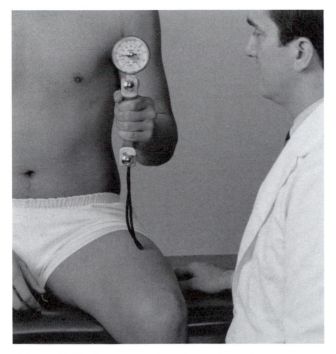

Figure 5–13. Grip strength testing using a dynamometer.

magnifies the load applied at the hand.[24] Examples of functional strength testing at the elbow include performing wall push–ups or holding a light weight in the hand of the involved limb while bringing that hand to the mouth (testing extension and flexion, respectively).

Neurological

The neurological examination is outlined in Chapter 2, Principles of Extremity Evaluation. Complaints of paresthesia, anesthesia, or weakness can indicate neurological impairment and thereby indicate neurological testing. The neurological examination includes motor function, light touch sensation, and deep tendon reflexes (DTR's). Motor function is assessed with resisted muscle testing as performed in the upper quarter screening examination. Light touch sensation should be tested in the upper limb, including the C4–T1 dermatomes and the regional cutaneous nerve fields (see Fig 2–13). Relevant DTR's include the biceps (C5–C6), brachioradialis (C6–C7), and triceps (C7–C8). With each of these neurological tests, the involved side should be compared to the contralateral limb and to normal. Elbow proprioception should also be assessed after any injury to the joint or its ligamentous structures.

Palpation

The palpation examination should proceed as described in Chapter 2, Principles of Extremity Evaluation. Palpation should begin with surface tissues and progress as tolerated to deeper structures. Bilateral comparisons should be made during palpation. The skin, bones, joints, ligaments, muscles, tendons, bursæ, and nerves of the elbow should be palpated. Any changes in temperature, color, and moisture may indicate reflex sympathetic dystrophy. The following structures should be palpated:

Anterior (Fig 5–14)

- musculocutaneous nerve
- median nerve
- cubital fossa
- brachioradialis
- pronator muscles
- biceps tendon
- brachial artery
- coronoid process of the ulna
- head of the radius
- biceps brachii
- brachialis

Posterior (Fig 5–15)

- triceps brachii
- anconeus
- olecranon process
- olecranon bursæ

Medial (Fig 5–16)

- ulnar collateral ligament
- cubital tunnel
- ulnar nerve
- medial epicondyle of the humerus
- wrist flexors

Lateral (Fig 5–17)

- radial and annular ligaments
- radial head
- lateral epicondyle of the humerus
- brachioradialis
- supinator
- wrist extensors
- radial nerve
- posterior interosseus branch of the radial nerve

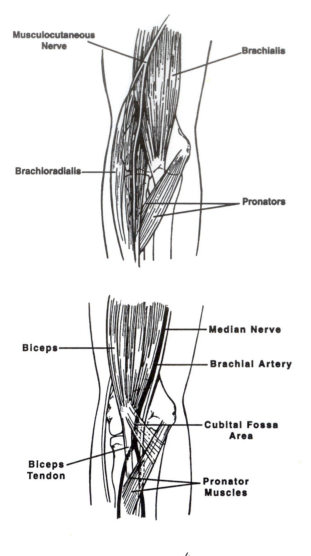

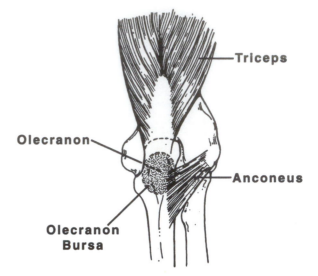

Figure 5–15. Structures to palpate at the elbow (right elbow; posterior view).

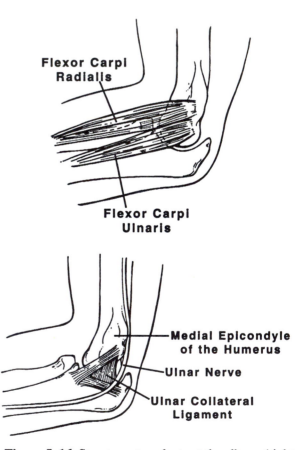

Figure 5–14. Structures to palpate at the elbow (right elbow; anterior view).

Figure 5–16. Structures to palpate at the elbow (right elbow; medial view).

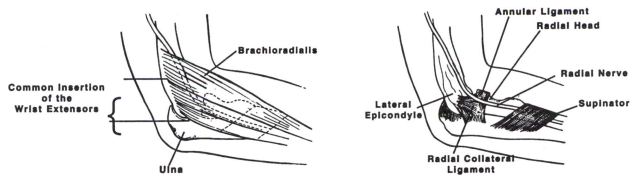

Figure 5–17. Structures to palpate at the elbow (right elbow; lateral view).

Special Tests

Special tests help the clinician rule out or confirm specific pathologies of the elbow. There are three types of special tests: neurological, musculotendinous, and joint and ligamentous. The special tests for the elbow are summarized in Table 5–3.

Neurological Tests

Pinch Test

The pinch test of the thumb–index finger increases pressure in the anterior compartment, testing for entrapment of the anterior interosseous branch of the median nerve as it passes through the interosseous membrane. The patient is told to pinch the tips of the thumb and index finger together. The normal response is a tip–to–tip pinch. The test is positive if the patient shows an abnormal pulp–to–pulp response (Fig 5–18).

Pronator Teres Syndrome Test

This tests for pronator teres syndrome (median nerve entrapment in the pronator teres muscle). The clinician strongly resists pronation of the elbow as the patient's elbow is extended from 90° flexion toward full extension. The test is positive if tingling or paresthesias are provoked in the forearm and hand in a median nerve distribution (Fig 5–19).

Elbow Flexion Test

The elbow flexion test assesses ulnar nerve entrapment at the cubital tunnel. The clinician asks the patient to completely flex the elbow and sustain flexion for up to 5 minutes. The test is positive when tingling or paresthesias are provoked in the forearm and hand in an ulnar nerve distribution (Fig 5–20).

Table 5–3. Special Tests for the Elbow

Test Type	Test Name	Purpose
Neurological	Pinch Test	Entrapment of anterior interosseous nerve in anterior interosseous membrane
	Pronator Teres Syndrome	Entrapment of median nerve by pronator teres
	Elbow Flexion Test	Entrapment of ulnar nerve in cubital tunnel
	Tinel's Test	Irritation of peripheral nerve
Musculotendinous	Golfer's Elbow	Medial epicondylitis
	Tennis Elbow	Lateral epicondylitis
Ligamentous	Varus Stress	Radial collateral ligament stability
	Valgus Stress	Ulnar collateral ligament stability

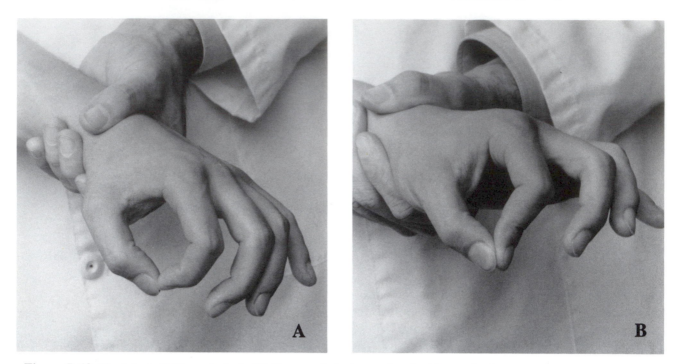

Figure 5–18. Pinch test. A) Normal pinch; B) Abnormal pinch associated with anterior interosseous nerve entrapment.

Tinel's Sign

This test assesses peripheral nerve entrapment. The test is administered by tapping at the cubital tunnel (ulnar nerve), the radial head and radial tunnel (radial nerve), and the carpal tunnel (median nerve)

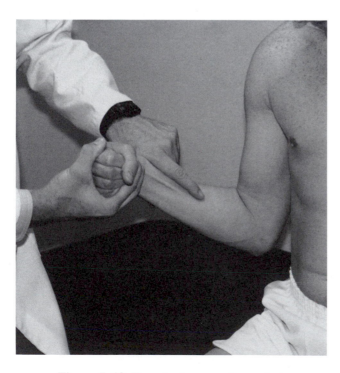

Figure 5–19. Pronator teres syndrome test.

(Fig 5–21). These tests are positive if they reproduce the patient's symptoms of sensory changes or pain.

Musculotendinous Tests

Tests for medial and lateral epicondylitis are administered in two steps: the muscle action is resisted, then the muscles are stretched.

Golfer's Elbow Test

For golfer's elbow (medial epicondylitis), wrist flexion is resisted. The stretch position of this test is full wrist extension with the elbow extended and the forearm in full supination (Fig 5–22). The test is positive if the resistance or the stretch position reproduces the patient's pain complaints.

Tennis Elbow Test

For tennis elbow (lateral epicondylitis), wrist extension is resisted. To stretch the muscles inserting at the lateral epicondyle, the wrist is moved into full flexion with the elbow straight and the forearm fully pronated (Fig 5–23). The test is positive if the stretch position or wrist extension resistance reproduces the patient's complaints. An additional test for lateral epicondylitis is resisted extension of the middle finger when the wrist is in full extension.

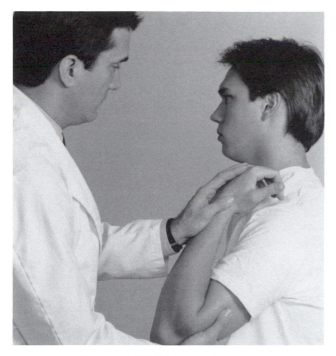

Figure 5–20. Elbow flexion test.

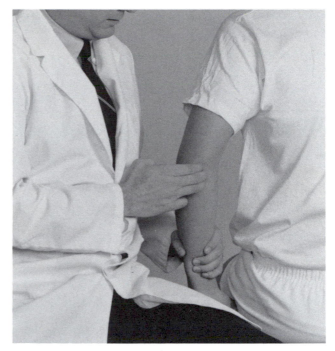

Figure 5–21. Tinel's Test at ulnar groove.

Joint and Ligamentous Tests

Varus Stress

To test the integrity of the radial collateral ligament, the clinician applies a varus stress to the elbow with the arm in a fully internally rotated

position (Fig 5–24). The test is positive if it shows signs of instability or symptom provocation.

Valgus Stress

To test the integrity of the ulnar collateral ligament, the clinician applies a valgus stress to the elbow with the arm in a fully externally rotated

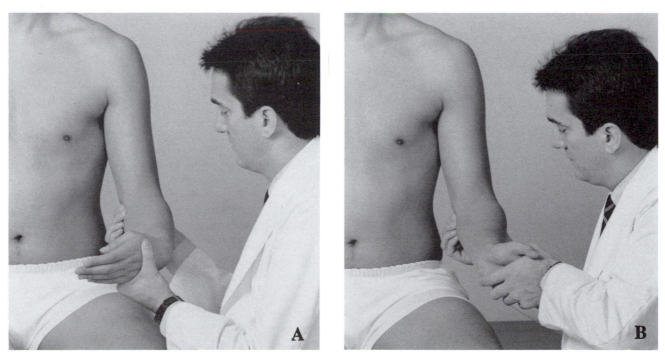

Figure 5–22. Golfer's elbow test. A) Resisting wrist flexion; B) stretching wrist flexors.

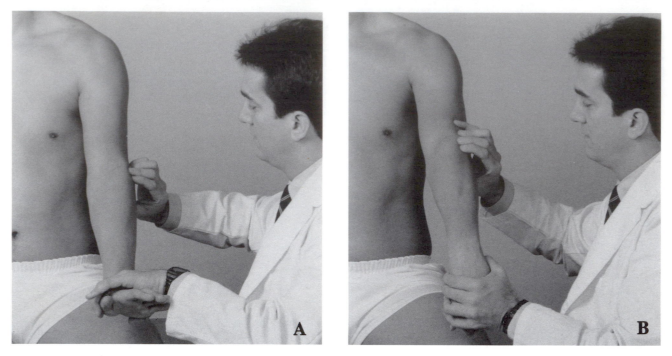

Figure 5–23. Tennis elbow test. A) Resisting wrist extension; B) stretching wrist extensors.

position (Fig 5–25). The test is positive if it shows instability or symptom provocation.

Objective Examination Summary

Many factors can contribute to the patient's complaints. The three joints of the elbow, the musculotendinous units, and the mechanical interfaces of the nerves as they enter the forearm are the areas most commonly involved. Other potential sources of elbow complaints include the shoulder, cervical spine, forearm, wrist, and hand. The initial evaluation must be geared toward screening these joints, and these potential contributors should be reconsidered during re–evaluation, especially if the patient is not benefiting from treatment.

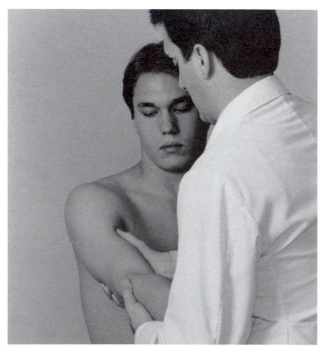

Figure 5–24. Varus stress test of the elbow.

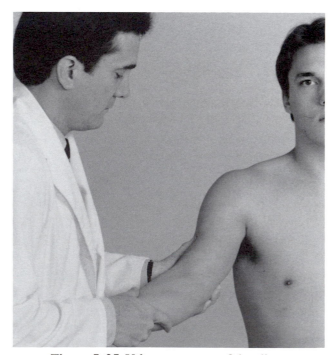

Figure 5–25. Valgus stress test of the elbow

At the conclusion of the evaluation, the clinician determines what problems the patient has and develops a problem list. The problem list helps the clinician set goals and plan treatments.

TREATMENT STRATEGIES

Elbow problems are frequently the result of overuse. Slings and braces can decrease stresses on the elbow during daily activities. Wrist braces can decrease the stresses on the muscles originating at the elbow. Night splints can eliminate stresses of certain sleep postures, such as hyperflexion at the elbow.

The goal of treatment is to teach the patient self–reliance and self–responsibility. This is particularly true for patients who have chronic elbow problems. These patients must be taught the early signs of overuse, protective mechanisms for acute injury, and basic principles of rehabilitation should minor injury recur. For example, patients who work in jobs with repetitive wrist extension and elbow flexion may be susceptible to lateral epicondylitis. Occasional breaks to stretch the wrist into flexion may help to prevent recurrence of this condition.

General treatment strategies are discussed in Chapter 3, Pathology and Treatment Principles. Chapter 11, Mobilization Techniques, and Chapter 12, Exercise, provide specific instructions for mobilization techniques, stretching, strengthening, and proprioceptive exercises for the elbow.

COMMON CLINICAL CONDITIONS

Lateral Epicondylitis

Problems with the lateral elbow are often diagnosed as lateral epicondylitis, inflammation at the origin of the wrist extensor muscles. The extensor carpi radialis brevis is usually implicated as the source of the complaints.[17] This muscle is susceptible to repetitive microtrauma, especially when the wrist is simultaneously flexed and ulnarly deviated with the forearm pronated and the elbow extended. The wrist extensors are often stressed in the backhand stroke for racquet sports, resulting in the lay term for this condition: "tennis elbow." However, many times lateral elbow symptoms arise from repetitive motions at work, where the patient performs repeated wrist motions or uses poor lifting techniques (Fig 5–26).

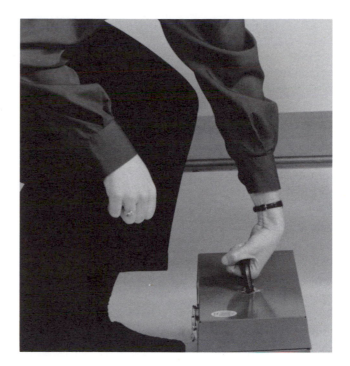

Figure 5–26. Lateral epicondylitis can be caused by lifting with the wrist flexed.

Lateral elbow pain may also arise from adverse mechanical neural tension (AMNT), a condition referred to as "radial tunnel syndrome."[6,19,20,25,27,31] The posterior interosseous branch of the radial nerve may become impinged or irritated as it passes through the supinator muscle via the radial tunnel. Another possible cause of lateral elbow pain is subluxation of the radial head from the annular ligament at the superior radioulnar joint. Careful examination is essential to differentiate between factors contributing to lateral elbow complaints.

History

Patients with lateral elbow complaints usually have a history of repetitive trauma or overuse of the wrist and forearm. The onset of symptoms is usually gradual. One specific incident can occasionally be identified, usually an unaccustomed activity such as lifting and carrying heavy loads. Other times there may be a direct blow to the lateral elbow resulting in acute symptoms. Patients with radial head subluxation usually have a history of a pull on the arm. This condition occurs most frequently in small children.

Signs and Symptoms

The primary site of symptoms is the lateral epicondyle, but some patients may also have symptoms proximal to the lateral elbow or distally in the forearm or hand. The patient complains of a dull aching pain at rest that increases with gripping, lifting, or repeated wrist and forearm movements. Some patients have no pain at rest but experience pain on these movements. Symptoms may be aggravated by sleeping with the wrist in extreme flexion, which may cause patients to complain of pain on awakening. The lateral epicondyle, radial head, and wrist extensor muscles are frequently tender to palpation. Combined passive movement into wrist and finger flexion with ulnar deviation, forearm pronation, and elbow extension provokes the symptoms. Testing the muscle strength of the wrist extensors with the fingers flexed and the wrist in increasing degrees of flexion (to increase muscle tension) will provoke the patient's symptoms. Pain may also be elicited during resisted tests of the finger extensors or the supinator muscle. Grip strength may be painful and weak, and the radial nerve bias form of the ULTT may be positive.[11]

Diagnostics

There are no standard diagnostic findings for lateral elbow pain. Radiographs can rule out radial head fractures (Fig 5–27) and may show extra space between the radius and ulna if there is a radial head subluxation. EMG is occasionally used to identify neurologic involvement (e.g., radial tunnel syndrome) when light touch and weakness are affected. Since soft tissues are most frequently involved, MRI can identify any specific anatomical pathology of the lateral elbow structures. Steroid injection at the lateral epicondyle—usually considered a treatment for lateral elbow pain—can identify the extensor muscles as the origin of the patient's complaints.

Problem List

Patients with lateral epicondylitis may present with any of the following clinical problems:

1. Tenderness to palpation at the lateral epicondyle.

2. Pain or weakness with gripping or repetitive supination.

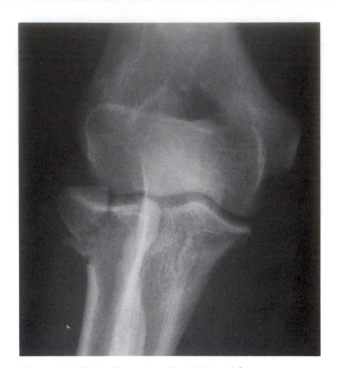

Figure 5–27. Radiograph of radial head fracture.

3. Poor wrist and elbow postures during daily activities.

4. Soft tissue tightness limiting motion into elbow extension when the wrists and fingers are flexed and ulnarly deviated.

5. Concurrent cervical or neurological symptoms in the radial nerve distribution.

Treatment

Treatment of lateral elbow pain can be challenging, especially if the condition is chronic.[17] If the symptoms are caused by radial head subluxation, surgery is usually indicated. Immobilization is the treatment of choice for simple fractures of the radial head. When the condition is caused by soft tissue problems, clinical trials have shown that early treatment is most effective.[17] Any cervical and neurological components of the injury should be treated initially.[6] Physical agents can control inflammation and relieve symptoms. The physician may choose to use steroid injections or oral anti-inflammatory medications as an adjunct to physical therapy. Friction massage to the site of a lesion in the extensor muscles should be used to stimulate healing, especially in chronic conditions.[9] Soft tissue mobilization to the lateral forearm may decrease symptoms and improve mobility.

The positions and motions that contribute to the condition should be limited by bracing as needed. Some modification of work activities is often needed to avoid repeated movements such as lifting and gripping. A wrist brace that stabilizes the joint in a neutral position facilitates the power grip position and will decrease the stress to the common extensor tendons at the lateral epicondyle. Counterforce bracing for lateral epicondylitis may help reduce symptoms and restore function (Fig 5–28).[10,28,33,38] Theoretically, these braces can decrease the forces applied to the extensor tendon or can limit the forces exerted by the muscles themselves.[10] The clinician should select any bracing based the positions and motions that aggravate the patient's condition. The brace may be used initially to decrease stresses during activity and strengthening exercises and is often gradually phased out; however, some patients may benefit from using a brace continuously to prevent injury.

After symptoms are reduced and the patient has been taught activity modification, treatment should progress to functional recovery. Exercise appears to be the most important factor in treating lateral epicondylitis. Physical agents and steroid injections are equally effective when combined with a home exercise program.[11] Flexibility exercises should be

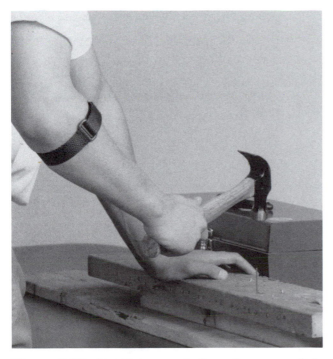

Figure 5–28. An elbow counterforce brace may help reduce symptoms and promote early return to work.

performed to improve wrist and finger flexion in ulnar deviation, with the forearm pronated and the elbow extended. Strengthening exercises should be incorporated into treatment as soon as tolerated, particularly if the patient shows weakness in the wrist extensors. The exercise program should be designed to build muscle endurance and increase tolerance to eccentric loading. Eccentric exercises improve the wrist extensor and supinator muscles' resistance to repetitive trauma;[8] therefore, exercise programs should include both eccentric and concentric exercises. When working with patients who have repetitive motion problems, exercises should be progressed cautiously to avoid aggravating the condition. Unless contraindicated, emphasis should be on high repetition–low resistance exercises using freeweights, elastic tubing, and so on. Grip strengthening exercises in the functional power grip position should be performed, increasing resistance as tolerated. Proper neck and shoulder postures should be emphasized during strengthening exercises and functional activities for all patients. Particular attention should be paid to the posture of those patients with cervical or neural tension signs.

When progressing a patient's therapy program, it is important to avoid aggravating the patient's condition. High repetition–low resistance activities often cause the initial injury, and the patient who continues to work will be subjected to these stresses at the work site. Under such circumstances, the patient's condition may be aggravated by a strengthening program that simulates the mechanism of injury; therefore, it is important to consider both the patient's strength needs and daily activities when developing an exercise program.

In addition to building strength and increasing flexibility, other means of preventing injury recurrence include checking and modifying the grip size of tools or racquets and modifying functional movement patterns at home or work. Ergonomic changes may need to be implemented. Gripping methods should also be checked and modified as needed. Braces that support the limb may also help reduce future injuries.

Medial Epicondylitis

The most common diagnosis associated with symptoms on the medial aspect of the elbow is medial epicondylitis, also known as "golfer's elbow" or "pitcher's elbow." This condition occurs far less frequently than lateral epicondylitis.[17] The symptoms arise from injury to the flexor muscle origins of the wrist and fingers. These muscles are susceptible to repeated trauma from using the wrist and finger flexors while they are simultaneously stretched into wrist extension, supination, radial deviation, and elbow extension. These stresses are common in golf and in throwing and racquet sports. They can also be found in the workplace. The wrist and finger flexors are stressed by turning tools clockwise (as when using a screwdriver) or by gripping and lifting with the forearm supinated and the wrist extended. AMNT should be considered as a potential source of symptoms at the medial elbow.[6] The above mentioned activities stretch the pronator muscle, causing pressure on the anterior interosseous branch of the median nerve.[42] The cubital tunnel and the ulnar collateral ligament may also be affected by these movements.

History

The most common mechanism of injury is repetitive motion, usually active wrist flexion and pronation from a position of wrist extension and supination with the elbow extended. Throwing sports or golf often provoke symptoms. Repeated use of hand tools such as screwdrivers or socket wrenches can also contribute to medial elbow pain. The onset of symptoms is usually gradual, but occasionally there will be a history of acute trauma (e.g., a direct blow to the medial epicondyle).

Signs and Symptoms

The site of the complaints is usually the medial epicondyle, occasionally accompanied by symptoms in the medial forearm. There is usually a dull aching pain at rest, but some patients do not experience discomfort until they begin to use the arm. Pain is provoked with gripping, lifting, and repeated wrist and forearm movements. Leaning on a desk, an armrest, or a workbench may aggravate symptoms. Most patients are tender to palpation of the medial epicondyle at the origin of the common flexor tendon. Some are tender in the muscle bellies of the wrist flexors and the pronators. Passive stretch into wrist and finger extension with the combination of radial deviation, supination of the forearm, and elbow

extension will aggravate the patient's symptoms. Pain may be provoked with resisted isometric wrist flexion and the combination of ulnar deviation, elbow extension, and forearm supination. Resisted pronation of the forearm with the elbow in extension may also aggravate symptoms. There will occasionally be pain during resisted finger flexion with the wrist and elbow extended. Grip strength may be weak and painful. The ULTT with a median or ulnar nerve bias may reproduce symptoms and may refer pain into the medial forearm and the hand (see Chapter 2, Principles of Extremity Evaluation).

Diagnostics

There are no definitive diagnostic findings for medial elbow pain. Radiographs will occasionally show calcification of the flexor aponeurosis.[1] If there is a history of acute trauma to the joint a radiograph may be used to rule out fracture of the medial epicondyle. If there are neurological signs of weakness and numbness in the medial or ulnar nerve distributions, EMG may be used to confirm nerve involvement. MRI can identify a specific anatomical pathology at the elbow. Although usually considered a treatment, steroid injection into the medial epicondyle can diagnose common flexor muscle origins of the patient's complaints.

Problem List

Patients with medial epicondylitis may present with any of the following problems:

1. Tenderness to palpation at the medial epicondyle.

2. Pain or weakness with gripping or repeated pronation.

3. Poor wrist and elbow postures during daily activities.

4. Tightness on stretching into wrist and finger extension.

5. Concurrent cervical or neurological symptoms in the median or ulnar nerve distribution.

Treatment

Treatment for medial epicondylitis is essentially the same as for lateral epicondylitis except location of treatment differs. Treatments may include physical agents or anti–inflammatory drug therapy to control symptoms initially. Splints, braces, or slings can reduce the stresses on the joint. Modification of daily activities may be necessary to allow healing. Flexibility exercises will help improve the pain free range at the wrist and fingers. Progressive high repetition–low load strengthening exercises should be introduced as tolerated, bearing in mind the patient's daily activities and the factors that caused the condition. The strengthening program should include eccentric exercises to improve the flexor mechanism's ability to withstand repetitive trauma. Grip strengthening in the power grip position should progress from low to high resistance as tolerated. If the patient continues to work under conditions that predispose epicondylitis, the strengthening program must not aggravate the patient's condition. Throughout the treatment progression, patient education should be incorporated to ensure modification of pertinent activities and correct shoulder and cervical positioning for exercise and work. It may be necessary to adjust the grip size of sport equipment or hand tools or make ergonomic changes to prevent recurrence of the injury.

Medial Collateral Ligament (MCL) Sprain

Injury to the ligaments of the elbow complex can be caused by a direct blow, elbow dislocation, or overuse. The ulnar collateral ligament is most commonly injured, especially in athletes who participate in throwing sports.[12] The throwing motion causes distractive forces at the medial elbow and stresses the ligament. With repeated throwing, the medial collateral ligament (MCL) may gradually become more lax, allowing compression of the lateral elbow at the radiohumeral joint. Increased lateral compression can cause articular cartilage changes of the radial head and eventual formation of loose bodies within the elbow joint.[12] Injury to the MCL with medial elbow muscle hypertrophy is common in the adolescent throwing athlete and is referred to as "little league elbow."

History

MCL sprain in the worker or the throwing athlete usually has a gradual onset after repetitive movements; however, some patients have a sudden onset of symptoms after a direct blow or a fall on the elbow with a valgus stress.

Signs and Symptoms

The chief complaint is progressive medial elbow pain and edema that usually improves with rest. The patient may have difficulty extending the arm and may show apprehension when throwing or when putting weight on the elbow by leaning on the outstretched arm. In more chronic cases, there may also be problems with lateral elbow pain, which could be caused by MCL laxity and increased lateral compression. Palpation may show tenderness over the medial epicondyle and, less frequently, over the wrist flexor tendons. Elbow extension may be limited and painful with overpressure. Passive wrist and finger extension will usually be painful. Resisted wrist and finger flexion may also cause pain due to the close anatomical relationship between the MCL and the wrist and finger flexor muscles. Stress testing the ligament with a valgus load may show increased ligamentous laxity when compared to the contralateral side and may provoke symptoms.

Diagnostics

Radiographs may show calcification at the proximal attachment of the ligament in adult patients. In adolescents there may be varying degrees of epiphyseal widening, possibly with a displaced fracture of the medial epicondyle. Additional radiographic changes such as fracture or dislocation may be present in patients who have suffered a direct blow to the joint or a fall on the elbow. If surgery is being considered, MRI can assess ligamentous integrity and determine viability of surgical repair. The ulnar nerve is occasionally affected in patients with MCL sprain. If neurological signs are present, an EMG may be used to identify nerve damage.

Problem List

Patients with an MCL sprain at the elbow may have any of the following problems:

1. Medial instability with valgus stress at the elbow

2. Swelling over the medial aspect of the elbow

3. Pain on palpation of the MCL attachments

4. Decreased functional activities (throwing, pushing, racquet sports, etc.) with pain

Treatment

Conservative management of MCL sprains is usually successful, except in cases of moderate to severe instability or functional limitations. Resting the joint by avoiding stressful activities is recommended. Immobilization is indicated if radiographs show evidence of osteochondritis dissecans of the capitulum. Immobilization can also be used after surgery to repair or reconstruct ligaments or if the patient has severe symptoms. Physical agents can be used as needed to decrease pain and inflammation. A progressive exercise program should be initiated with the goal of restoring full pain free mobility and normal strength of the hand, wrist, and elbow. A high repetition–low load strengthening program should be initiated as tolerated. Proprioception exercises will help treatment progression and prevention of injury recurrence. Functional progression to throwing and other activities should be introduced gradually while avoiding symptom recurrence. Athletes in contact sports may benefit from preventive taping or bracing upon return to sport. Throwing mechanics or work postures that exacerbate the problem may need to be modified.

Surgical repair of the ligament is usually the first option in cases of acute instability; however, if the ligament is not viable at the time of surgery, reconstruction using autogenous grafts (e.g., the palmaris longus tendon) may be attempted. The clinician should work closely with the surgeon to determine the most appropriate progression for rehabilitation based on the specific procedure performed and the healing constraints. Harrelson outlines a common protocol for treatment of the post-operative ulnar collateral ligament instability patient.[12]

Cubital Tunnel Syndrome

The cubital tunnel is formed by the ulnar collateral ligament and the arcuate ligament (the tendon expansion of the flexor carpi ulnaris muscle) after the ulnar nerve passes through the ulnar groove of the medial humeral epicondyle (Fig 5–6). Elbow flexion places tension on the ulnar nerve,[6] and the nerve is compressed within the tunnel by the arcuate ligament when the joint is flexed past 90°.[35,36] The ulnar nerve can be injured by direct trauma; ligament laxity; hyperflexed elbow posturing; compression from muscular hypertrophy; recurrent subluxation or dislocation of the nerve out of the ulnar groove; or from restriction of the nerve by adhesions in the cubital tunnel.[12,35,36,39,40,41] Ulnar nerve injury occurs commonly in the throwing athlete and in manual laborers. Prolonged postures that place pressure on the nerve, such as leaning on a workbench or desk, could lead to problems. Repeated use of tools leading to forearm muscle hypertrophy may cause intermittent nerve compression.

History

The onset of symptoms is usually gradual, aggravated by activity and relieved by rest. The symptoms often become more severe if overuse continues. Patients may report such predisposing activities as throwing; racquet sports; repeated tool use with gripping and supination–pronation; or leaning on a desk or workbench.

Signs and Symptoms

Symptoms are felt at the medial elbow and may be referred to the forearm and hand. Less commonly, symptoms are felt proximal to the ulnar groove. There may be a dull ache at rest or after activity. In more advanced stages, symptoms include tingling in the fourth and fifth digits, decreased light touch sensation, and weakness in the ulnar nerve distribution. Sleeping with the elbow hyperflexed will provoke symptoms on waking. Complaints of crepitus or popping at the cubital tunnel with flexion–extension movements are common in patients with a subluxing ulnar nerve. Palpation during active flexion–extension may reveal subluxation. Patients with intermittent compression due to muscle hypertrophy may complain of muscle cramping sensations. Palpation of the cubital tunnel may cause tenderness, which may spread into the flexor carpi ulnaris muscle. There will be a positive Tinel's sign at the tunnel, indicting the ulnar nerve. Elbow hyperflexion will elicit symptoms, and the ULTT for an ulnar nerve bias will be positive (see Chapter 2, Principles of Extremity Evaluation).[6] Light touch sensation and MMT should be used to rule out true ulnar nerve damage. Cubital tunnel syndrome can mimic thoracic outlet syndrome (TOS); therefore, tests for TOS should be included in a thorough examination (see Chapter 4, The Shoulder).

Diagnostics

EMG can confirm involvement of the ulnar nerve and the site of entrapment. Radiographs are not usually necessary. If surgical transposition of the nerve is being considered, MRI can identify specific anatomic involvement at the tunnel (Fig 5–29).

Problem List

Common problems associated with Cubital Tunnel Syndrome include:

1. Pain at medial elbow with repetitive daily activities

2. Subluxing ulnar nerve with elbow flexion and extension

3. Muscle weakness in C8–T1 distribution

4. Concurrent cervical or thoracic outlet symptoms

5. Decreased functional ability due to pain or weakness

Treatment

Conservative management of this condition is challenging. Initial treatment consists of symptom relief with physical agents and rest from aggravating postures and movements. If necessary, night splints can be used to prevent elbow hyperflexion. Exercises to increase flexibility of the forearm muscles, especially the wrist and finger flexors, should be introduced as tolerated. Functional activities should be introduced slowly. Strengthening exercises can be used as needed as long as wrist and finger flexors hypertrophy is avoided and symptoms are not increased. The clinician should consider concurrent treatment of cervical and neural tension components if TOS elements are suspected. Neck, upper back, and shoulder girdle postures should be considered throughout the rehabilitation process. The physician may include anti–inflammatory medications to help control symptoms and aid healing. Surgical transposition of the ulnar nerve is used in severe cases

in which conservative treatment has failed. After surgery, the clinician should work closely with the surgeon to establish the rehabilitation progression. Any rehabilitation protocol should address the prevention of post–surgical scarring or adhesions that can cause re–impingement of the nerve.[21] Early mobility of the elbow and the ulnar nerve in the ulnar groove and cubital tunnel is an essential follow–up to surgery.

Elbow Contracture

A patient with a chief complaint of loss of elbow range of motion is often referred for physical therapy. Loss of mobility is a common complication of elbow dislocation; supracondylar humeral or radial head fractures; moderate to severe contusions; and osteochondritis dissecans. Other related injuries of the arm or forearm that cause prolonged immobilization can also lead to elbow stiffness. The elbow complex is susceptible to flexion contractures, and early mobilization after injury is necessary to prevent loss of range. Immobilization longer than two weeks after surgery or injury can affect the long–term outcome.[21] The cause of restricted motion—whether capsular, bony, or soft tissue—must be determined to

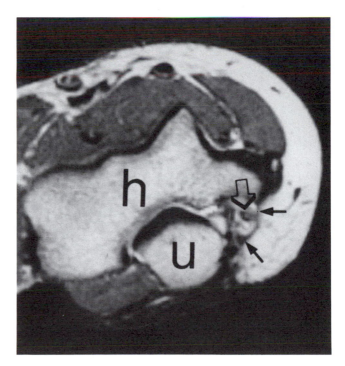

Figure 5–29. MRI showing normal cubital tunnel. Small arrows indicate the cubital tunnel; "H" is the humerus; "U" is the ulna; and the open arrow indicates the ulnar nerve.

form an appropriate treatment plan. Although the primary goal is to regain full range of motion, functional movements in daily activities can occur in a range of motion slightly less than the full range.[37]

History

The clinician should note onset date, and surgical and immobilization history. Onset is usually an acute trauma, but stiffness may occur in post–traumatic arthritis.

Signs and Symptoms

The patient's chief complaint will be restricted use of the elbow because of decreased range of motion. Pain may limit the patient's self–stretching attempts; if pain occurs before the limit of range, there may be inflammation provoking the symptoms. Specific functional motion limitations should be noted and reassessed frequently to determine treatment effectiveness. There may be muscle weakness caused by disuse during immobilization. Neurological symptoms may be present since restricted movement for prolonged periods can affect nerve tissue mobility. The patient may have decreased joint play in a capsular pattern (see Chapter 11, Mobilization Techniques).

Diagnostics

Diagnostic tests are usually of little value in determining treatment for elbow contracture. Radiographs may reveal bony growths or malalignments that cause the motion restriction. Since joint contracture is most commonly caused by immobilization, radiographs, MRI's, or EMG's taken when the initial injury occurred should be reviewed to determine if any additional pathologies are causing the motion restriction.

Problem List

Common problems include:

1. Pain with stretch and with activity
2. Decreased joint play
3. Decreased function
4. Decreased soft tissue mobility
5. Muscle atrophy

Treatment

Symptom relief measures such as physical agents or anti–inflammatory drugs should be used throughout the rehabilitation process to prevent inflammation. Inflammation will increase symptoms, prevent motion gains and possibly cause motion loss.

When capsular tightness is the limiting factor, joint mobilization techniques performed at end range will probably provide the greatest gains in range of motion. Joint mobilization should be followed by low intensity–long duration stretches of physiological motions. High intensity–short duration stretches are contraindicated at the elbow because they may stimulate ossification in traumatic myositis ossificans, cause motion loss, increase pain, and ultimately worsen the patient's condition.[12,13,23,26] Heat can be used to increase the connective tissue extensibility before stretching or joint mobilization. Dynamic elbow splints can be used to provide a low–load, prolonged stretch.[13] Wall push–ups, biking, upper body ergometers, and other closed kinematic chain exercises can be used for functional strengthening. It is important to set reasonable and attainable goals to motivate the patient and prevent discouragement if progress is slow.

SUMMARY

The integrated approach to problems at the elbow complex has been presented. The elbow's three joints and four muscle groups function synergistically, and are influenced by the shoulder proximally and the wrist and hand distally. Symptoms felt at the elbow may be referred from the cervical spine, shoulder, wrist or hand. Patients with elbow problems cannot be assumed to have isolated problems from acute trauma. Often elbow symptoms are caused by repetitive trauma and arise from complex interactions with other joints in the upper limb and cervical spine. Effective elbow management includes consideration of related neuromusculoskeletal structures in an appropriate, functional manner.

Refer to Chapter 11, Mobilization Techniques, Chapter 12, Exercise, and Chapter 13, Prevention of Extremity Injuries, for expanded information on joint mobilization techniques; flexibility; strengthening; proprioceptive exercises; and prevention of elbow problems.

REFERENCES

1. Advisory Panel on Standard Nomenclature of Athletic Injuries. American Medical Association: Standard Nomenclature of Athletic Injuries, 1976.

2. Basmajian J, Griffin W: Function of the Aconeous Muscle: An EMG Study. JBJS 54:1712-1714, 1972.

3. Basmajian J, Latif A: Integrated Actions and Functions of the Chief Flexors of the Elbow: A Detailed EMG Analysis. JBJS 39:1106-1118, 1957.

4. Basset FH, Numley HA: Comparison of the Musculocutaneous Nerve at the Elbow. JBJS 64A: 1050, 1982

5. Boissonnault W, Janos S: Screening For Medical Disease: Physical Therapy Assessment and Treatment Principles. Examination in Physical Therapy Practice: Screening For Medical Disease. Churchill-Livingstone, New York NY 1991.

6. Butler D: Mobilisation of the Nervous System. Churchill-Livingstone, Melbourne Australia 1991.

7. Chao E, Morrey B: Three Dimensional Rotation of the Elbow. Joul of Biomechanics 11:57-73, 1978.

8. Curwin S, Standish WD: Tendinitis: Its Etiology and Treatment. Collamire Pren. Lexington MA 1984.

9. Cyriax J, Coldham M: Treatment By Management, Manipulation, and Injection. Textbook of Orthopaedic Medicine. Volume 2, 11th ed. Bailliere-Tindall, London England 1984.

10. Groppel JL, Nirschl PP: A Mechanical and EMG Analysis of the Effects of Various Joint Counterforce Braces on the Tennis Player. AM J Sports Med 14(3):195-200, 1986.

11. Halle JS, Franklin RJ and Karalfa BL: Comparison of Four Treatment Approaches for Lateral Epicondylitis of the Elbow. JOSPT 8(2):62-68, 1986.

12. Harrelson GL: Shoulder Rehabilitation. Physical Rehabilitation of the Injured Athlete. JR Andrews and GL Harrelson, ed. WB Saunders, Philadelphia PA 1991.

13. Hepburn GR, Crivelli RJ: Use of Elbow Dynasplint for Reduction of Elbow Flexion Contractures: A Case Study. JOSPT 8(2)62-68, 1984.

14. Hollinshead WH: Anatomy For Surgeons. The Back and Limbs, Vol 3, 2nd ed. Harper and Row, New York NY 1982.

15. Jobe FW, Fanton GS: Nerve Injuries. The Elbow and its Disorders. BF Morrey, ed. WB Saunders, Philadelphia PA 1985.

16. Kapanji I: The Physiology of the Joints, 5th ed. Churchill-Livingstone, New York NY 1982.

17. Leach RE, Miller JK: Lateral and Medial Epicondylitis of the Elbow. Clin Sports Med 6(2):259-272, 1987.

18. Lehmkuhl L, Smith L: Brunnstrom's Clinical Kinesiology, 5th ed. FA Davis, Philadelphia PA 1983.

19. Lister GD, Belsole RB, Kleinert HE: The Radial Tunnel Syndrome. Journal of Hand Surgery 4A:52-60, 1979.

20. Lundborg G, Dahlin LB: Pathophysiology of Nerve Compression. Nerve Compression Syndromes. RM Szabo, ed. Slack, Thorofare, London 1989.

21. Melhoff TL, Noble PC, Bennett JB, and Tullos HS: Simple Dislocation of the Elbow in the Adult. JBJS 70:244-249, 1988.

22. Morrey BF: Anatomy and Kinematics of the Elbow. American Academy of Orthopaedic Surgeons Instructional Course Lectures XL. HS Tullos, ed. CV Mosby, St. Louis MO 1991.

23. O'Donoghue DF: Treatment of Injuries to Athlete, 2nd ed. WB Saunders, Philadelphia PA 1970.

24. Palmer M, Epler M: Clinical Assessment Procedures in Physical Therapy. JB Lippincott Co, Philadelphia PA 1990.

25. Peimer CA, Wheeler DR: Radial Tunnel Syndrome/ Posterior Interoseus Nerve Compression. Nerve Compression Syndromes. RM Szabo, ed. Slack, Thorofare, London 1989.

26. Raney RB, Brasher HR: Shand's Handbook of Orthopaedic Surgery. CV Mosby, St. Louis MO 1971.

27. Roles NC, Maudsley R: Radial Tunnel Syndrome: Resistant Tennis Elbow as a Nerve Entrapment. JBJS 54B:449-508, 1972.

28. Snyder-Mackler L, Epler M: Effect of Standard and Aircast Tennis Elbow Hands on Integrated EMG of Forearm Extensor Musculative Proximal to the Hands. AM J of Sports Med 17(2):278-281, 1989.

29. Soderberg G: Kinesiology - Application to Pathological Motion. William and Wilkins, Baltimore MD 1986.

30. Spinner M, Kaplan EB: The Relationship of the Ulnar Nerve to the Medial Intermuscular Septum and Its Clinical Significance. Hand 8:239-246, 1976.

31. Spinner M, Linshied RL: Nerve Entrapment Syndromes. The Elbow and its Disorders. BF Morrey, ed. WB Saunders, Philadelphia PA 1985.

32. Spinner M, Spencer PS: Nerve Compression Lesions of the Upper Extremity: A Clinical and Experimental Review. Clin Orthop and Rel Res 104:46, 1974.

33. Stonecipher DR, Catlin PA: The Effect of a Forearm Strap on Wrist Extension Strength. JOSPT 6(3):184-189, 1984.

34. Stroyan M, Wilk K: The Functional Anatomy of the Elbow Complex. JOSPT 17(6):279-288, 1993.

35. Tullos HS, Bryan WJ: Examination of the Throwing Elbow. Injuries to the Throwing Athlete. B Zarins,

JR Andrews and WG Carson, ed. WB Saunders, Philadelphia PA 1985.

36. Vanderpool DW, et al: Peripheral Compression Lesion of the Ulnar Nerve. JBJS 50:792-803, 1968.

37. Volz R, Morrey B: The Physical Examination of the Elbow. The Elbow and its Disorders. B Morrey, ed. WB Saunders, Philadelphia PA 1985.

38. Wadsworth CT, Nelson DH, Burns LT, et al: Effect of the Counterforce Armband on Wrist Extension and Grip Strength and Pain in Subjects With Tennis Elbow. JOSPT 11(5):192-197, 1989.

39. Wadsworth TG: Entrapment Neuropathy in the Upper Limb. Operative Surgery, The Hand. R Birch and R Brook, ed. Butterworth, London England 1984.

40. Wadsworth TG: The External Compression Syndrome of the Ulnar Nerve at the Cubital Tunnel. Clin Orthop 124:189-204, 1977.

41. Wadsworth, TG: The Cubital Tunnel Syndrome. Elbow Joint. D Kashiwagi, ed. Elsevier Science Publishers, Amsterdam 1985.

42. Wiens E, Lane S: The Anterior Interosseus Nerve Syndrome. Can J Surg 21:354, 1978.

43. Youm Y, Dryer R, et al: Biomechanical Analyses of Forearm Pronation-Supination and Elbow Flexion-Extension. Joul of Biomechanics 12:245-255, 1979.

CHAPTER 6

THE WRIST AND HAND

INTRODUCTION

The forearm, wrist, and hand provide a large variety of functional movements unique to humans.[61] These movements range from fine motor control (such as threading a needle) to gross motor control (such as turning a doorknob).

The forearm, wrist, and hand function together, and the position of each influences the capabilities of the others. For example, consider the power grip position of the wrist. Its slight extension increases tension in the finger flexors, facilitating flexion of the interphalangeal (IP) joints.

A large part of the central nervous system is devoted to control of the hand,[61] reflecting its importance in functional activities. The wrist and hand are rich in neurovascular supply and contain intricate mechanical relationships. Consequently, injury to the wrist and hand can be devastating to function.

Symptoms felt at the forearm, wrist, and hand may be referred from the shoulder, elbow, and cervical spine. Effective problem management in the distal extremity joints must include consideration of the related neuromusculoskeletal structures.

FUNCTIONAL ANATOMY

Osseous and Capsuloligamentous Components

The wrist, hand, and fingers are made up of 29 bones and 31 joints (Fig 6–1). Although wrist, hand, and fingers will be discussed separately, they function together to carry out the vast number of movements and functions available. Special consideration should be given to the thumb, which contributes up to 40% of the hand's function.[61,66]

The bony structures of the wrist and hand form three arches. These arches support the hand for strength and allow the hand to cup for prehension. The three arches are 1) the longitudinal arch; 2) the metacarpal phalangeal transverse arch; and 3) the carpal transverse arch (Fig 6–2).

Wrist

The wrist is composed of a) the distal radioulnar joint; b) the radiocarpal joint; c) the intercarpal joints; and d) the mid carpal joints. The carpal tunnel, a common site of pathology, is formed by wrist bones and ligaments. The main ligaments of the wrist are shown in Figure 6–3.

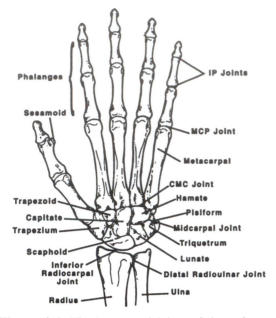

Figure 6–1. The bones and joints of the wrist and hand (right hand, posterior view).

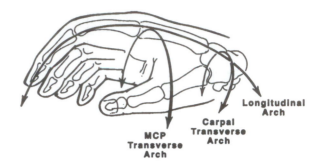

Figure 6–2. The arches of the hand.

joint is frequently limited after injury to the mid or distal forearm.

Distal Radioulnar Joint

The distal radioulnar joint is a uniaxial pivot joint between the distal portions of the radius and ulna. It is a synovial joint and is important in supination and pronation. These motions occur as the radius moves over a relatively stationary ulna: the ulna moves slightly proximally and laterally during pronation; and distally and medially during supination. The distal radioulnar joint contributes to ≈15° of supination and ≈15° of pronation. Movement at this

Radiocarpal Joint

The radiocarpal joint is a biaxial ellipsoid joint between the radius and the scaphoid and lunate carpal bones. The joint is stabilized medially by the radial collateral ligament. The radiocarpal joint contains a triangular–shaped disc located at the ulnar side of the distal radius. It attaches to the ulna at the base of the ulnar styloid process. This disc articulates with the lunate and triquetrum carpal bones. It adds stability to the wrist by connecting the carpal bones to the ulna and by securing the distal ends of the ulna and radius. The disc is also a shock absorber, cushioning forces transmitted across the wrist. When intact, the load bearing ratio between the radius and the ulna is 60:40. If the disc is removed, the ratio becomes 95:5.[53]

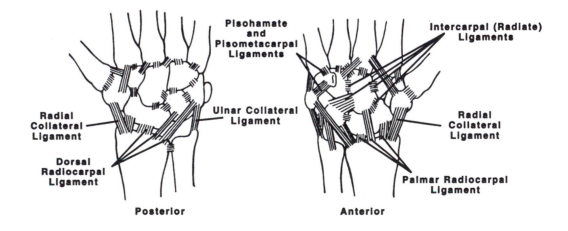

Figure 6–3. Wrist ligaments (right hand).

This joint and disc are commonly injured in a forced extension trauma such as attempting to break a fall on an outstretched arm. The motions available at the radiocarpal joint are wrist flexion, extension, ulnar deviation, radial deviation, and circumduction.

Intercarpal Joints

The intercarpal joints are formed between the individual bones in the proximal row of carpal bones: scaphoid, lunate, triquetrum; and in the distal row: trapezium, trapezoid, capitate, hamate. These joints allow only a small amount of gliding motion and are held together by the dorsal, palmar, and interosseous intercarpal ligaments. Simultaneous movements must occur at multiple intercarpal joints to achieve normal function.[33] A special joint exists between the pisiform and triquetrum bones. The pisiform rests on the triquetrum but does not participate in intercarpal motion.

The intercarpal joints can be the site of restricted motion after a period of immobilization. The intercarpal ligaments are commonly sprained in acute trauma.

Mid Carpal Joints

The mid carpal joints are formed between the proximal and distal rows of the carpal bones, excluding the pisiform. There are two functional joints. *Medially,* the scaphoid, lunate, and triquetrum in the proximal row articulate with the capitate and hamate in the distal row. *Laterally,* the scaphoid in the proximal row articulates with the trapezoid and trapezium in the distal row. Both of these compound joints act like sellar joints, allowing much greater mobility than the intercarpal joints. The mid carpal joints are stabilized by the dorsal and palmar ligaments.

The center of rotation for the wrist during flexion/extension and radial/ulnar deviation is approximately at the base of the capitate (Fig 6–4).[72] The scaphoid functions with the distal row of carpal bones during extension and with the proximal row during flexion.[60] Wrist extension occurs predominantly at the radiocarpal joint. Wrist flexion occurs primarily at the mid carpal joint.

Fracture or ligamentous injury of the mid carpal joints can cause many problems in functional wrist motion. Instability can lead to pain and dysfunction in daily activities. Carpal bone fractures are notorious for poor healing and occasionally result in avascular necrosis.

Carpal Tunnel

The carpal tunnel is a common site of neural entrapment. The carpal tunnel has the following anatomical boundaries in the wrist.[48]

1. Roof (volar surface): transverse carpal ligament.

2. Floor (dorsal surface): volar radiocarpal ligament and volar intercarpal ligament expansions. The carpal bones form a concave arch. These bones are (lateral to medial): scaphoid, lunate, triquetrum, and pisiform.

3. Medial wall (ulnar surface): pisiform and the hook of the hamate.

4. Lateral wall (radial surface): tuberosity of scaphoid and tubercle of trapezium.

Nine flexor tendons and the median nerve pass through this tunnel.

Hand

The hand includes the junction of the wrist and fingers at the carpometacarpal (CMC) joints; the intermetacarpal joints; the metacarpophalangeal (MCP) joints; and the proximal and distal (PIP and DIP) joints of the fingers.

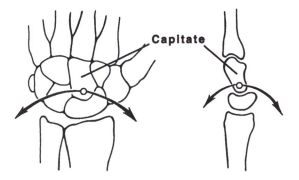

Figure 6–4. The center of rotation of the wrist is the base of the capitate (left hand, posterior and lateral views).

Carpometacarpal (CMC) Joints

The CMC joints lie between the distal row of carpal bones and the metacarpal bones of the hand. The second through fourth joints are plane synovial joints supported by dorsal, palmar, and interosseous ligaments. Gliding is the only movement allowed at these joints. The fifth CMC joint resembles a saddle-shape joint, but it has less mobility than true sellar joints.[59] The thumb has a sellar CMC joint. It is supported by dorsal and palmar ligaments and a lateral ligament that runs from the radial side of the first metacarpal to the lateral side of the trapezium. All CMC joints are susceptible to sprains.

The shape of the first CMC joint lets the thumb be placed in a variety of positions; however, this wide range of positions and stresses in daily activities predisposes this joint to degenerative arthritis. The planar motions available to the CMC joint include palmar abduction and adduction, radial abduction and adduction, opposition and retroposition.[2] Retroposition can be considered the opposite of opposition (Fig 6–5). The motions of the thumb are illustrated in the "Passive Mobility" section of this chapter.

Intermetacarpal Joints

The intermetacarpal joints are the joints formed between the second through fourth metacarpal bones. They are plane joints held together by dorsal, palmar, and interosseous ligaments. A small amount of gliding motion occurs between the bones, providing for hand flexibility when the thumb opposes the palm in gripping. The ligamentous support stabilizes the transverse arch of the hand while allowing flexibility. Receiving a firm handshake with a limp hand will quickly remind of the play between these joints.

Metacarpophalangeal (MCP) Joints

The MCP joints are formed between the distal end of the metacarpal bones and the proximal end of the proximal phalanx. These are condyloid joints supported by palmar, transverse, and collateral ligaments (Fig 6–6). The available motions at the second through fifth MCP are flexion–extension, and abduction–adduction. The first MCP has only flexion–extension available. Due to the shape of the head of the metacarpals, the collateral ligaments become tight on flexion.[24,61] The amount of abduction–adduction is greatest in neutral. The ligamentous restraints allow more radial and ulnar deviation when the fingers are in extension than when

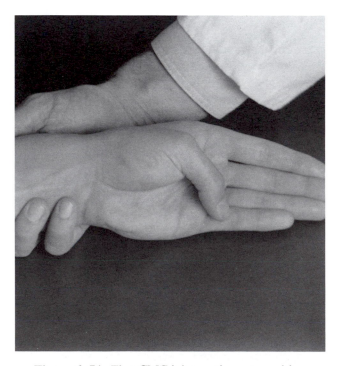

Figure 6–5A. First CMC joint motions: opposition.

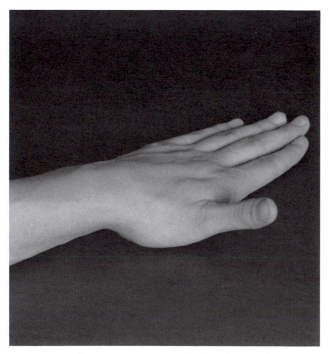

Figure 6–5B. First CMC joint motions: retroposition.

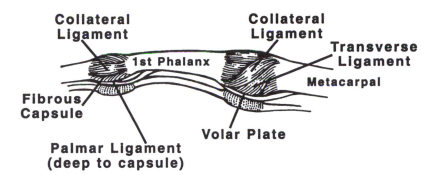

Figure 6–6. MCP and IP ligaments.

in flexion.[71] The first MCP joint can rotate, augmenting the function of the first CMC joint. Injuries to the MCP joints are common, ranging from fractures and dislocations to simple sprains.

Interphalangeal (IP) Joints

There are two IP joints in each finger, except for the thumb, which only has one IP joint. These joints are the proximal interphalangeal joint (PIP) and the distal interphalangeal joint (DIP). The PIP lies between the proximal phalanx and middle phalanx of the fingers. The DIP lies between the middle and distal phalanx. They are uniaxial hinge joints that allow flexion and extension. They are stabilized by palmar and collateral ligaments and a fibrous capsule (Fig 6–6). Unlike the collateral ligaments at the MCP joints, the IP collateral ligaments do not become tight on flexion. The proximal ends of the proximal phalanxes are unequal in length; thus, as the fingers flex, there is an oblique motion toward the thumb that maximizes the gripping function of the hand.[27]

The IP joints are commonly injured in daily activities, ranging from the occasional "jammed" or sprained finger to volar plate injuries.

Table 6–1 summarizes the movements and range of motion available at the forearm, wrist, and hand.

Neuromuscular Components

Muscular Structures

Many of the muscles that act on the forearm, wrist, and hand cross several joints. The muscles of

this region are shown in Figure 6–7. Table 6–2 summarizes their actions and peripheral and segmental nerve innervations. The muscles will be discussed here according to their functions at the wrist

Table 6–1. Movements and Range of Motion at the Forearm, Wrist, and Hand

Forearm	Pronation	80-90°
	Supination	90°
Wrist	Flexion	80-90°
	Extension	70-90°
	Ulnar Deviation	30-45°
	Radial Deviation	15-20°
Fingers	MCP Flexion	85-90°
	MCP Extension	30-45°
	MCP Abduction	20-30°
	MCP Adduction	0°
	PIP Flexion	100-115°
	PIP Extension	0°
	DIP Flexion	80-90°
	DIP Extension	20°
Thumb - 1st digit	MCP Flexion	50-55°
	MCP Extension	0°
	IP Flexion	85-90°
	IP Extension	0-5°
	CMC Palmar Abduction	70°
	CMC Radial Abduction	50°
	CMC Adduction	30°

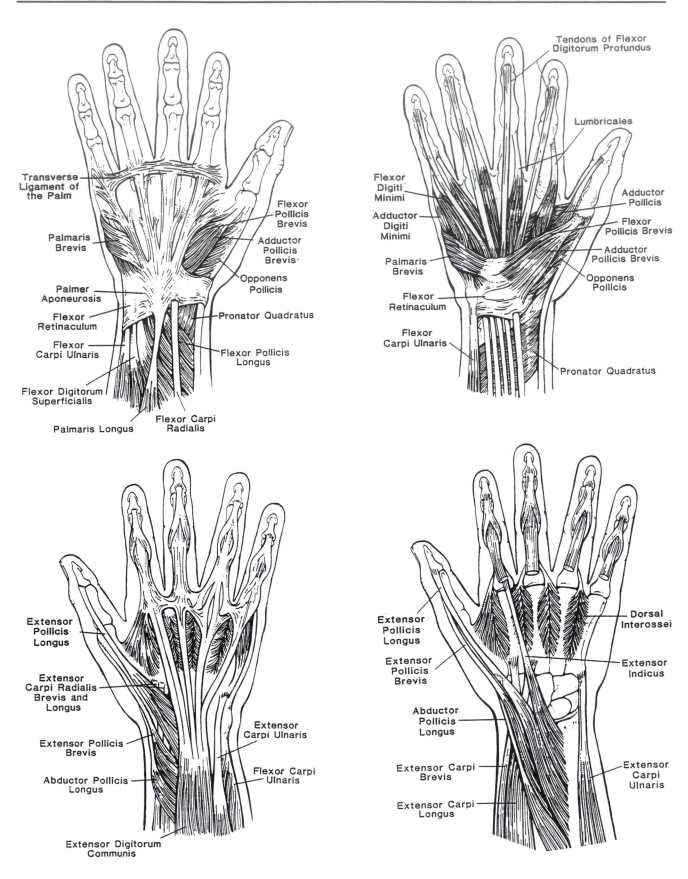

Figure 6-7. Muscles of the wrist and hand. Top: anterior view; bottom: posterior view.

Table 6–2. Wrist and Hand Muscles, Actions and Innervations

Muscles	Actions	Peripheral Nerve Supply	Spinal Segment
Supinator	Supination	Posterior interosseous (radial)	C5, C6
Biceps	Supination	Musculocutaneous	C5, C6
Pronator quadratus	Pronation	Anterior interosseous	C8, T1
Pronator teres	Pronation	Median	C6, C7
Flexor carpi radialis	Pronation	Median	C6, C7
Extensor carpi radialis longus	Wrist extension, radial deviation	Radial	C6, C7
Extensor carpi radialis brevis	Wrist extension	Posterior interosseous (radial)	C7, C8
Extensor carpi ulnaris	Wrist extension, ulnar deviation	Posterior interosseous (radial)	C7, C8
Flexor carpi radialis	Wrist flexion, radial deviation	Median	C6, C7
Flexor carpi ulnaris	Wrist flexion, ulnar deviation	Ulnar	C7, C8
Abductor pollicis longus	Wrist radial deviation	Posterior interosseous (radial)	C7, C8
Extensor pollicis brevis	Wrist radial deviation	Posterior interosseous (radial)	C7, C8
Extensor digitorum communis	Finger extension	Posterior interosseous (radial)	C7, C8
Extensor indices	Index finger extension	Posterior interosseous (radial)	C7, C8
Extensor digiti minimi	5th finger extension	Posterior interosseous (radial)	C7, C8
Flexor digitorum profundus	Finger flexion	Anterior interosseous (median)	C8, T1
Flexor digitorum superficialis	Finger flexion	Median	C7, C8, T1
Lumbricals	Finger flexion	1st-2nd, Median; 3rd-4th, Ulnar	C8, T1
Dorsal interossei	Finger flexion, abduction	Ulnar	C8, T1
Flexor digiti minimi	5th finger flexion	Ulnar	C8, T1
Palmar interossei	Finger flexion, adduction	Ulnar	C8, T1
Abductor digiti minimi	5th finger abduction	Ulnar	C8, T1
Extensor pollicis longus	Thumb extension/retroposition	Posterior interosseous (radial)	C7, C8
Extensor pollicis brevis	Thumb extension/retroposition, radial abduction	Posterior interosseous (radial)	C7, C8
Abductor pollicis longus	Thumb radial abduction	Posterior interosseous (radial)	C7, C8
Flexor pollicis brevis	Thumb flexion, opposition	Superficial head, median; Deep head, ulnar	C8, T1
Flexor pollicis longus	Thumb flexion	Anterior interosseous (median)	C8, T1
Opponens pollicis	Thumb flexion/opposition	Median	C8, T1
Abductor pollicis longus	Thumb palmar abduction	Posterior interosseous (radial)	C7, C8
Abductor pollicis brevis	Thumb palmar abduction, opposition	Median	C8, T1
Adductor pollicis	Thumb palmar and radial abduction	Ulnar	C8, T1
Opponens digiti minimi	5th finger opposition	Ulnar	C8, T1

and hand. Muscles that control forearm movements are discussed in Chapter 5, The Elbow.

Wrist

Effective hand function is dependent on positioning the wrist in slight extension.[61] Normally, the most active muscle in grasping is the extensor carpi radialis brevis, which holds the wrist in extension.[56] All wrist extensor muscles are innervated by the radial nerve. Injury to this nerve can have devastating results for effective hand function.

Radial and ulnar deviations of the wrist result from the synergistic action of the wrist flexors and extensors. An example is the simultaneous action of the extensor carpi radialis and flexor carpi radialis muscles as they radially deviate the wrist. This synergistic movement helps control wrist positions for various hand functions. Dynamic wrist stability is provided by three muscles that are active during both flexion and extension: the extensor carpi ulnaris, the extensor pollicis brevis (EPB), and the abductor pollicis longus.[33]

All muscles acting on the wrist can be cyclically contracted to perform wrist circumduction. This is one example of functional movement produced by serial synergistic muscle activity. Other examples of serial synergistic activity of the wrist and hand include typing and playing the piano.

Hand

Two special digits—the index finger and the thumb—give the hand unique functional capabilities of the hand. The thumb is controlled by four intrinsic (thenar) and four extrinsic (forearm) muscles.[66] These eight muscles let the thumb move to oppose the tips of any of the fingers for grasping.

The intrinsic muscles of the hand—the interossei and lumbricals—place tension on the extensor expansion, allowing the extensor digitorum to extend the IP joints. The extensor digitorum is also the primary extensor of the MCP joints.[71] The lumbricals and interossei assist the flexor digitorum superficialis in MCP flexion. The interossei also abduct and adduct the digits. The extensor pollicis longus (EPL) causes IP and MCP extension and CMC retroposition.

The flexor digitorum superficialis and flexor digitorum profundus muscles flex the MCP. When the MCP is stable, the flexor digitorum superficialis flexes the PIP joints. When the PIP joints are stable, the flexor digitorum profundus flexes the DIP joints. The fifth digit has special functions. The opponens digiti minimi hollows the palm for cupping the hand (for example, to drink water) or helps grasp a cylindrical object.

Integrated Function

Generally, functional power is provided by the extrinsic muscles, and fine control is provided by the intrinsic muscles. These functions are all dependent on holding the wrist in the optimal position of 20–30° of extension. This functional position lets the hand muscles maintain or develop the required tension (Fig 6–8).[61]

There are two types of functional grip: power and precision (prehension). The power grip is generally used to exert force or pressure on an object where the digits maintain the object against the palm. This requires the combined positions of finger flexion and wrist extension with ulnar deviation. Four types of power grip are shown in Figure 6–9. The precision grip is generally used when precise and accurate

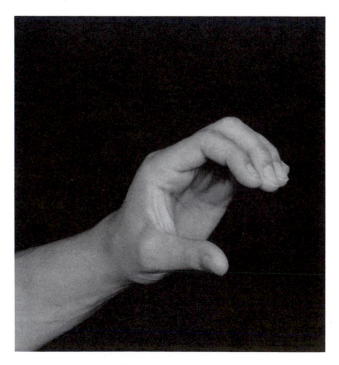

Figure 6–8. Functional position of the hand.

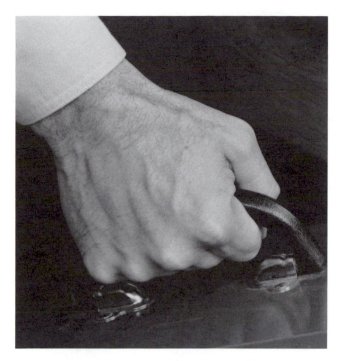

Figure 6–9A. Power grip positions: hook.

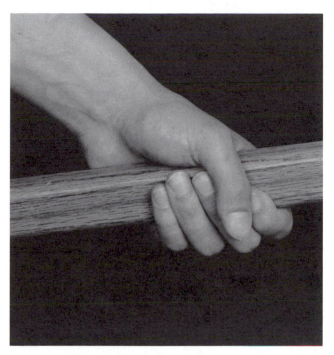

Figure 6–9B. Power grip positions: fist.

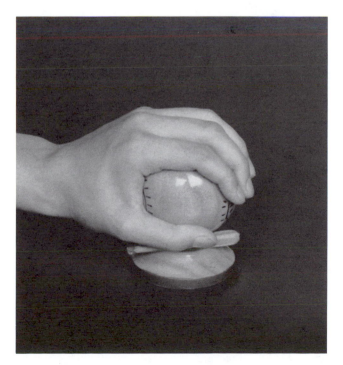

Figure 6–9C. Power grip positions: sphere.

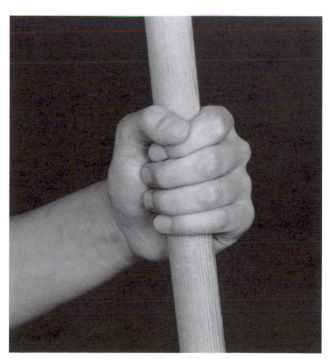

Figure 6–9D. Power grip positions: cylinder.

grasps are needed. Three types of precision grip are shown in Figure 6–10.

Neural Structures

Median Nerve

The median nerve pierces the flexor digitorum superficialis after passing between the heads of the pronator muscle (see Chapter 5, <u>The Elbow</u>). The nerve courses distally toward the wrist between the flexor digitorum superficialis and flexor digitorum profundus muscles. About 5–8 cm distal to the lateral epicondyle, the anterior interosseus nerve branches off the median nerve. The anterior interosseus nerve is primarily motor, but supplies some sensory fibers to the wrist joint and can contribute to wrist pain.[21] The median nerve continues distally, giving off a sensory branch that innervates the thenar eminence. The main portion of the nerve passes under the transverse carpal ligament and through the carpal tunnel. The nerve branches again, sending motor fibers to the thenar eminence and the first two lumbricals. Sensory branches supply the volar aspect of the first three digits and the radial aspect of the fourth digit.[57]

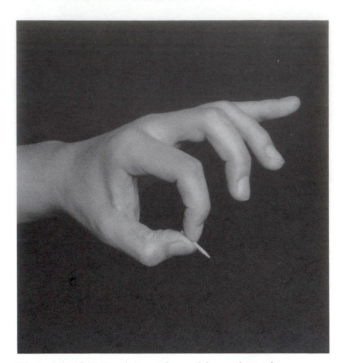

Figure 6–10A. Precision grip positions: tip to tip prehension.

The median nerve is subject to compression or entrapment at three sites distal to the elbow. These sites are 1) at the pronator teres or flexor digitorum superficialis; 2) the carpal tunnel; and 3) the thenar eminence (Fig 6–11).

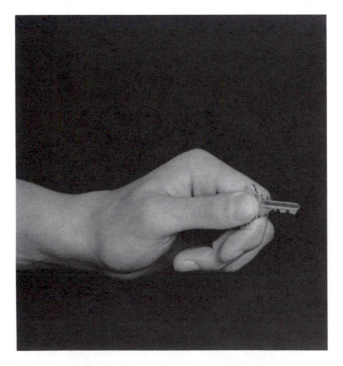

Figure 6–10B. Precision grip positions: lateral prehension.

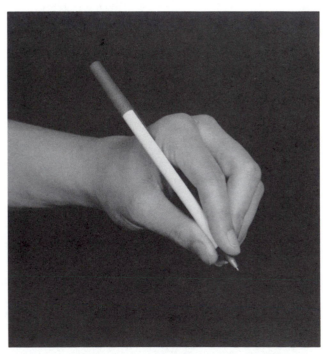

Figure 6–10C. Precision grip positions: digital prehension or "chuck" position.

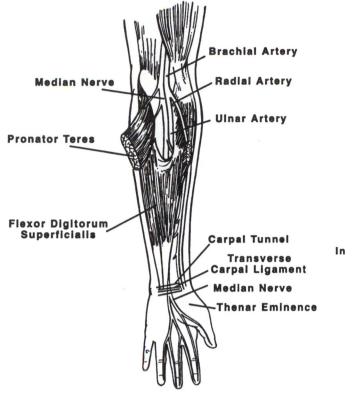

Figure 6–11. Median nerve pathway, with possible compression sites at the pronator teres or flexor digitorum superficialis, the carpal tunnel, and the thenar eminence (left arm, anterior view).

Radial Nerve

While there are anatomical anomalies, in most people the radial nerve branches into two nerves just distal to the elbow. These nerves are the posterior interosseus nerve and the superficial radial nerve.

The superficial radial nerve runs beneath the brachioradialis muscle to the distal third of the forearm. It passes between the tendons of the extensor carpi radialis longus and the brachioradialis. There it moves dorsally to course along the radius just beneath the skin. This nerve supplies sensation to the posterior radial aspect of the hand. The posterior interosseus branch pierces the supinator muscle at the Arcade of Froshe distal to the elbow. It is primarily a motor nerve.

The radial nerve can be subject to compression or entrapment at three areas distal to the elbow. These are 1) the Arcade of Froshe; 2) between the tendons of the extensor carpi radialis longus and the brachioradialis; and 3) along the radius (Fig 6–12).

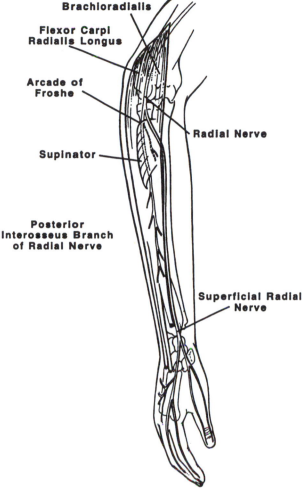

Figure 6–12. Radial nerve pathway, with possible entrapment sites at the Arcade of Froshe and between the tendons of the extensor carpi radialis longus and the brachioradialis (right arm, posterolateral view). The superficial radial nerve is also subject to compression from external forces as it runs superficially along the distal third of the radius.

Ulnar Nerve

The ulnar nerve passes through the cubital tunnel at the elbow. Two sensory nerves branch off the ulnar nerve in the forearm: the palmar cutaneous branch and the dorsal cutaneous branch. The palmar cutaneous branch innervates the hypothenar eminence. The dorsal cutaneous branch innervates the posterior surface of the fourth digit and the radial half of the fifth digit.

The main portion of the ulnar nerve continues distally to the base of the hand and enters Guyon's Tunnel. Guyon's Tunnel lies superficially and medially to the carpal tunnel. It is bordered medially by the hook of the hamate and laterally by the pisiform bone. The pisohamate ligament forms the roof of the tunnel, and the flexor retinaculum forms its floor. The ulnar nerve and artery pass through Guyon's Tunnel. The ulnar nerve then bifurcates into the superficial branch and the deep motor branch. The superficial branch supplies sensation to the distal border of the palm. It divides into two palmar digital nerves that supply sensation to the anterior surfaces of the fifth digit and half of the fourth digit. The deep motor branch takes an abrupt turn around the hook of the hamate. This branch supplies motor fibers to the muscles of the hypothenar eminence and portions of the thenar eminence. The ulnar nerve can be compressed or entrapped at only one site distal to the cubital tunnel: Guyon's Tunnel (Fig 6–13).

There are four stages of gripping:[8,54] 1) opening the hand; 2) closing the fingers; 3) exerting force; and 4) releasing the object. The thumb, wrist, hand, and fingers control these actions in a coordinated sequence, with varying ranges of precision or power. Injuries to the nerve structures of the wrist and hand can significantly affect tissue sensation and the ability to grip objects. Damage to the radial nerve affects the ability to maintain a functional wrist position, open

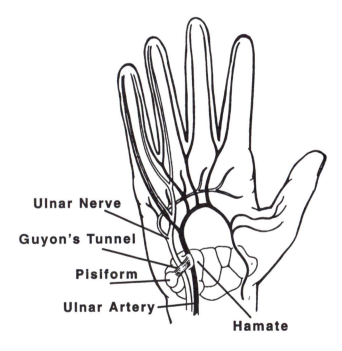

Figure 6–13. Ulnar nerve pathway with possible entrapment site at Guyon's tunnel (right arm, anterior view).

the hand, and release the object. Median nerve injury affects flexion and sensation of the digits on the radial side of the hand, ultimately affecting precision grip. Injury to the ulnar nerve affects flexion and sensation of the digits on the ulnar side of the hand, affecting the power grip. Thumb function in both types of grips can be affected by injury to either the median or ulnar nerves.

EVALUATION

Subjective Examination

The subjective examination should proceed as outlined in Chapter 2, Principles of Extremity Evaluation. The patient's main complaints give the clinician valuable clues about the patient's current problems and help plan the objective examination. In acute conditions, the mechanism of injury helps determine the possible structures involved. For example, a patient with a hyperextension injury to an IP joint may have capsuloligamentous injury. A fall on the hand may cause a hyperextension injury to the wrist, and ligamentous sprain and fractures need to be ruled out. Lacerations to the hand and wrist may involve serious injury to the tendons or nerves. Chronic problems caused by repetitive wrist and finger movements can involve the muscles, tendons, and nerves. Determining the specific aggravating factors will help the clinician identify which structures contribute to the complaints.

If the problem is long standing, the patient may have reflex sympathetic dystrophy (RSD). This condition is characterized by chronic pain, skin changes, and swelling. Acute, insidious onset of swelling in the IP joints may be caused by an arthritic condition. Complaints of weakness and sensation changes may have their origin at the cervical spine or other proximal areas of the upper limb. Many disorders, including vascular, arthritic, and neurological problems, can affect the posture, shape, and function of the wrist and hand.

Planning the Objective Examination

The objective examination of the forearm, wrist, and hand is based on the subjective clues found during the interview. The clinician should consider the degree to which distal problems are caused by cervical or proximal limb factors. Tests that screen for proximal involvement should be included in the evaluation of the wrist and hand.

The fragile nature of the neuromusculoskeletal tissues of this area requires careful and systematic inspection; however, excessive symptom provocation may preclude a complete and accurate assessment. Therefore, before beginning the objective examination, it helps to plan which tests to perform based on the severity, irritability and nature (SIN) of the problem. Patients with unstable fractures or recent crush injuries may be harmed by excessive testing; therefore, only the most essential tests should be performed.

Objective Examination

The objective examination should proceed as outlined in Chapter 2, Principles of Extremity Evaluation. The cervical spine, shoulder, and elbow should be screened to see if further examination is warranted. The quadrant test (see the "Clearing Tests" section of Chapter 2) can rule out cervical spine involvement as the source of complaints. Wrist symptoms easily provoked by neck movements or positions warrant a complete examination of the cervical spine. The shoulder and elbow should be examined to confirm or rule out their contribution to the patient's problem. This is particularly important if the patient complains of pain radiating from these areas. Screening tests for these joints are described in Chapter 2.

Structural Observation

Many disorders manifest themselves in changes in the appearance of the hand.[8] The mannerisms of the hand at rest or during movement can give clues about neurological involvement. The clinician should observe the posture and use of the patient's hands when greeting the patient, during the subjective examination, and while the patient is undressing. Structural asymmetries of the soft tissue contours of the forearm, wrist, and hand should be noted. Specific muscle wasting of the hand, especially the thenar and hypothenar eminences, may reflect injury to the nerves innervating these areas (median and ulnar nerves, respectively). Changes in color, temperature, and sweating may signify peripheral vascular problems caused by Raynaud's disease, RSD, or diabetes mellitus. Any swelling should be noted.

Swelling is commonly found on the posterior aspects of the wrist, hand, and fingers. The appearance of the fingernails may reflect systemic problems.

There are many common deformities of the wrist and hand, including:

Neurological deformities (Fig 6–14)

- Wrist Drop (radial nerve palsy)
- Claw Hand (combined median and ulnar nerve palsy)
- Ape Hand (median nerve palsy)
- Bishop's Hand (ulnar nerve palsy)

Arthritic deformities (Fig 6–15)

- Heberden's Nodes
- Bouchard's Nodes
- Ulnar Drift
- Swan Neck
- Boutonnière's
- Z–Thumb

Tendon deformities (Fig 6–16)

- Dupuytren's Contracture
- Trigger Finger
- Mallet Finger

Mobility

Physiological Mobility

Physiological mobility refers to the movement of the forearm, wrist, and hand in standard planar movements and functional movements.

Active Mobility

Active mobility is examined to assess the patient's ability and willingness to move the forearm, wrist, and hand. The number and order of the motions tested is determined by the subjective clues. Those motions suspected to cause severe symptoms or irritability should be checked last, and the examination should only include the motions the clinician feels won't exacerbate symptoms. Bilateral

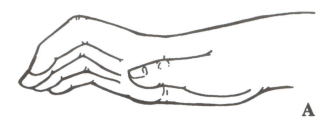

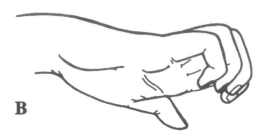

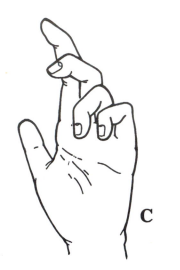

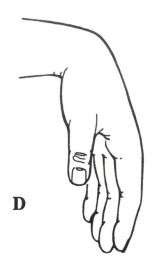

Figure 6–14. Neurological deformities of the hand. A) ape hand; B) claw hand; C) bishop's hand; D) wrist drop.

and normal comparison should be noted. The following motions should be tested:

Thumb:

- IP: flexion–extension

- MCP: flexion–extension

- CMC: palmar abduction–adduction
            radial abduction–adduction
            opposition–retroposition

Fingers:

- MCP: flexion–extension
            abduction–adduction

- PIP/DIP: flexion–extension

Functional movements should also be checked since these combine many movements of the wrist, hand, and forearm. For example, the thumb can circumduct, which is a combination of motions at both the CMC and MCP joints. Simple functional tests include daily activities such as tying shoelaces,

buttoning a shirt, zipping a jacket, shuffling and dealing cards, or writing.

Active mobility can be limited for many reasons, including post–traumatic or post–surgical stiffness, contracture, edema, and pain. Arthritic conditions, RSD, and neurological disorders can also affect active mobility.

Active mobility testing is usually performed in sitting, but other positions can be used if necessary. Overpressure should be applied at end range if tolerated. The clinician should consider the fragile nature of the tissues of the wrist and hand when determining the amount of overpressure to apply.

Passive Mobility

Passive mobility testing assesses the integrity of the non–contractile structures of the forearm, wrist, and hand. Passive testing should include any active motions that are not within the normal limits of motion or where the clinician is unable to test the end–feel. When testing passive mobility, the clinician

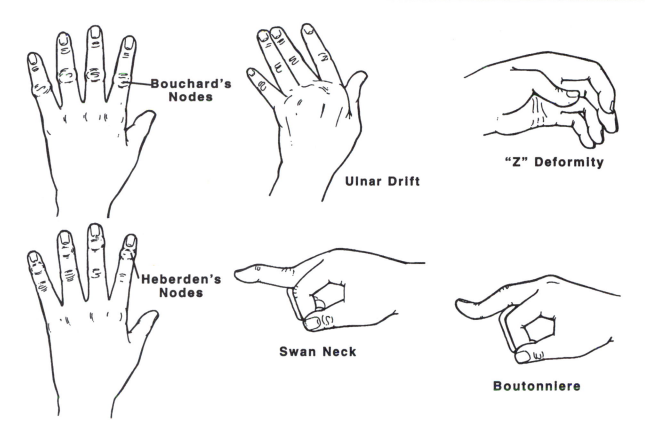

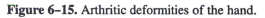

Figure 6–15. Arthritic deformities of the hand.

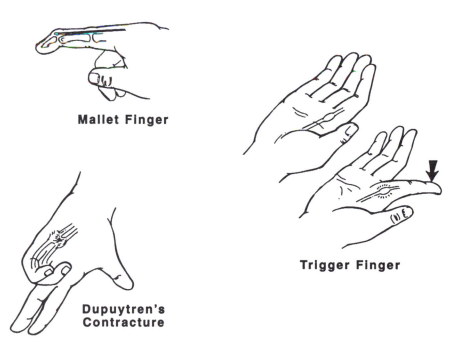

Figure 6–16. Tendon deformities of the hand.

note the available range of motion, symptom response to movement, end–feel, and pattern of motion restriction. Bilateral and normal passive mobility comparison should be noted.

The pattern of motion restriction can be considered capsular or non—capsular. The combined capsular patterns of the forearm, wrist, and hand are: *mild limitation of supination and pronation at the distal radioulnar joint; equal limitations of wrist flexion and extension; abduction limited more than retroposition at the first CMC joint;* and *flexion limited more than extension at the MCP and IP joints.*

The symptom response to passive motion can reveal the stage of the problem (see Chapter 2, Principles of Extremity Evaluation). Patients can be tested while they are sitting or supine (Fig 6–17).

Accessory Mobility

Accessory mobility of the joints refers to component motions and joint play.[46] Joint play movements of the forearm, wrist, and hand can be examined with the patient in sitting or supine (see Chapter 11, Mobilization Techniques).

The accessory mobility findings should be compared bilaterally and to normal. These findings include the resistance encountered, the end–feel, any crepitus noted, and any symptoms provoked. The results should be consistent with the physiologic mobility examination. For example, limited extension at the first MCP would correlate with a limitation in volar glide at the same joint.

Strength

Manual muscle tests (MMT) assess the status of the contractile structures of the forearm, wrist, and hand. The tests are performed in the mid–range of motion to avoid stress on the non–contractile structures. To avoid substitution of synergistic muscles, the patient is told to gradually increase effort to a voluntary maximum contraction. The clinician resists isometrically. The muscle strength should be graded, and any symptom response noted. Any muscle acting on, acting across, or influencing the forearm, wrist, or hand should be tested. Cyriax's four patterns of response (see the "Strength Examination"

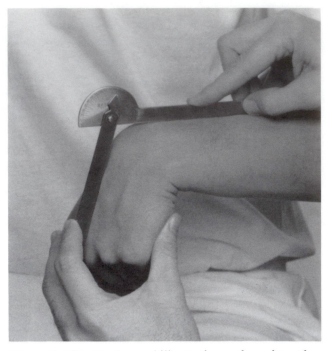

Figure 6–17A. Passive mobility testing at the wrist and hand: wrist flexion.

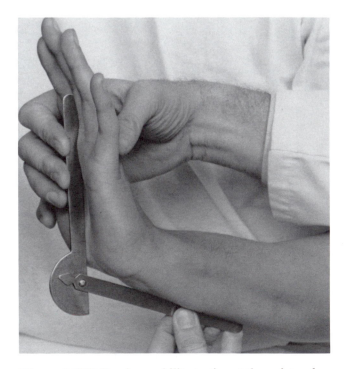

Figure 6–17B. Passive mobility testing at the wrist and hand: wrist extension.

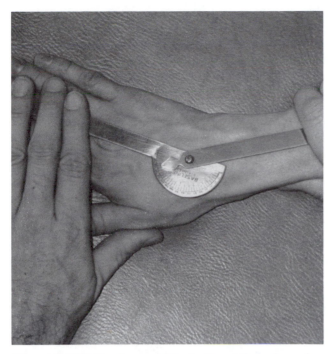

Figure 6–17C. Passive mobility testing at the wrist and hand: wrist ulnar deviation.

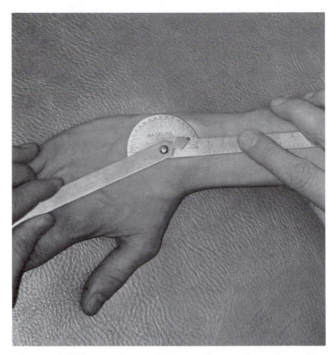

Figure 6–17D. Passive mobility testing at the wrist and hand: wrist radial deviation.

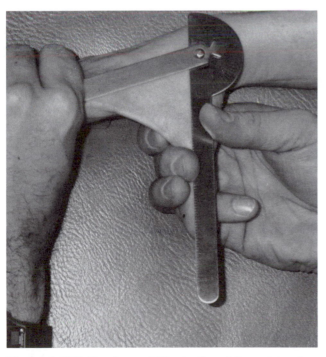

Figure 6–17E. Passive mobility testing at the wrist and hand: 1st CMC palmar abduction.

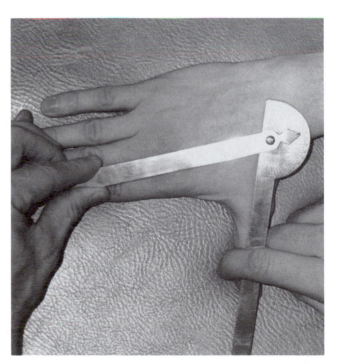

Figure 6–17F. Passive mobility testing at the wrist and hand: 1st CMC radial abduction.

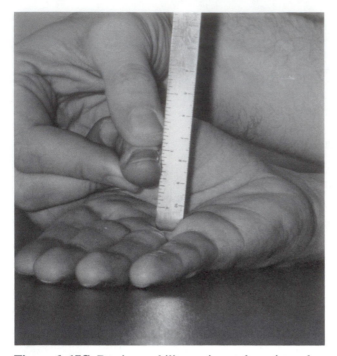

Figure 6–17G. Passive mobility testing at the wrist and hand: 1st CMC opposition.

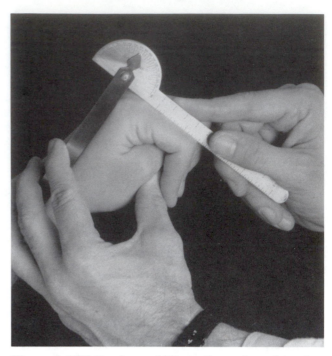

Figure 6–17H. Passive mobility testing at the wrist and hand: MCP flexion.

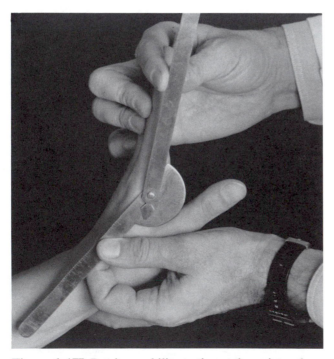

Figure 6–17I. Passive mobility testing at the wrist and hand: MCP extension.

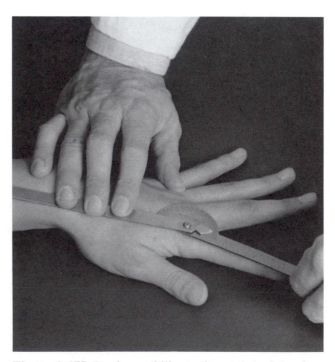

Figure 6–17J. Passive mobility testing at the wrist and hand: MCP abduction.

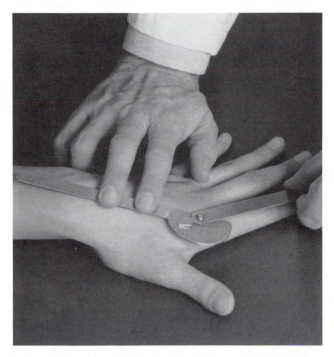

Figure 6–17K. Passive mobility testing at the wrist and hand: MCP adduction.

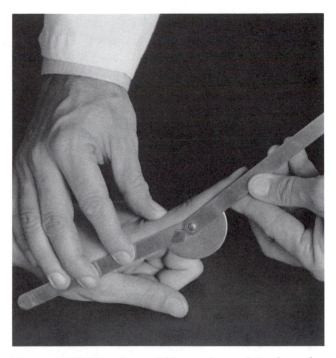

Figure 6–17M. Passive mobility testing at the wrist and hand: IP extension.

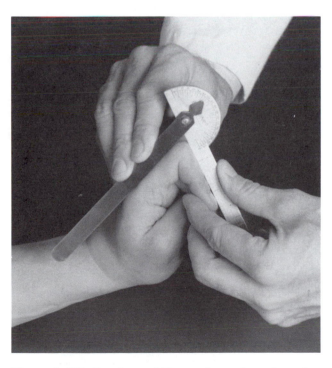

Figure 6–17L. Passive mobility testing at the wrist and hand: IP flexion.

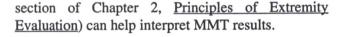

section of Chapter 2, Principles of Extremity Evaluation) can help interpret MMT results.

Some clinicians advocate functional strength testing of the forearm, wrist, and hand.[54] This may include simple tasks such as grasping and holding objects for a specified time, using elastic resistance against repetitive thumb movements, and lifting 1–5 lb weights with the wrist.

Resisted muscle testing should include a measure of power and precision grip for the hands and fingers. Hand dominance should be noted. A difference of 5–10% between dominant and non–dominant power grip strength is normal in adult subjects.[43]

The power grip strength test is usually performed with a hand–held grip dynamometer (Fig 6–18); however, a sphygmomanometer can also measure grip strength (Fig 6–19).[28] The "repeated measures" reliability of sphygmomanometer grip measurements in normal subjects is considered acceptable.[28]

The sphygmomanometer method has three advantages over dynamometer testing. First, it is readily available for other purposes in most clinics. Second, it uses a scale with smaller increments,

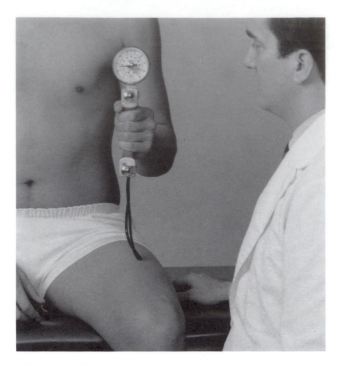

Figure 6–18. Grip strength testing with a dynamometer.

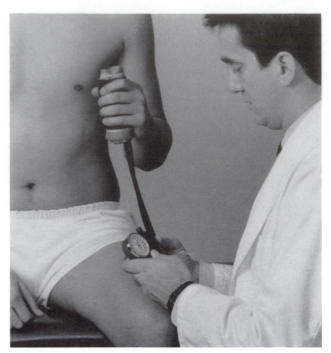

Figure 6–19. Grip strength testing with a sphygmomanometer.

improving the sensitivity to small changes in strength. Finally, the compliant surface of the sphygmomanometer decreases discomfort during testing.[28] The sphygmomanometer should be inflated at 20 mm Hg at a circumference of ≈7 in. The patient should be told to grip the device three times; the average of the three trials should be calculated. Maximum effort should be encouraged, but fatigue should be avoided by allowing a 1–2 minute rest between efforts. The standard position for hand strength testing should be used, as shown in Figure 6–19.[23] To convert sphygmomanometer readings (SR) to equivalent dynamometer values (DV), use this formula: DV = (0.54 x SR) - 45.12.

The hand–held dynamometer should be set at the third setting, a common position for measurement.[6] Some authors advocate testing using the dynamometer at each of the five adjustable hand spacings.[6,43] A graph of the results should resemble a bell curve (Figure 6–20), with the highest forces generated at the middle spacings and the weakest forces generated at the ends. An injury should not affect the shape of the curve but will show lower values. An abnormal curve shape or test–retest discrepancies >20% indicate the patient may not be giving maximal effort.[5,44] There are many normative value tables of grip strength based on gender, age, and handedness.[14,43,45,58]

The three types of precision grip can be measured using a pinch meter (Figure 6–21). The average of three trials is used; bilateral and normal comparison should be noted.[43,45]

Neurological

The neurological examination should be carried out as outlined in Chapter 2, <u>Principles of Extremity Evaluation</u>. Indications for neurological testing include patient complaints of paresthesia, anesthesia, or weakness. The examination includes resisted muscle tests, light touch sensation tests, and deep tendon reflexes (DTR) tests. Motor function is assessed in the upper extremity myotomes per the upper quarter screening examination. Light touch sensation should be tested in the upper limb, including the C4–T1 dermatomes and the regional cutaneous nerve fields (see Fig 2–12 on pages 24 and 25).

The hand has many different types of sensation besides light touch that can be tested. Stereognosis is the ability to identify common objects by touch. To test stereognosis, an object is placed in the patient's

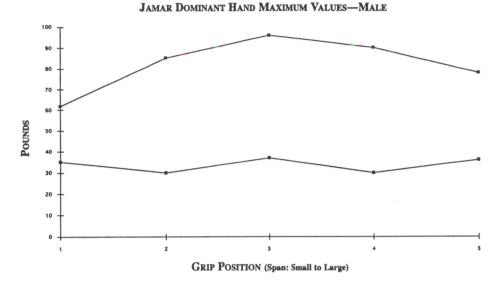

JAMAR DOMINANT HAND MAXIMUM VALUES—MALE

GRIP POSITION (Span: Small to Large)

Figure 6–20. Grip strength testing results. A bell-shaped curve (upper line) is expected. A flat or irregular curve (lower line) may indicate submaximal effort.

hand, and the patient is not permitted to see the object. Patients with normal stereognosis should be able to name the object within 3 sec of touching it.[32] Light touch can be tested using a pressure esthesiometer (Semmes–Weinstein). This instrument consists of varying thicknesses of nylon monofilament, which are applied to the skin perpendicularly until the filament bends (Fig 6–22). The patient is not

permitted to watch and is asked to identify when the filament bends. Normal values are 2.36–$2.83\,g/mm^2$ pressure.[13] Pain sensation can be tested with a pinprick. Vibration sense, which is closely allied with position sense, is tested using a 256 Hz tuning fork.[47] The fork is struck, and the single prong end is placed over a bony prominence. The resulting sensation is usually described as "buzzing." Unilateral and

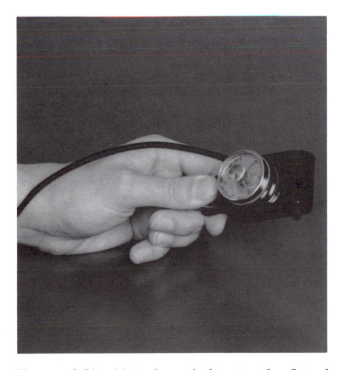

Figure 6–21. Measuring pinch strength. Lateral prehension, or "key pinch" is shown.

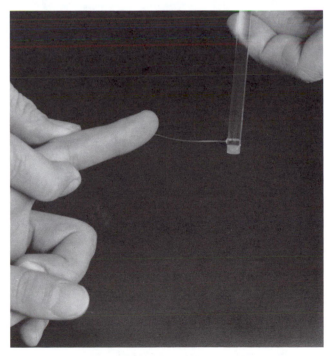

Figure 6–22. Light touch measured with a pressure esthesiometer.

bilateral differences in sensation should be noted. Proprioception or position sense is tested by positioning one extremity and having the patient assume the same position with the other extremity. Two–point static discrimination is tested using a two–point discriminator (Fig 6–23). The goal is to find the minimal distance at which the patient can distinguish between two stimuli. Patients with normal sensation should be able distinguish between points 3 mm apart on the pulps of the fingers.[47] Temperature sensation can be tested by applying warm or cold objects to the skin and asking the patient to discriminate between the two temperatures. Unilateral, bilateral, and normal comparisons should be noted.

There can be many reasons for sensation changes in the forearm, wrist, hand, and fingers. The clinician should correlate the findings to patterns of cervical disc, nerve root, peripheral nerve entrapment, or other peripheral neurovascular problems that coincide with the patient's complaints and examination.

The relevant DTR's include the biceps (C5–6), brachioradialis (C6–7), and triceps (C7–8). Unilateral and bilateral comparison for symmetry should be noted. Patients should also be examined for signs of adverse mechanical neural tension (AMNT). This testing includes the base ULTT and the more specific tests for median, ulnar, and radial nerve bias (see Chapter 2, Principles of Extremity Evaluation).[12]

Palpation

The palpation examination should proceed as discussed in Chapter 2, Principles of Extremity Evaluation. The process should be consistent with layered palpation, gradually proceeding from surface to deeper tissues. Bilateral comparisons should be made.

When palpating, the clinician should start proximally with the forearm structures, which may cause problems distally into the hand. The tendons of the forearm muscles should be followed distally toward the wrist and hand, and the radius and ulna should be palpated starting proximally and moving distally toward the wrist and hand. The remainder of the palpation examination can proceed from the posterior to the anterior surfaces.

The first through fifth metacarpals, MCP joints, phalanges, and IP joints should be palpated in a posterior–to–anterior and medial–to–lateral manner. The clinician should look and feel for tenderness, edema, or temperature changes. Many patients with traumatic injuries or arthritic diseases will have findings at these areas.

The overlying palmar creases can be related to the anatomical structures underneath.[41,65] These creases are formed at the point of least mobility at the skin–to–fascia interface and are caused by movements of the underlying joints.

The following structures should be palpated:

Anterior surface (Fig 6–24)

- flexor tendons
- median nerve at the carpal tunnel
- ulnar nerve at Guyon's Tunnel
- thenar eminence (intrinsic muscles of the thumb)
- hypothenar eminence (intrinsic muscles of the fifth digit)
- flexor carpi ulnaris tendon insertion at the pisiform bone
- hook of the hamate
- carpal bones: scaphoid, lunate, triquetrum, pisiform, trapezium, trapezoid, capitate, and hamate bones
- metacarpals
- MCP joints
- phalanges
- IP joints

Posterior surface (Fig 6–25)

- radius and ulna
- superficial branch of radial nerve
- distal radioulnar joint
- abductor pollicis longus
- extensor digitorum tendons
- extensor carpi radialis longus and brevis

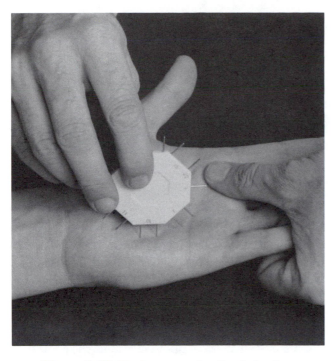

Figure 6–23. Testing two point discrimination.

- extensor pollicis longus tendon

- anatomical "snuff box"

- wrist and finger extensor tendon tunnels

Special Tests

Special tests help the clinician gather more information to identify the specific structures that contribute to the patient's problem. There are five types of special tests at the wrist and hand: neurological, vascular, musculotendinous, ligamentous, and coordination/dexterity. The special tests are summarized in Table 6–3.

Neurological Tests

Tinel's Sign

Nerve compromise can be tested by tapping the nerves near the surface in the wrist and hand. This can be checked at the carpal tunnel (median nerve), at Guyon's Tunnel (ulnar nerve), and proximal to the radial styloid (superficial radial nerve) (Fig 6–26A, B & C). These tests are positive if they cause pain and tingling distal to the site being tapped.

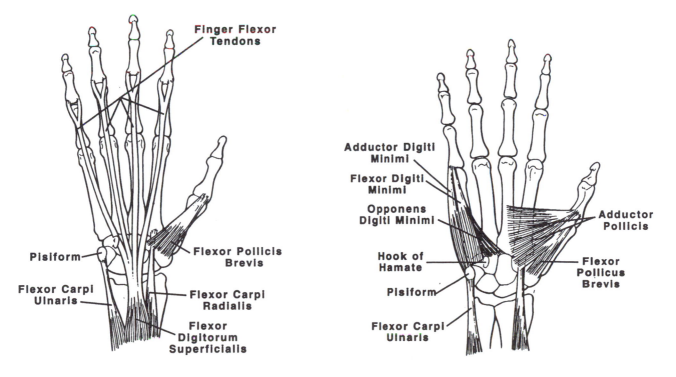

Figure 6–24. Musculotendinous structures to palpate on the anterior surface of the wrist and hand. Bony structures to palpate are shown in Figure 6–1; neural structures are shown in Figures 6–11, 6–12, and 6–13.

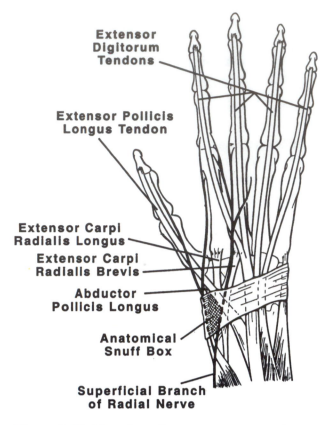

Extensor
Digitorum
Tendons

Extensor Pollicis
Longus Tendon

Extensor Carpi
Radialis Longus

Extensor Carpi
Radialis Brevis

Abductor
Pollicis Longus

Anatomical
Snuff Box

Superficial Branch
of Radial Nerve

Figure 6–25. Musculotendinous structures to palpate on the posterior surface of the wrist and hand (right hand, posterior view). Bony structures are shown in Figure 6–1.

Phalen's Test

This test identifies median nerve entrapment at the wrist. For Phalen's Test, the wrists are held in maximum flexion for one minute (Fig 6–27). The test is positive if there is tingling into the thumb, index, and middle fingers and into the radial side of the ring finger.

Pinch Test

A thumb–index finger pinch test increases pressure in the anterior compartment, testing for entrapment of the anterior interosseous branch of the median nerve as it passes through the anterior interosseous membrane. The patient is told to pinch the tips of the thumb and index finger together. The normal response is a tip–to–tip pinch. The test is positive if the patient shows an abnormal pulp–to–pulp response (Fig 6–28A&B).

Table 6–3. Special Tests for the Forearm, Wrist and Hand

Test Type	Test Name	Purpose
Neurological	Pinch Test	Entrapment of anterior interosseous branch of the median nerve
	Phalen's Test	Carpal Tunnel Syndrome
	Tinel's Sign	Peripheral nerve compromise
Musculotendinous	Finkelstein's Test	De Quervain's syndrome
	Trigger Finger Test	Flexor tenosynovitis
Ligamentous	Bunnel-Littler Test	Tight capsule vs. tight intrinsic muscles
	Retinacular Test	Retinacular ligament tightness
	Watson's Test	Scapulolunate ligament stability
	Triquetrolunate Test	Triquetrolunate stability
	Ulnar Snuff Box Test	Triquetrum or radiocarpal disc injury
	Lunate Displacement Test	Lunate dislocation
Vascular	Allen Test	Blood supply to hand
	Modified Allen Test	Blood supply to the fingers
	Volumetric Measures	Swelling
	Capillary Refill	Cutaneous circulation

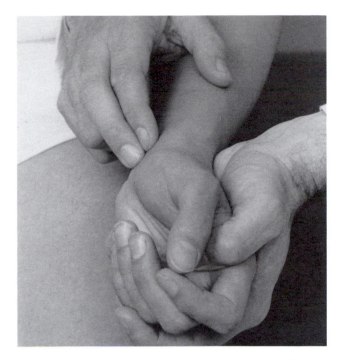

Figure 6–26A. Tinel testing at carpal tunnel.

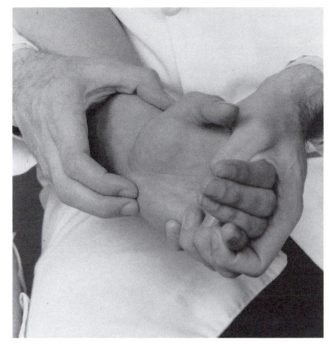

Figure 6–26B. Tinel testing at Guyon's Tunnel.

Vascular Tests

Allen Test

The Allen Test is used to identify circulatory impairment in the hand. The blood supply to the hand and fingers is tested by simultaneously compressing the radial and ulnar arteries while the patient squeezes and opens the fist several times (Fig 6–29). The compression of the arteries is alternately released to allow return of blood flow. The flushing responses of the radial and ulnar arteries should be noted and compared unilaterally and bilaterally. The test is positive if there is an uneven flushing response.

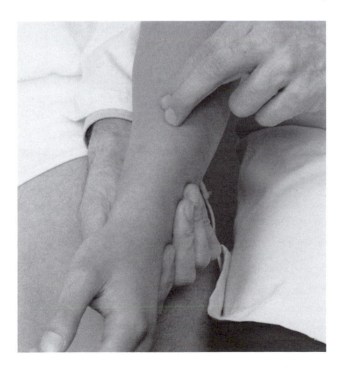

Figure 6–26C. Tinel testing along the distal radius.

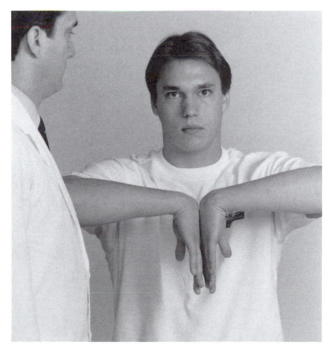

Figure 6–27. Phalen's Test.

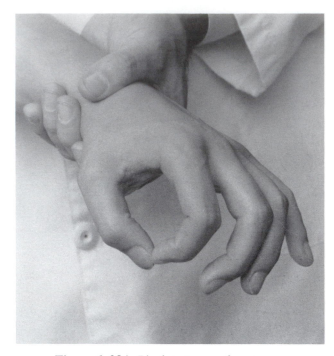

Figure 6–28A. Pinch test normal response.

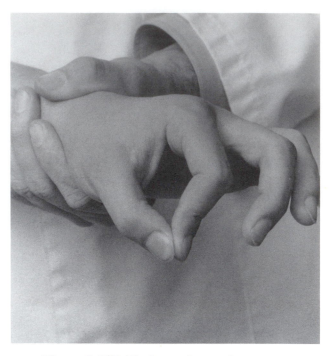

Figure 6–28B. Pinch test abnormal response.

Modified Allen Test

A simple test to check distal blood flow to the fingers requires that the patient open and close the hand several times. With the hand in a fist, the clinician then applies pressure on the sides of finger at the proximal phalanx to occlude the digital arteries (Fig 6–30). When the fist is opened, the finger should be paler than the other digits. When the pressure is released, the finger should flush. The test is positive if there is an abnormal normal flush response. Comparison should be made between fingers unilaterally and bilaterally.

Volumetric Measures

While not truly a vascular test, volumetric measurement is included here because it identifies swelling. A special container called a volumometer is filled with water to the level of a spout. The patient inserts a hand into the volumometer, causing water to spill out of the spout (Fig 6–31). The volume of water displaced is the volume of the hand. Bilateral comparison should be noted. When taking volumetric measurements, it is important for the patient to position the hand in the same manner from one test to another. Inserting the hand at a different angle can affect the amount of water displaced. When making bilateral comparisons, there may be normal differences between the dominant and non–dominant hands of ≈5–10ml.[9] The test is positive for swelling if there is greater than a 10ml difference in water displacement when compared bilaterally.

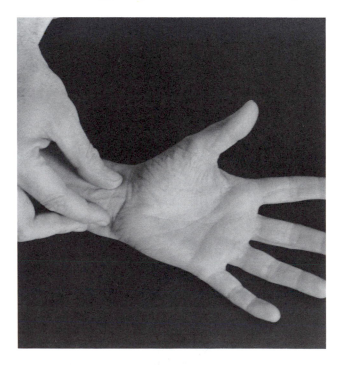

Figure 6–29. Allen Test.

Musculotendinous Tests

Flexor/Extensor Tenosynovitis Test

The flexor and extensor tendons of the wrist and fingers can be tested individually for tenosynovitis. To test for involvement of these structures, the muscle's action is isometrically resisted while palpating the tendon (Fig 6–32). The test is positive if it provokes pain or crepitus.

Finkelstein's Test

The classic test for the first extensor compartment tenosynovitis—de Quervain's Disease—is called Finkelstein's Test. The patient closes his or her fist with the thumb enclosed. The clinician moves the wrist into passive ulnar deviation while maintaining the closed fist position (Fig 6–33). The test is positive if it provokes pain at the first extensor compartment. This test is not definitive for de Quervain's Disease. The clinician should note that this test stretches the superficial radial nerve and may cause symptoms due to AMNT.

Trigger Finger Test

The trigger finger test assesses flexor tenosynovitis. This condition has usually progressed to the stenosis or "triggering" phase by the time the symptoms are noticed. Triggering is caused by roughness in the retinacular sheath, resulting in an abrupt catch in the movement. The patient is asked to hold the digit extended. The clinician palpates over the anterior surface of the IP joints. The patient is asked to actively flex and extend the IP (Fig 6–34). The test is positive if there is a palpable snapping or "triggering."

Ligamentous Tests

Bunnel–Littler Test

The Bunnel–Littler Test differentiates between tight intrinsic muscles and contracture of the joint capsule when flexion of the PIP is limited. PIP flexion is compared with the MCP in slight extension. If PIP flexion is limited, either the capsule or the intrinsic muscles are tight (Fig 6–35). Then the MCP joints are flexed, and PIP flexion is repeated. The test is positive for capsular tightness if there is decreased PIP flexion with the MCP joints fully flexed.

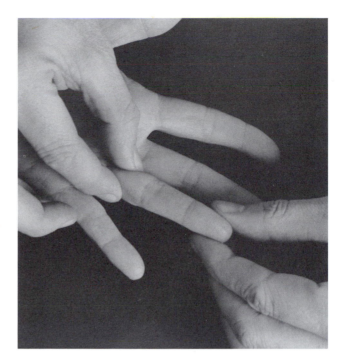

Figure 6–30. Modified Allen Test.

Retinacular Test

The retinacular test is similar to the Bunnel–Littler Test and can be performed at the DIP when flexion is limited. If the DIP exhibits limited flexion with the PIP in neutral, either the capsule or the

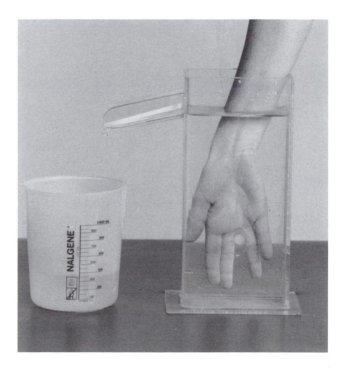

Figure 6–31. Measurement of hand volume.

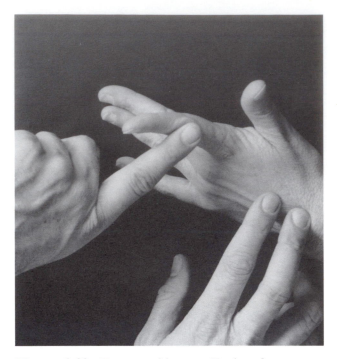

Figure 6–32. Tenosynovitis test. Testing for extensor tenosynovitis is shown.

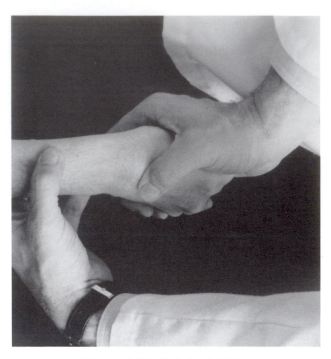

Figure 6–33. Finkelstein's Test.

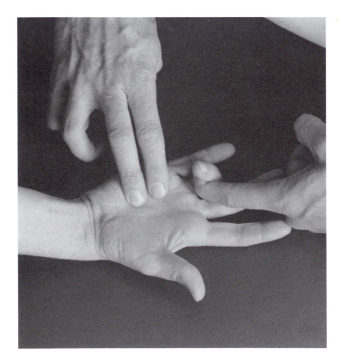

Figure 6–34. Trigger finger test.

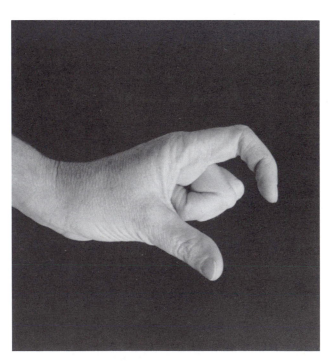

Figure 6–35. Bunnell-Littler Test.

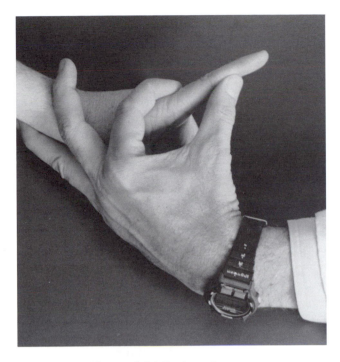

Figure 6–36. Retinacular test.

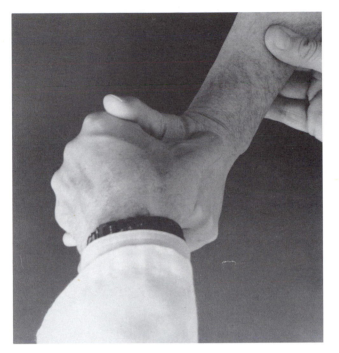

Figure 6–37. Watson's Test.

retinacular ligaments are tight (Fig 6–36). The test is positive for retinacular ligament tightness if the DIP flexes easily when the PIP is flexed.

Watson's Test

Watson's Test assesses scapholulolunate ligament stability. The scaphoid is palpated anteriorly and posteriorly on its distal aspect as the wrist is moved from ulnar deviation to radial deviation (Fig 6–37). The test is positive if there is pain or a palpable displacement of the scaphoid posteriorly, which sometimes occurs with a "clunk."[67]

Triquetrolunate Test

The integrity of the triquetrolunate ligament can be tested by immobilizing the lunate and moving the triquetrum and pisiform up and down on the lunate (Fig 6–38). The test is positive if it produces pain or excessive mobility.

Ulnar Snuff Box Test

This test identifies injury to the triquetrum or the radiocarpal joint disc. The ulnar snuff box is formed between the flexor and extensor carpi ulnaris tendons. The triquetrum can be palpated here (Fig 6–39). The test is positive if there is tenderness on palpation.

Ligamentous Instability

All joints of the wrist and hand can be checked for instability. Any of the accessory mobility tests (see Chapter 11, Mobilization Techniques) can be used to assess stability. At the wrist, the radial collateral ligament can be checked by ulnarly deviating the

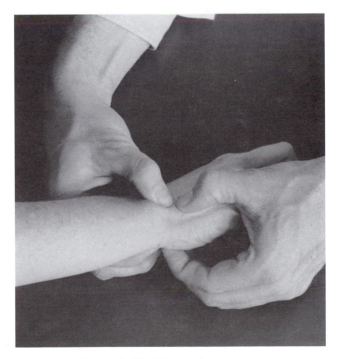

Figure 6–38. Triquetrolunate test.

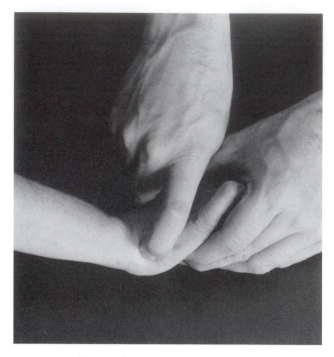

Figure 6–39. Ulnar snuff box test.

wrist in a neutral position. The ulnar collateral ligament is tested by radially deviating the wrist in neutral (Fig 6–40A&B). The integrity of collateral ligaments in the fingers can be assessed by applying ulnar and radial stresses (Fig 6–41). Overpressure can be applied to any of the carpal joints to test their

stability. The scaphulolunate and triquetrolunate joints are commonly affected.[1,64] These tests are positive if there is excessive joint mobility or pain.

Coordination/Dexterity Tests

There are many tests to assess the coordination and manual dexterity of the wrist and hand. These are standardized tests to assess a patient's functional abilities.

The Jebsen–Taylor Hand Function Test

This test measures gross coordination of the forearm, wrist, and hand. Manipulative skills and prehension are assessed by performing seven functional tests:

1. picking up large objects (light)
2. picking up large objects (heavy)
3. picking up small objects
4. stacking objects
5. turning cards
6. writing
7. feeding simulation

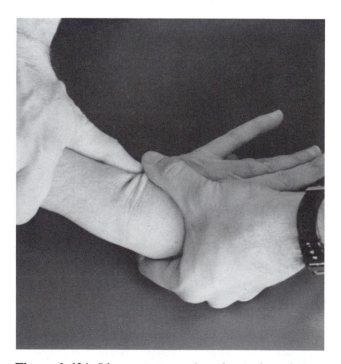

Figure 6–40A. Ligamentous stress testing at the wrist: radial collateral stress test.

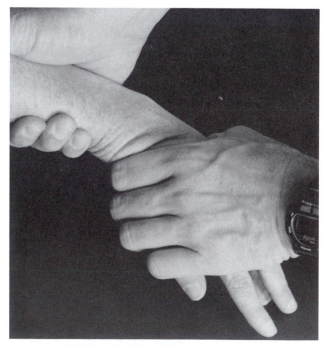

Figure 6–40B. Ligamentous stress testing at the wrist: ulnar collateral stress test.

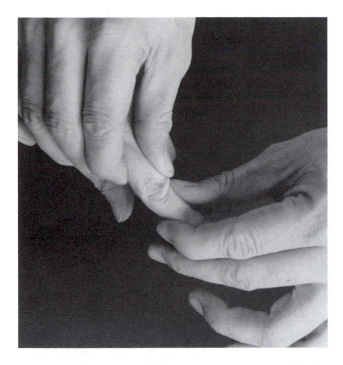

Figure 6–41. Collateral ligament testing at the IP joint. Radial collateral ligament testing is shown.

The objects manipulated in this test are standardized. The patient performs these tasks a standard number of times, and each trial is timed.

The Minnesota Rate of Manipulation Test

This test measures dexterity and gross coordination of the forearm, wrist, and hand. Five activities are timed and compared bilaterally and to normal.[41] The activities are:

1. placing objects
2. turning objects
3. displacing objects
4. one–hand turning and placing objects
5. two–hand turning and placing objects

Purdue Peg–Board Test

The Purdue Peg–Board Test measures fine coordination. Small objects such as pins and washers are used in five categories of activities:

1. manipulation with the right hand
2. manipulation with the left hand
3. manipulation with both hands

4. transfer of objects from right to left hand
5. assembly of small objects

These tests are timed. The patient's scores are compared to normative values, based on the patient's gender and occupation.[41]

Simulated ADL Test

This test measures the patient's functional level while performing simulated daily activities. There are 19 activities, ranging from standing and walking to threading a needle and using eating utensils. Each task is timed and compared to normal values.[41]

Selection of these or any other standardized tests should be based on the patient's functional needs.

Objective Examination Summary

There are many structures that can contribute to the patient's complaints. Signs and symptoms may arise from injuries to joints, muscles, or nerves. Repetitive trauma can manifest as tendinitis, nerve entrapment, compartment syndromes, or neural tension problems. Sprains, dislocations, and fractures are common. Crush injuries or lacerations can cause severe trauma. Arthritic deformities can debilitate hand function.

There are many challenges that face the clinician when developing treatment plans for rehabilitation of the forearm, wrist, and hand. The initial examination must be geared to identify the structures contributing to the patient's signs and symptoms. The clinician should be willing to look beyond the wrist and hand to identify these contributing factors.

At the conclusion of the evaluation, the clinician develops a problem list based on the patient's signs and symptoms. This problem list reminds the clinician to consider all the patient's problems when planning treatments. It also helps set goals and prioritize treatments.

TREATMENT STRATEGIES

The hand's unique role in functional activities makes injuries to this region particularly problematic. Traumatic injuries are common, and edema in this area can be difficult to resolve. Compression wraps and proper positioning should be used to prevent the formation of dependent edema. Wrist and hand postures may need to be modified, especially when the problem stems from cumulative trauma.

Functional strengthening exercises should begin as soon as possible. These should emphasize functional power and precision grips and combined motions that mimic wrist and hand function. Proprioception exercises and simulation of daily activities can promote functional recovery.

General treatment strategies are discussed in Chapter 3, Pathology and Treatment Principles. See Chapter 11, Mobilization Techniques, and Chapter 12, Exercise, for the sections relating to mobilization techniques, stretching and strengthening exercises for the forearm, wrist, and hand. Injury prevention is discussed more fully in Chapter 13, Prevention of Extremity Injuries.

COMMON CLINICAL CONDITIONS

Carpal Tunnel Syndrome

Carpal Tunnel Syndrome (CTS) is the most researched peripheral nerve entrapment neuropathy. CTS occurs in women more than men, usually after the age of 40.[55,70] There is some evidence that women have smaller wrists but not correspondingly smaller tendons, making them more susceptible to CTS for purely mechanical reasons.[3] Obesity has been shown to be a risk factor.[49] A higher incidence of CTS has recently been found in younger persons, especially those involved in work at a computer keyboard and in repetitive manual labor.[50,51] This increased incidence of CTS in younger people may be due to increased awareness of the problem and improved sensitivity of diagnostic tests. There is a high incidence of bilateral CTS (>50%),[63] which indicates systemic or physiologic disorders may cause the problem. In fact, many patients with unilateral complaints have bilateral nerve conduction abnormalities.[7]

The carpal tunnel is formed by the concave arch of the carpal bones and the transverse carpal ligament. Nine tendons and the median nerve pass through this tunnel (Fig 6–42). During wrist and finger movement, these tendons and the median nerve must slide relative to each other and relative to the tunnel itself. CTS is thought to occur when there is an imbalance between the size of the tunnel and its contents. This imbalance prevents normal sliding movements and puts pressure on the median nerve. Some authors have measured the mean pressure in the carpal tunnel and found a marked increase in pressure (up to 10 times normal) in patients diagnosed with CTS.[26,68] Maximal sustained contractions elicited by tetanic stimulation can at least triple the pressures in the carpal tunnel.[68]

Three potential causes of CTS have been identified: 1) changes in anatomical structures; 2) underlying systemic or physiological disorders; and 3) cumulative patterns of trauma from overuse. Many patients with CTS may have a combination of these factors.[63]

Concurrent involvement of the cervical spine (C6–C7 levels), neurovascular compression (thoracic outlet syndrome), and adverse neural tension proximal to the wrist should be confirmed or ruled out. It has been postulated that even the thoracic spine can contribute to symptoms in the hand by irritating the sympathetic trunk.[11]

History

Acute onset of problems may be caused by vigorous overuse in unaccustomed activity or by trauma. Chronic CTS can occur insidiously, brought on by repeated microtrauma, underlying disease, or other unknown causes. The symptoms typically occur after specific activities but often occur at night. It is common for a proximal lesion of the median nerve to coexist with a compressive problem at the carpal tunnel.[63] A thorough medical history is needed to identify contributing factors.

Signs/Symptoms

CTS resulting from trauma has a rapid and intense onset, with symptoms of pain and paresthesia into the hand and fingers in the distribution of the median nerve. Progressive numbness and weakness are cause for concern, as they may indicate nerve damage. The symptoms usually occur after a specific activity and at night. There are no signs of true numbness or weakness on physical examination. As the problem progresses, the patient may have complaints of constant pain and paresthesias, motor weakness, and sensory changes in the median nerve distribution. Atrophy of the thenar eminence may be

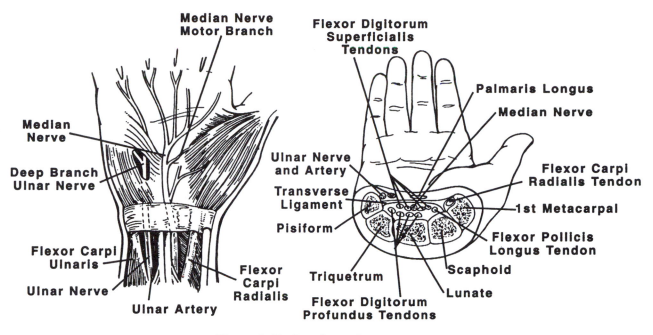

Figure 6–42. Carpal tunnel structures.

present. There may be overlapping symptoms from other problems such as ulnar nerve entrapment in Guyon's Tunnel. This may make it difficult to identify the source of symptoms. Tinel's Sign and Phalen's Test may be positive in all stages of the problem. The ULTT may be positive, and the use of a more specific median nerve bias can be helpful.[12] Sensory testing using the Semmes–Weinstein monofilaments (see the "Neurological" examination section of this chapter) can be useful. Motor weakness may present more subtly since only 6% of the median nerve fibers at the wrist are motor fibers.[63]

Diagnostics

Electromyography (EMG) may be inconclusive; conservative treatment may be initiated before such testing. Some authors recommend EMG testing after activity, when the most symptoms are present.[63] Others have advocated work simulation before testing to help diagnose chronic CTS in the early stages.[17] Repeated testing on different occasions lets the clinician monitor progress of CTS or of recovery.[63] Routine radiographs of the wrist can be taken, looking for malunited fractures, calcifications, or other bony problems that may decrease the size of the carpal tunnel. MRI of the wrist has been used to diagnose CTS (Fig 6–43); however, CTS can usually be diagnosed and managed without an MRI scan.[17,30,31,58]

Problem List

Patients with carpal tunnel syndrome may present with the following problems:

1. Pain and paresthesias in the hand and fingers. Problems are intermittent in early stages and constant in later stages.

2. Positive signs of median nerve compression

3. Decreased sensation

4. Weakness in thenar muscles

5. Daily activities limited by pain, paresthesias, and weakness

6. Concurrent signs of cervical involvement

Treatment

Early intervention is critical in the management of CTS. The acute onset of CTS after unaccustomed activity will usually resolve with rest. The use of anti–inflammatory drugs and PRICE helps resolve symptoms rapidly. The post–traumatic acute CTS patient should be managed in the same way, but treatment of the pathology that causes the symptoms is a priority. These patients must be monitored closely. If there is a rapid progression of symptoms, they may require surgical release of the transverse carpal ligament. The patient in the early stages of

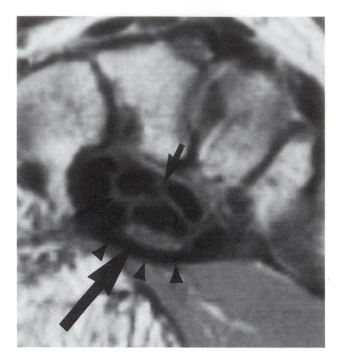

Figure 6–43. MRI of carpal tunnel syndrome. Axial image through the carpal tunnel at the level of the hook of the hamate, showing thickening and increased signal intensity involving the median nerve (large arrow) which is interposed between the transverse carpal ligament (arrowheads) and the superficial row of flexor tendons. Note the thickening of soft tissues between the flexor tendons of the carpal tunnel, consistent with associated synovial hyperplasia.

chronic CTS should respond well to conservative measures. The underlying pathophysiology at this stage is transient epineural ischemia and impaired axonal transport, which are thought to be reversible.[62] Resting splints for use at work and at night can relieve pressure on the carpal tunnel. Modifying positions or movements that contribute to CTS will help control symptoms and promote healing. Steroid injections into the carpal tunnel provide temporary relief in <80% of patients; however, <22% of patients have lasting relief a year after injection.[25] Physical agents have been used to treat CTS, but their effectiveness has not been measured. Clinically, iontophoresis appears effective for the patient in the early stages of chronic CTS, but controlled studies of its effectiveness have not been conducted. Soft tissue mobilization, joint mobilization, and neural mobilization may help increase the mobility of the structures in the carpal tunnel.

Surgery has been advocated as an effective treatment for the patients with long term chronic CTS,

but some patients experience no relief after surgery.[20,29] After surgery, early mobilization is essential to prevent any adhesions from compromising the mobility of or the space around the median nerve in the tunnel. Treatment may include passive mobilization of the wrist and hand; soft tissue mobilization to the skin incision and the transverse carpal ligament; mobilization of the carpal bones; and neural tissue mobilization.[12,39] Endoscopic carpal tunnel release is being studied as a new method of treatment, and it may improve the post–operative results by inducing less surgical trauma.

Patients must be taught ways to modify repetitive stresses to the carpal tunnel. Early treatment and education will help reduce treatment time, optimize function, and prevent recurrence. Modification of stresses may include changing work heights; altering wrist and hand postures; taking short, frequent breaks from stressful activities; and early treatment when symptoms are recognized. Permanent modification of adverse ergonomic factors at work may be necessary. Unfortunately, these changes are often ignored in favor of prolonged passive treatments.

Colles' Fracture

Fracture of the distal radius, with or without concurrent fracture to the distal ulna, is called a Colles' Fracture. It is one of the most common fractures of the wrist. The incidence is higher in older women than men, possibly due to the prevalence of osteoporosis. Malunion of the fracture site with resulting deformity is common. The most common complication after injury is the development of neural related problems such as RSD and CTS.[4] A recent study has suggested that the nervous system may be responsible for range of motion limitations in up to 35% of Colles' Fracture patients.[4] Rarely, the EPL tendon may be ruptured as a result of the tendon being stressed at or near a malunion fracture site.

History

Generally the mechanism of injury is a fall on an outstretched hand, with the shoulder mildly externally rotated and abducted and the elbow extended. The fracture involves the distal radius and can include the distal ulna. Closed reduction is commonly performed unless surgical intervention is indicated. Some type of immobilization (usually a cast) is required for up to six weeks. Patients may be progressed through a number of successively smaller casts that allow early movement in the hand and fingers, ending with a soft brace. The patient may not be referred to physical therapy until fracture complications, such as RSD or decreased range of motion, become bothersome.

Signs/Symptoms

The Colles' fracture patient may complain of stiffness in the elbow, wrist, and hand. Intermittent pain and paresthesias into the hand may signify developing neural complications, such as CTS and RSD. Pain complaints out of proportion to the problem may indicate the development of RSD. If RSD is present or is developing after a Colles' Fracture, any of the following signs may be present:

- moderate restriction of movement in all directions

- moderate edema

- moist and cool skin

- smooth and shiny skin

- hypersensitivity to light touch

- weak grip strength

Diagnostics

Radiographs can identify fracture malunions and osteoporosis (Fig 6–44).[34] Osteoporosis is a common finding in the forearm, wrist, and hand after Colles' fracture. If the patient shows progressive neural signs, an EMG may be needed to clarify any nerve impairment.

Problem List

Common problems associated with Colles' Fracture include:

1. Pain and stiffness with wrist and hand use

2. Residual range of motion limitations after immobilization

3. Decreased functional use of the hand and wrist in ADL

4. Concurrent median nerve involvement at the carpal tunnel

5. Concurrent RSD

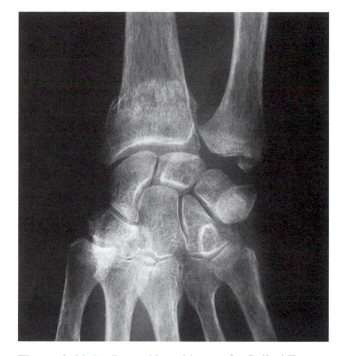

Figure 6–44. Radiographic evidence of a Colles' Fracture involving the distal portions of the radius and ulna.

Treatment

After the fracture is healed, early mobilization is essential to optimize function and reduce treatment time. Accessory motions at the wrist and hand should be mobilized if they are limited. Early stress loading to the forearm, wrist, and hand is recommended to prevent or treat RSD.[15] Stress loading is progressive longitudinal loading of the limb to increase weight bearing tolerance (Fig 6–45). The patient should be encouraged to use the limb in daily activities. When edema and pain are under control, the patient should gradually begin functional strengthening and proprioceptive activities. These should simulate daily activities. Early treatment and education will help reduce treatment time and optimize function.

If RSD develops as a complication to Colles' Fracture, sympathetic nerve blocks may be used to reduce sympathetic activity to the limb and break up the pain cycle. Treating associated findings in the thoracic spine may indirectly reduce sympathetic activity.[11]

Wrist Sprains

Wrist ligament sprains are common injuries in the workplace and in recreational activities. Sprains can occur when the wrist is overstretched, especially

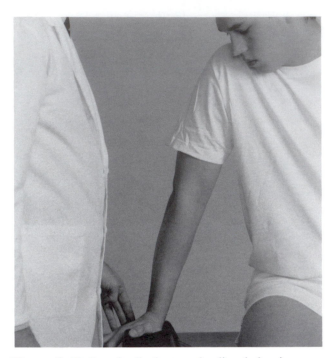

Figure 6–45. Longitudinal stress loading helps increase weight-bearing tolerance.

when it is loaded. A hyperextension injury is the most common.

The interplay between carpal bones during wrist movement is complex. The center of motion in the wrist is the capitate, and the other carpal bones rotate and translate around it as the wrist moves.[19] The distal row of carpals is rigidly fixed to the metacarpals and to each other. The tendons of the wrist flexors and extensors attach to this row. The wrist is predisposed to ligamentous sprains because the proximal row of carpal bones has no direct tendinous attachments. The movements of the proximal row of carpals are controlled by indirect forces and modified by ligamentous restraints.[35] In neutral, the scaphoid rests in a flexed position and the triquetrum is slightly extended; thus, the ligamentous restraints tend to flex the scaphoid and extend the triquetrum. As long as the triquetrolunate and scaphulolunate ligaments are intact, the proximal row of carpal bones remains in balance. If there are instabilities between the carpal bones, the wrist will not have normal synchronous motion.

History

Patients with wrist sprains should be evaluated carefully. The history and mechanism of injury

should be noted. Commonly, the patient falls on an outstretched hand and hyperextends the wrist. Hyperflexion is less common. Another common mechanism of injury is a forceful twisting action, such as turning a screwdriver against resistance. The patient often hears a pop or a snap in the wrist. This is common for an injury to the scaphulolunate ligament.[35] Some patients may have a history of gradually increasing wrist problems without specific injury.

Signs/Symptoms

Patients may complain of sudden pain, weakness, snapping, clicking, or clunking of the wrist with movement or with a forcible grip.[1] Swelling depends on the acuteness of the injury. Motion may be limited. Structural examination is difficult because the wrist ligaments are not directly palpable.[1] The key is to try to localize the signs and symptoms with a thorough examination. The severity and irritability of the condition should be considered when performing palpation and mobility tests. The anatomic "snuff box" should be palpated for tenderness—particularly the scaphoid bone, which is commonly fractured. Watson's test for scaphulolunate ligament injury may be positive. The triquetrolunate stability, ulnar snuff box, and lunate displacement tests may be positive, depending on the specific ligaments involved in the injury. Palpation of the hook of the hamate may cause pain if this bone was fractured. The other carpal bones should also be palpated. Carpal joint play motions should be tested as shown in Chapter 11, Mobilization Techniques. Ligamentous injury may result in pain or excessive mobility on testing.

Diagnostics

Routine radiographs of the wrist usually rule out fracture or abnormal carpal position. If these are negative, but the examination is consistent with instability signs, then cineradiography can be considered. This may include videotape cineradiograph while the patient performs the motion that reproduces the complaints or while the clinician stresses the wrist. This test is particularly useful if the patient complains of "clunking" with wrist motion.

Arthrography can also identify ligament injury (Fig 6–46). Bone scans can be used as a screening test if the radiographs were negative. A follow up

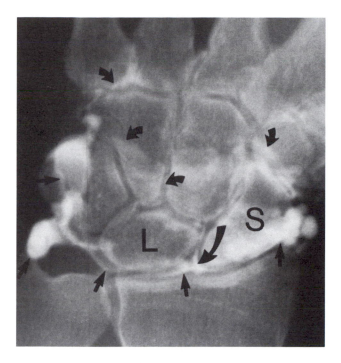

Figure 6–46. Wrist arthrogram showing a scaphulolunate ligament tear. After injection of iodinated contrast into the radiocarpal joint, contrast is seen throughout normal recesses of the radiocarpal joint (straight arrows), as well as extending through a tear of the scaphulolunate ligament (large curved arrow) into the mid carpal and carpometacarpal joints (small curved arrows).

tomogram may be performed if the bone scan is positive. The tomogram can identify a fracture site. Finally, an arthroscopic examination can identify specific ligament injury and inspect the articular cartilage.

Problem List

Patients with wrist sprains can have the following problems:

1. Wrist pain with activity
2. Limited wrist range of motion
3. Joint noise during functional movement of the wrist (clunking)
4. Swelling
5. Temporary weakness or the wrist "giving way"

Treatment

Mild wrist sprains may require immobilization during strenuous activities. PRICE and activity

modification are often useful. If instability is present, treatment will depend on the site, severity, and functional disability from the injury. Less severe sprains can be immobilized with a cast or brace. After immobilization, it is important to begin range of motion and stretching exercises to restore function and prevent reinjury. Friction massage may be used to promote healing and to increase the mobility of the collagen fibers without stressing the ligament longitudinally. If the patient has post–immobilization tightness, it may be necessary to stretch the joint. Ultrasound can be used before or during stretching. Progressive functional activities should be included in treatment. These should include progressive strengthening and stress loading activities. A wrist brace may help reduce the chance of reinjury.

There are many surgical procedures used to stabilize the unstable wrist. They range from primary ligament repair and reconstruction to internal fixation and even arthrodesis. The clinician should work closely with the surgeon to establish reasonable post–operative guidelines for restoring mobility and functional ability. Generalized treatment guidelines for these problems have not been established. Some degree of permanent impairment may occur after any severe wrist ligament injury.[1]

Finger Sprains

Purely ligamentous injuries or sprains occur frequently in the hand. These injuries deserve special attention, but many people treat them casually. Improper treatment may result in prolonged impairment or even permanent disability.[22,52] These injuries are very common in the workplace and in sport or recreational activities. They are often referred to as a "jammed" finger. These sprains may occur at the CMC, MCP, PIP, and DIP joints. Sprains at any of these joints present with similar appearances but differing degrees of severity. The goal of therapy to identify the specific injury and follow up with treatment aimed at restoring functional movement. Chip fractures must be ruled out because a displaced intra–articular fracture may require surgical intervention. Injury to the volar plate is common in dislocation injuries of the MCP and IP joints. Recurrent injury is very common. The CMC joint of the thumb is particularly prone to subtle reinjury and stresses. These repetitive traumas may lead to arthritic changes, which are commonly found at this joint. An injury to the ulnar collateral ligament of the thumb at the MCP joint is sometimes called "skier's thumb" because of the high incidence of this injury in skiers. Early intervention and specific diagnosis are critical to appropriate management of these problems. Prompt attention can spare many patients from unnecessary impairment.[22,52]

History

Most of these injuries have an acute traumatic history, but sprain of the CMC at the thumb may present more subtly. Recurrent injury is common in these finger joints. The joints are usually injured by a twisting and jamming force on the end of the finger. Other mechanisms include hyperextension or overstretching by radial or ulnar forces. The mechanism of the injury directs the examination toward the specific structures involved. Many patients ignore the initial injury and continue daily activities, without interruption, at the expense of prolonged symptoms and dysfunction. Dislocations are sometimes "relocated" by a lay person; however, improper relocation may displace a fracture within the joint.

Signs/Symptoms

The patient complains of pain, stiffness, and easy aggravation of the problems with activity. Physical examination may show edema and limited mobility, depending on the severity of the injury. Crepitus in an acutely injured joint may indicate a fracture. Specific ligament testing is needed to identify the injured structures. Likewise, specific palpation for tenderness and instability helps locate the involved ligaments. The eraser end of a pencil can help palpate the exact location of ligament injury. The collateral ligaments of the MCP joints should be tested in their tightened positions: MCP flexion, IP joints in <20° of flexion. Any patient who may have a fracture that has not been ruled out by standard radiographs or who has moderate to severe instability should be referred to an orthopædic hand specialist.

Diagnostics

Standard radiographs are done routinely to confirm or rule out a fracture. Radiographs with oblique views, tomograms, and CT scans can clarify the specific injury. Stress views are occasionally taken to further clarify the injury.

Problem List

Common problems associated with finger sprains include:

1. Pain with active movement limiting functional hand use

2. Swelling around the involved joint

3. Range of motion limitation

4. Ligamentous instability

5. Grip weakness due to pain and dysfunction

Treatment

Treatment of the minor sprains may only involve a simple "buddy" taping (taping one finger to its neighbor) to provide some stabilization (Fig 6–47). PRICE treatment is recommended and activity modification advised. Recurrent injury can delay healing and may progress to instability. The common positions for immobilization are:

- MCP joints: 60–75° flexion

- IP joints: 10–30° flexion

- Thumb: functional attitude of opposition.[52]

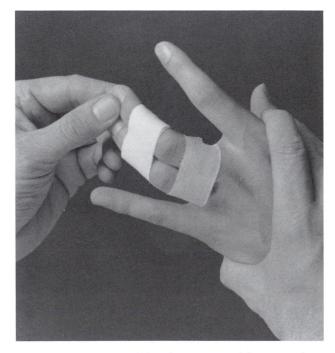

Figure 6–47. Buddy taping for support of finger sprains.

The preferred immobilization position may vary based on specific injuries. There are a variety of MCP shell splints (Fig 6–48) and IP splints available to immobilize the joints. The period of immobilization can be 2–6 weeks; some severe injuries require longer immobilization.

Joint motion should be encouraged as soon as possible to prevent contractures. Joint mobilization techniques are commonly used to regain mobility after immobilization. Joint mobilization after immobilization for an MCP fracture has been shown to significantly increase joint active range of motion and decrease joint stiffness.[57] Dynamic splints can augment the passive mobility treatments. Ultrasound can be used with prolonged physiological stretching to help regain normal joint mobility. Strengthening exercises and exercises that simulate functional activities should be added as the symptoms allow.

de Quervain's Disease

The most common tendinitis at the wrist is inflammation of the tendon sheaths of the abductor pollicis longus and extensor pollicis brevis. This inflammation occurs at the first extensor compartment, where the tendons pass over the radial aspect of the distal radius (Fig 6–49). This condition is called de Quervain's Disease, named after the Swiss surgeon who first reported it in 1895. These tendons lie in a bony groove in the radial styloid and are covered by the fibrous extensor retinaculum. The superficial radial nerve is close to the first extensor compartment. Concurrent problems with entrapment or irritation of this nerve[39] should be assessed.

Problems with pain in the area of the first extensor compartment are frequently misdiagnosed.[68] de Quervain's Disease usually results from repetitive overuse in activities that require simultaneous thumb and wrist movements (e.g., wringing motions or gripping tools in ulnar deviation). With these movements, the tendon sheaths of the first extensor compartment are stressed in the bony groove and under the retinaculum. They may become 2–4 times thicker than normal, and the tendons may become inflamed, swollen, and frayed from stresses inside the sheath.[16] Repetitive forearm pronation may squeeze the superficial radial nerve between the tendons of the extensor carpi radialis longus and the brachioradialis.[18] External compression from

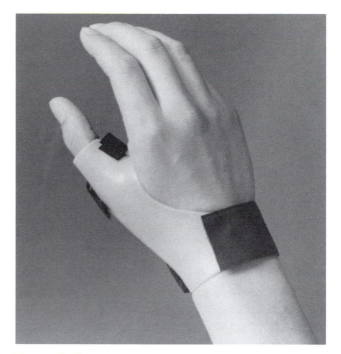

Figure 6–48. Thumb immobilization in an MCP shell splint.

wristwatches and handcuffs may also irritate the nerve.[36,42] Superficial radial nerve compression results in pain and paresthesias from the distal third of the forearm to the wrist. Differentiation between these conditions followed by early intervention is critical to preventing the chronic tissue changes associated with them.

History

The patient usually reports a gradual onset of pain related to repetitive movements. Occasionally, acute trauma is the aggravating factor. The patient may

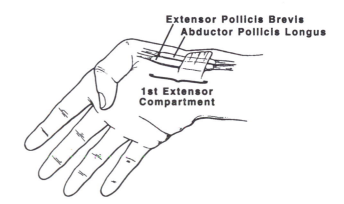

Figure 6–49. de Quervain's Disease occurs at the first extensor compartment.

have difficulty gripping objects due to pain, and many functional activities may be affected. There may be a history of intermittent complaints that led to a constant problem.

Signs/Symptoms

The main complaint is wrist pain near the radial styloid that may radiate proximally up the forearm or distally into the thumb. Swelling may be present near the radial styloid, over the first extensor compartment. There may be tenderness to palpation in this area. The patient may hold the wrist in radial deviation due to pain or constriction in the compartment. Finkelstein's Test will be positive and motion into ulnar deviation may be limited. The clinician must be careful when interpreting Finkelstein's Test because it can give false positive results.[40,69] Symptoms referred into the thumb or up the forearm on testing may indicate involvement of the superficial radial nerve. A simple way to confirm involvement of the superficial radial nerve is to perform the Finkelstein's Test and, while holding the test position, pronate the forearm and extend the elbow; depress the shoulder girdle; and abduct the arm. If the shoulder movements alter the symptoms, the patient's condition has a neural tension component.[11] Tapping the nerve along the radius above the radial styloid may refer symptoms into the thumb if the neural component is present.

Diagnostics

Standard radiographs are invariably negative.[16] They are typically taken only if there is a traumatic onset. Symptom relief after corticosteroid injection into the tendon sheath implicates the first extensor compartment.

Problem List

Patients with de Quervain's Disease may present with any of the following problems:

1. Wrist pain with daily activities
2. Swelling at the first extensor compartment
3. Decreased ulnar deviation with pain
4. Concurrent neural tension signs

Treatment

The treatment of this problem is similar to treatment of other tendinitis and tenosynovitis problems. Initial conservative care includes modifying daily activities, taking anti–inflammatory drugs, and PRICE. Friction massage and ultrasound can decrease inflammation and stimulate healing. Iontophoresis may help decrease the symptoms and allow progression to an improved functional level. Patients with persistent cases may benefit from a corticosteroid injection and temporary use of a resting splint. If neural tension problems are suspected, soft tissue mobilization can increase mobility of the nerve. This treatment should be directed to the area where the superficial radial nerve emerges between the extensor carpi radialis and brachioradialis tendons. Other proximal areas that may cause neural tension problems should be considered for treatment. Mild stretching should be included in the treatment program to improve mobility of the involved tendons at the wrist. It is essential to teach patients to prevent injury and modify aggravating positions.

In severe chronic cases, surgical release of the first extensor compartment may be considered. Common complications after surgery include excessive scar tissue formation on the superficial radial nerve and subluxation of the tendons out of the radial styloid groove on wrist flexion.[10,37]

SUMMARY

The evaluation, treatment, and prevention of problems at the forearm, wrist, and hand has been presented. Complaints in these areas frequently arise from acute trauma or cumulative repetitive trauma. The symptoms felt in the forearm, wrist, and hand can originate in the cervical spine, the shoulder, the elbow, or in the distal areas themselves. The hand depends on the proximal structures for optimal neuromusculoskeletal function. The wrist and hand are rich in vascular supply and contain many intricate mechanical relationships. Injury to this area can devastate function in daily activities. Effective management of problems in the forearm, wrist, and hand should include treatment of all involved neuromusculoskeletal structures.

REFERENCES

1. Amadio P: Ligament Injuries of the Wrist. In Occupational Hand and Upper Extremity Injuries and Diseases. M Kasdan, ed. Hanley & Belfus, Philadelphia PA 1991.

2. American Society for Surgery of the Hand: In The Hand- Examination and Diagnosis, 2nd ed. Churchill-Livingston, New York 1983

3. Armstrong TJ, Chaffin DB: Some Biomechanical Aspects of the Carpal Tunnel. J Biomech 12:567, 1979.

4. Aro H, et al: Late Compression Neuropathics After Colles' Fracture. Clin Orthop and Rel Res 233:217-225, 1988.

5. Aulcine PL, DuPuy TE: Clinical Examination of the Hand. Rehabilitation of the Hand; Surgery and Therapy. J Hunter, et al, ed. CV Mosby, St Louis MO 1990.

6. Bechter CO: The Use of a Dynamometer with Adjustable Handle Spacings. JBJS 36A(4):820-824, 1954.

7. Bendler EM, Greenspun B, et al: The Bilaterality of Carpal Tunnel Syndrome. Arch Phys Med Rehabil 58:362, 1977.

8. Berry TJ: The Hand as a Mirror of Systemic Disease. FA Davis, Philadelphia PA 1963.

9. Blair SJ, et al: Evaluation of Impairment in the Upper Extremity. Clin Orthop and Rel Res 221:42-58, 1987.

10. Burman M: Stenosing Tendovaginitis of the Dorsal and Volar Compartments of the Wrist. Arch Surg 65:752-762, 1952.

11. Butler D: Adverse Neural Tension Disorders Centered in the Limbs. In Mobilisation of the Nervous System. D Butler, ed. Churchill-Livingstone, Melbourne Australia 1991.

12. Butler D: Tension Testing of the Upper Limb. In Mobilisation of the Nervous System. D Butler, ed. Churchill-Livingstone, Melbourne Australia 1991.

13. Callahan AD: Sensibility Testing. In Rehabilitation of the Hand: Surgery and Therapy. J Hunter, ed. CV Mosby, St Louis MO 1990.

14. Canadian Standardized Test of Fitness Operative Manual. Ottawa Fitness and Amateur Sport. Canada, 1986.

15. Carlson LK, Watson HK: Treatment of Reflex Sympathetic Dystrophy Using the Stress-Loading Program. J Hand Ther 1:149-154, 1988.

16. Chipman JR, et al: Tendinitis of the Upper Extremity. In Occupational Hand and Upper Extremity Injury and Disease. M Kasdan, ed. Hanley & Belfus, Philadelphia PA 1991.

17. Cone RO, Szabo R, Resnick D, et al: Computed Tomography of the Normal Soft Tissues of the Wrist. Invest Radiol 18:546, 1983.

18. Dellon SE, Mackinson SE: Susceptibility of the Superficial Sensory Branch of the Radial Nerve to Form Painful Neuromes. J Hand Surg 9B:42-45, 1984.

19. deLunge A, Kauer JMG, and Huiskes R: Kinematic Behavior of the Human Wrist Joint: A Roentgen-Stereo-Photogrammatic Analysis. J of Orthop Res 3:56-64, 1985.

20. Eason SY, Belsole RJ, and Greene TL: Carpal Tunnel Release: Analysis of Suboptimal Results. Journal of Hand Surgery 10-B(3):365-369, 1985.

21. Elvey RL, Quinter JL, Thomas AN: A Clinical Study of Repetitive Strain Injury (RSI). Australian Family Physician 15:1314-1319, 1986.

22. Falconer DP, et al: Occupational Hand Fractures and Dislocations. In Occupational Hand and Upper Extremity Injuries and Diseases. M Kasdan, ed. Hanley & Belfus, Philadelphia PA 1991.

23. Fess EE, Moran CA: Clinical Assessment Recommendation. American Society of Hand Therapists. 1002 Van Dora Springs Rd, Suite 101, Garner NC 27529. Booklet.

24. Flatt AE: Kinesiology of the Hand. American Academy of Orthopaedic Surgery Instructional Course Lectures XVIII. CV Mosby, St. Louis MO 1961.

25. Gelberman RH, et al: Carpal Tunnel Syndrome-Results of Prospective Trial of Steroid Injection and Splinting. JBJS 62A:1181, 1980.

26. Gelberman RH, Hergenroeder PT, et al: The CTS: A Study of Carpal Tunnel Pressures. JBJS 63A:380-383, 1981.

27. Gigis PI, Kuczynski K: The Distal Interphalangeal Joints of Human Fingers. Joul of Hand Surgery 7:176-182, 1982.

28. Hamilton GF, McDonald C, and Chenier TC: Measurement of Grip Strength: Validity and Reliability of the Sphygmomanometer and Jamar Grip Dynamometer. JOSPT 16(5):215-219, 1992.

29. Inglis AE, Straub LR, and Williams CS: Median Nerve Neuropathy at the Wrist. Clin Orthop and Rel Res 83:48-54, 1972.

30. Jetzer TC, Webb AG: The Use of Computer Assisted Tomography in the Analysis of CTS in VDT Users and Assemblers. Cumulative Trauma Syndrome, 1986. Abstract.

31. John V, Nau HE, et al: CT of Carpal Tunnel Syndrome. AJNR 4:770-772, 1983.

32. Jones LA: The Assessment of Hand Function: A Critical Review of Techniques. Joul of Hand Surgery 14A:221-228, 1989.

33. Kauer JMG: Functional Anatomy of the Wrist. Clin Orthop 149:9-20, 1980.

34. Lankford LL: Reflex Sympathetic Dystrophy. In Rehabilitation of the Hand: Surgery and Therapy,

3rd ed. CV Mosby Co 1990.

35. Linscheid RL, Dobyns JH, et al: Traumatic Instability of the Wrist: Diagnosis, Classification, and Pathomechanics. JBJS 54A:1612-1632, 1972.

36. Linscheid RL: Injuries to the Radial Nerve at the Wrist. Arch of Surg 91:942-946, 1965.

37. Lister B: The Hand: Diagnosis and Indications, 2nd ed. Churchill-Livingstone, New York NY 1984.

38. MacConaill MA, Basmajian JV: Muscles and Movement: A Basis for Human Kinesiology. Williams & Wilkins, Baltimore MD 1969.

39. MacKinnon SE, Dellon AL: Surgery of the Peripheral Nerve. Thieme, New York NY 1988.

40. MacKinnon SE: Nerve Compression Syndromes. In Current Therapy in Plastic and Reconstructive Surgery. JL Marsh, ed. BC Decker, Philadelphia PA 1989.

41. Magee D: Forearm, Wrist, and Hand. In Orthopaedic Physical Assessment, 2nd ed. WB Saunders, Philadelphia PA 1992.

42. Massey EW, Pleet AB: Handcuffs and Cheiralgia Paresthetica. Neurology 28:1312-1313, 1978.

43. Mathiowetz V, Kashman N, Volland G, et al: Grip and Pinch Strength: Normative Data For Adults. Arch Phys Med Rehabil 66:69-74, 1985.

44. Mathiowetz V, Weber K, et al: Reliability and Validity of Grip and Pinch Strength Evaluations. Joul of Hand Surgery 9A:222-226, 1984.

45. Mathiowetz V, Weimer D, and Freeman S: Grip and Pinch Strength: Norms for 6-19 Year Olds. Am J Occup Ther 40:705-711, 1986.

46. Mennell J: Joint Pain. Little-Brown, Boston MA 1964.

47. Mitchell F, Moran P, Pruzzo N: An Evaluation and Treatment Manual of Osteopathic Muscle Energy Procedures. Mitchell, Moran and Pruzzo Associates, Valley Park MI 1979.

48. Mosley LH, et al: Cumulative Trauma Disorders and Compression Neuropathies of the Upper Extremities. In Occupational Hand and Upper Extremity Injuries. M Kasdan, ed. Hanley & Belfus, Philadelphia PA 1991.

49. Nathan P, et al: Obesity as a Risk Factor For Slowing of Sensory Conduction of the Median Nerve in Industry. Joul of Occ Med 34(4):379-383, 1992.

50. Nathan PA, et al: Occupation as a Risk Factor For Impaired Sensory Conduction of the Medican Nerve at the Carpal Tunnel. J of Hand Surg 13B:167, 1988.

51. Nathan PA, et al: Relationship of Age and Sex to Sensory Conduction of the Median Nerve at the Carpal Tunnel and Association of Slowed Conduction with Symptoms. Muscle Nerve 11:1149, 1988.

52. Noellert RC, Hankin FM: Ligament Injuries of the Hands. In Occupational Hand and Upper Extremity Injuries and Diseases. M Kasdan, ed. Hanley & Belfus, Philadelphia PA 1991.

53. Palmer AK, Werner FW: The Triangular Fibrocartilage Complex of the Wrist: Anatomy and Function. Joul of Hand Surgery 6:152, 1981.

54. Palmer ML, Epler M: Clinical Assessment Procedures in Physical Therapy. JB Lippincott, Philadelphia PA 1990.

55. Phalen GS: The Carpal Tunnel Syndrome. Seventeen Years Experience in Diagnosis and Treatment of 654 Hands. JBJS 48A:211, 1966.

56. Radonjic D, Long CL: II. Kinesiology of the Wrist. Am J of Phys Med 50:57-71, 1971.

57. Randall T, et al: Effects of Joint Mobilization on Joint Stiffness and Active Motion of the MCP Joint. JOSPT 16(1):30-36, 1992.

58. Robertson A, Dietz J: A Description of Grip Strength in Pre-school Children. Am J Occup Ther 42:647-652, 1988.

59. Sandzen SC: Atlas of Wrist and Hand Fractures. PSG Publishing, Littleton MA 1979

60. Sarrafian SK, Melamed JL, and Goshgarian GM: Study of Wrist Motion in Flexion and Extension. Clin Orthop 126:153-159, 1977.

61. Soderberg G: Wrist and Hand. In Kinesiology - Application to Pathological Motion. Williams & Wilkins, Baltimore MD 1986.

62. Szabo RM, Gelberman RH: The Pathophysiology of Nerve Entrapment Syndromes. J Hand Surg 12A:880, 1987.

63. Szabo RM, Madison M: Management of Carpal Tunnel Syndrome. In Occupational Hand and Upper Extremity Injuries and Diseases. M Kasdan, ed. Hanley & Belfus, Philadelphia PA 1991.

64. Taleisnik J: Carpal Instability. JBJS 70A:1262-1268, 1988.

65. Tubiana R: The Hand. WB Saunders, Philadelphia PA 1981.

66. Wadsworth CT: Clinical Anatomy and Mechanics of the Wrist and Hand. JOSPT 4:206-216, 1983.

67. Watson HK, et al: Limited Triscaphoid Intercarpal Arthrodesis For Rotary Subluxation of the Scaphoid. JBJS 68A:345-349, 1986.

68. Werner CD, et al: Pressure and Nerve Lesions in the Carpal Tunnel. Acta Orthop Scand 54:312-316, 1983.

69. Wood MB, Dobyns JH: Sports-related Extra-articular Wrist Syndromes. Clin Orthop 202:93-102, 1978.

70. Yamaguchi DM, Lipscomb PR and Soule EH: Carpal Tunnel Syndrome. Minnesota Medicine 48:22-33

71. Youm Y, Gillespie TE, et al: Kinematic Investigation of Normal MCP Joints. J Biomech 11:109-118, 1978.

72. Youm Y, McMurty RY, et al: Kinematics of the Wrist: 1. An Experimental Study of Radial-Ulnar Deviation and Flexion-Extension. JBJS 60:423-431, 1978.

SECTION 3
The Lower Quarter

CHAPTER 7

THE HIP

INTRODUCTION

The hip joint is the proximal joint in the kinematic chain of the lower limb. It stabilizes and controls the position of the lower limb. The hip is responsible for handling large joint forces from repetitive loads and from muscular contractions, so it is very susceptible to joint pathology.

The hip exerts a mechanical influence on the pelvis and the lumbar spine. Pain felt in the hip can be referred from either of these areas. Pelvic obliquity is frequent cause of hip pain and arthritis.[4,8] Abnormal mechanics or pathology in the knee, foot, and ankle can affect symptoms and joint integrity at the hip. Effective management of hip problems needs to include these related neuromusculoskeletal structures.

FUNCTIONAL ANATOMY

Osseous and Capsuloligamentous Components

The hip joint is a multiaxial ball and socket joint formed between the femoral head and the acetabulum. The acetabulum is the fused portion of the pelvis and consists of the ilium, ischium, and pubic bones (Fig 7–1). It faces anterolaterally in an inferior direction. A labrum attaches to the acetabulum and effectively deepens the socket. The functional articular surface of the acetabulum is called the lunate surface.[46] (Fig 7–2). It is covered by articular cartilage that is thick superiorly and is absent inferiorly.[25] The femoral head forms the shape of 2/3 of a sphere and is largely covered with articular cartilage.

The hip joint is covered by an extensive capsule blended with three strong ligaments: the iliofemoral or "Y" ligament, which resists extension; the ischiofemoral ligament, which resists extension and internal rotation; and the pubofemoral ligament, which resists abduction (Fig 7–3). The femoral neck forms a 135° angle with the shaft of the femur. The femoral head is anterior to the frontal plane so that the long axis of the femoral neck is rotated ≈15° anterior to the long axis of the femur. This is called *anteversion* and the reverse is called *retroversion* (Fig 7–4). Excessive anteversion will position the lower limb in internal rotation. Retroversion will position the limb in external rotation.

The capsule, the ligaments and the deep acetabulum provide stability; however, due to the superincumbent body weight (compression) and muscular forces across this joint (Table 7–1), large shear forces are generated. The motions available at the hip are flexion, extension, abduction, adduction, internal rotation, and external rotation. Table 7–2 summarizes the movements and range of motion at the hip.

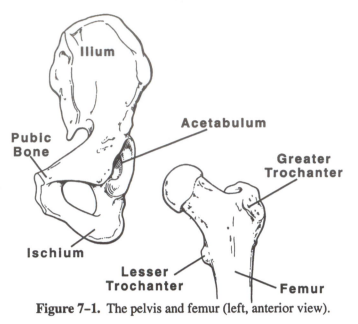

Figure 7–1. The pelvis and femur (left, anterior view).

Neuromuscular Components

Muscular Structures

The muscles of the hip are classified according to their function: flexors and extensors; abductors and adductors; and internal and external rotators. Hip position can greatly influence the actions of the muscles around the hip (Table 7–3).[13] Many of the muscles that cross the hip also affect other joints. Some of these will be discussed in this section, and others will be discussed in Chapter 8, The Knee. The muscles that act on the hip are shown in Figure 7–5.

Extensors

The most powerful hip extensors are the gluteus maximus and the hamstrings. They function in a closed kinematic chain in many daily activities, such as getting up from a chair, lifting, stair climbing, running, and jumping. The hamstrings also flex the knee in an open kinematic chain.

Flexors

The two prime movers of hip flexion are the iliacus and psoas major muscles, collectively referred to as iliopsoas. In an open kinematic chain, the iliopsoas flexes the hip. In a closed kinematic chain, iliopsoas contraction tilts the pelvis anteriorly, increases lumbar lordosis, and can help flex or extend the lumbar spine. If the trunk is already flexed, iliopsoas contraction causes further flexion. If the

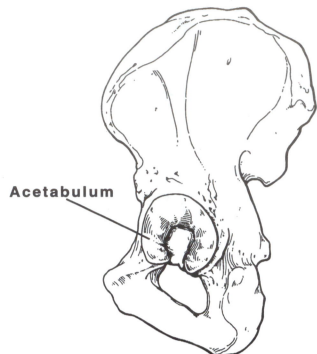

Figure 7–2. The lunate surface of the acetabulum.

trunk is already extended, iliopsoas contraction causes further extension.[12]

Abductors

The hip abductors are important in weightbearing at the hip and pelvis. The most important abductors are the gluteus medius and gluteus minimus muscles. Their primary weightbearing function is to pull the pelvis toward the ipsilateral femur when standing on one leg (and at the mid–stance phase in the gait cycle; see Chapter 10, Gait Evaluation). This prevents the pelvis from dropping on the opposite side. Weakness in these muscles often causes a lack of control of the pelvis, presenting as a Trendelenburg gait pattern (see Chapter 10). The medius and the minimus work with the tensor fascia latæ and piriformis to abduct the femur from the midline in an open kinematic chain.

Adductors

The adductor muscles have a much less important role than the abductors. They contract during the swing phase of gait (see Chapter 10) and can participate as accessory muscles in rotation and extension, depending on the position of the thigh.[46]

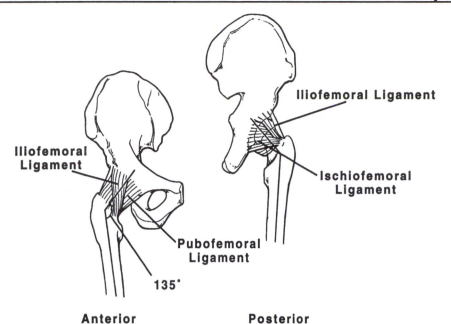

Figure 7–3. Ligaments of the hip. The normal angle of inclination at the hip is 135° (right hip).

Internal/External Rotators

The prime movers of internal rotation are the anterior fibers of the gluteus medius and gluteus minimus muscles.[16] As many as nine muscles can contribute to this motion.[46] The prime movers of external rotation are the obturator externus and quadratus femoris, but other muscles contribute to this movement.[46] The rotators fine–tune the position of the femur in the gait cycle in both the open and closed kinematic chains.

In summary, movement of the hip is a result of joint configuration and the forces created by the muscles crossing the joint. These forces are affected by weightbearing status and the position of the hip. The hip muscles, their actions, and their segmental and peripheral nerve innervations are shown in Table 7–4.

Neural Structures

Two neural structures are subject to entrapment in the hip region: the lateral femoral cutaneous nerve (anteriorly) and the sciatic nerve (posteriorly).

Lateral Femoral Cutaneous Nerve (LFCN)

The lateral femoral cutaneous nerve (LFCN) is an entirely sensory nerve that originates as a branch of the upper lumbar nerve roots (L2 and L3) in the lumbar plexus. The lumbar plexus is imbedded in the psoas major muscle at its origin, and the nerves arising from the plexus (including the LFCN) must exit from the psoas muscle.[28] The LFCN emerges from the lateral margin of the psoas major and passes through the pelvis. It then courses beneath the inguinal ligament near its attachment to the anterior

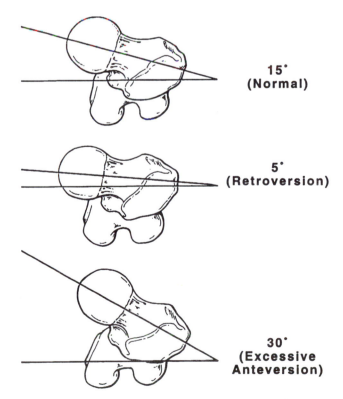

Figure 7–4. Anteversion and retroversion at the hip.

Table 7–1. Forces at Hip under Different Loading Conditions[37]

Standing	0.33 x TBW
Single leg stance	2.40 to 2.60 x TBW
Walking	1.30 to 5.80 x TBW
Climbing stairs	3.00 to 6.00 x TBW
Running	≈4.50 x TBW

TBW = total body weight

superior iliac spine (ASIS) and into the tensor fascia latæ tissue (Fig 7–6).

The inguinal ligament is the main source of compression or irritation of the LFCN, resulting in anterolateral thigh aching, burning, and paresthesia.[15,29,40,49] The common term for symptoms caused by LFCN entrapment is "meralgia paresthesias."

Sciatic Nerve

The sciatic nerve originates from the sacral plexus and forms as the fibers pass through the sciatic foramen of the pelvis. The nerve then passes under the piriformis muscle, occasionally splits the muscle, courses distally to enter the thigh via the sciatic notch near the ischial tuberosity, and then passes through the hamstring muscles. The anterior portion of the nerve arises from anterior branches of the ventral rami of L4–S3 and forms the tibial nerve. The posterior portion of the nerve, which arises from the posterior branches of the lumbosacral trunk (L4–S2), forms the common peroneal nerve. The pathway of the sciatic nerve at the hip is shown in Figure 7–7.

Table 7–2. Movements and Range of Motion at the Hip

Flexion	110-120°
Extension	10-15°
Abduction	30-50°
Adduction	30°
Internal rotation	30-40°
External rotation	40-60°

The piriformis muscle is a common site of sciatic nerve entrapment;[52] however, the hamstring muscles can be involved in sciatic nerve compression and irritation, as evidenced by positive neural tension signs (positive Slump test) in athletes with diagnoses of Grade I hamstring strains.[2,5,32,34] There is also surgical evidence that myofascial bands of the biceps femoris muscle can entrap the sciatic nerve.[2,5,32,34,53]

EVALUATION

Subjective Examination

The subjective examination should proceed as described in Chapter 2, Principles of Extremity Evaluation. The patient's main complaints provide valuable clues that help the clinician plan the objective examination. Knowing the mechanism of injury can help the clinician identify the structures involved. For example, complaints of anterior hip pain after performing unaccustomed running are probably caused by a hip flexor muscle strain and not a capsular injury; however, anterior hip pain caused by an acute fall probably involves the joint and its capsular structures rather than the muscles. Acute falls can cause a femoral fracture. In some cases, however, a pathological fracture causes a fall, especially in the elderly. Gradual onset of symptoms and loss of motion is consistent with the progression of osteoarthritis. The symptoms of joint injuries are usually made worse in weightbearing because of the large forces transmitted across the hip (Table 7–1).

A thorough medical history should be obtained to rule out systemic arthritic conditions, cancer, or other non–musculoskeletal etiologies. Symptoms felt in the hip can be referred from the pelvis, knee, or lumbar spine. Symptoms from the hip can refer to the thigh, knee, and lower leg. Asking about the specific postures, movements, and activities of work, sport, home, and recreation will help the functional assessment. The patterns of the symptoms should guide the objective examination.

Planning the Objective Examination

The objective examination of the hip should be based on the information gained from the subjective examination. Excessive provocation of the problem can lead to an inaccurate picture of the patient's condition; therefore, it helps to prioritize the tests to

Table 7–3. Primary and Secondary Muscle Actions at Different Angles of Hip Flexion

	0° Primary	0° Secondary	40° Primary	40° Secondary	90° Primary	90° Secondary
Adductor brevis	Ad		Ad		Ad	E
Adductor longus	Ad	F	Ad		Ad	E
Adductor magnus (middle fibers)	Ad	E	E	Ad	E	Ad
Adductor magnus post. fibers)	E	Ad	E		E	Ad
Adductor minimus	Ad		Ad		Ad	E
Biceps femoris	E		E		E	
Gemellus inferior	ER		ER			
Gemellus superior	ER		ER	Ab	Ab	
Gluteus maximus	E					
Gluteus medius (anterior fibers)	Ab		IR	Ab	IR	
Gluteus medius (middle fibers)	Ab	Ab		IR	IR	
Gluteus medius (post. fibers)	Ab	ER	Ab		IR	
Gluteus minimus (anterior fibers)	Ab		IR	Ab	IR	
Gluteus minimus (middle fibers)	Ab		Ab	IR	IR	
Gluteus minimus (post. fibers)	Ab		Ab		IR	
Gracilis	Ad		Ad		Ad	E
Iliopsoas	F		F		F	
Obturator externus	Ad		Ad	ER	ER	
Obturator internus	ER	ER			Ab	
Pectineus	Ad	F	Ad		Ad	
Piriformis	ER	Ab	Ab		Ab	IR
Quadratus femoris	Ad	ER	ER	E	E	ER
Rectus femoris	F	Ab	F		F	Ab
Sartorius	F	Ab	F		F	Ab
Semimembranosus	E		E		E	
Semitendinosus	E		E		E	
Tensor fasciæ latæ	Ab	F	F	Ab	F	Ab

E = extension; F = flexion; Ad = adduction; Ab = Abduction; ER = external rotation; IR = internal rotation

ensure that the most useful information is gained without exacerbating the patient's symptoms. If the patient is unable to sustain certain hip positions, especially in weightbearing, these positions may need to be avoided during the examination. In cases where severe weightbearing symptoms are felt, sinister pathology should be ruled out. Establishing whether or not the patient's symptoms are entirely mechanical is important but not always easy. If it is clear during the subjective examination that the patient's condition is easily provoked, the condition is considered irritable, so the number of motions tested during the examination should be limited. Evaluation of a patient with total hip arthroplasty will be limited to the extent that the motions do not compromise the prosthesis. For this patient, the nature of the problem limits the extent of the examination.

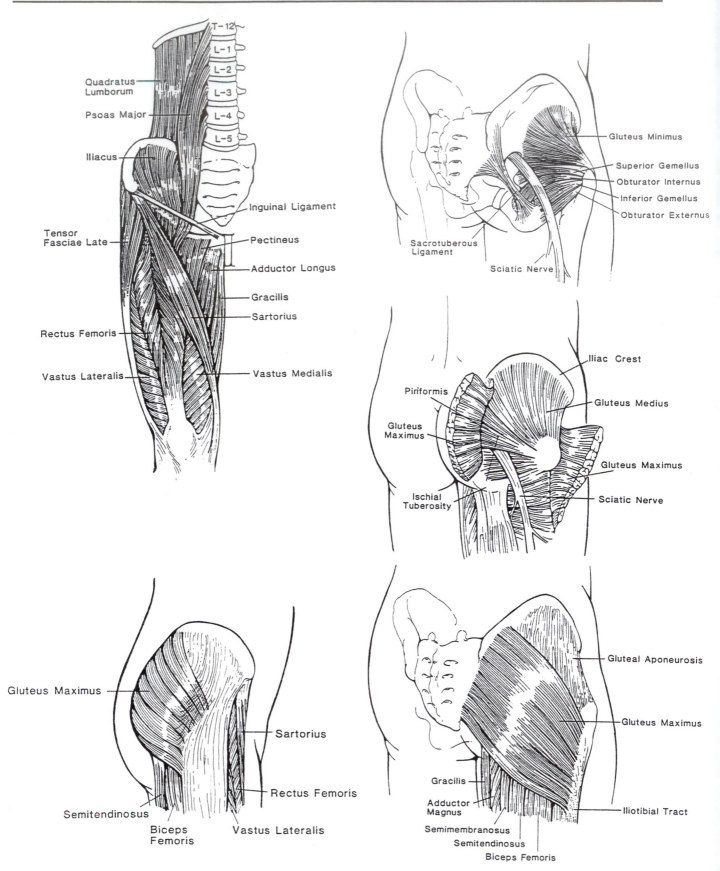

Figure 7–5. Hip muscles.

Table 7–4. Muscles of the Hip: Their Actions, Peripheral Nerve Supplies and Nerve Roots

Muscles	Actions	Peripheral Nerve Supply	Spinal Segment
Adductor brevis	Flexion/adduction/internal rotation	Obturator	L2-L3, L5/L2-L4
Adductor longus	Flexion/adduction/internal rotation	Obturator	L2-L4
Adductor magnus	Abduction/internal rotation	Obturator/Sciatic	L2-L4
Add. magnus (ischiocondylar part)	Extension/adduction	Obturator/Sciatic	L2-L4
Biceps femoris	Extension	Sciatic	L5, S1-S2
Gemellus inferior	External rotation	N. to quadratus femoris	L5, S1
Gemellus superior	External rotation	N. to obturator internus	L5, S1
Gluteus maximus	Extension/abduction/ext. rotation	Inferior gluteal	L5, S1-S2
Gluteus medius	Abduction	Superior gluteal	L5, S1
Gluteus medius (anterior part)	Extension/abduction/int. rotation	Superior gluteal	L5, S1
Gluteus medius (posterior part)	Extension/external rotation	Superior gluteal	L5, S1
Gluteus minimus	Abduction	Superior gluteal	L5, S1
Gluteus minimus (anterior part)	Abduction/internal rotation	Superior gluteal	L5, S1
Gracillus	Flexion/adduction/internal rotation	Obturator	L2-L3
Iliacus	Flexion	Femoral	L2-L3
Obturator externus	External rotation	Obturator	L3-L4
Obturator internus	External rotation	N. to obturator internus	L5, S1
Pectineus	Flexion/adduction/internal rotation	Femoral	L2-L3
Piriformis	External rotation	L5, S1-S2	L5, S1-S2
Psoas	Flexion	L1-L3	L1-L3
Quadratus femoris	External rotation	N. to quadratus femoris	L5, S1
Rectus femoris	Flexion	Femoral	L2-L4
Sartorius	Flexion/abduction/external rotation	Femoral	L2-L3
Semimembranosus	Extension	Sciatic	L5, S1-S2
Semitendinosus	Extension	Sciatic	L5, S1-S2
Tensor fasciæ latæ	Abduction/internal rotation	Superior gluteal	L4-L5

Objective Examination

The objective examination should proceed as outlined in Chapter 2, <u>Principles of Extremity Evaluation</u>. The screening examination should include the lumbo–pelvic area, especially if the patient complains of symptoms radiating from this area to the hip. The quadrant test for the lumbar spine will help clear spinal structures as a cause of hip symptoms (see "Clearing Tests" in Chapter 2, <u>Principles of Extremity Evaluation</u>). The test is positive if it provokes hip pain or lumbo–pelvic signs on the side of the patient's complaints. Hip symptoms that are easily provoked by lumbo–pelvic movements or positions warrant a complete lumbo–pelvic examination before evaluating the hip itself. Any significant findings on the screening examination should be noted and analyzed to identify their contributions to the current complaints at the hip.

Structural Observation

The structural observation begins as the patient walks into the examination room. The gait pattern should be observed, noting the patient's willingness to bear weight on either limb; any side to side differences in stride length; knee position; trunk position; and the quality of active motions (see Chapter 10, <u>Gait Evaluation</u>). The patient's reaction to

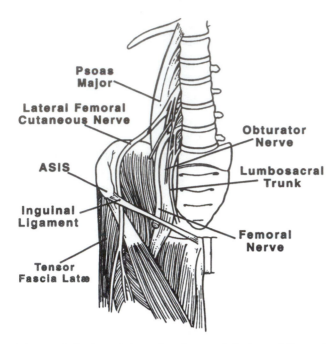

Figure 7–6. The origin and pathway of the lateral femoral cutaneous nerve with potential entrapment site beneath the inguinal ligament

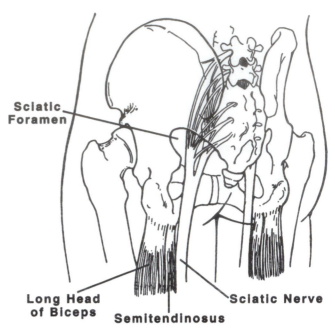

Figure 7–7. The pathway of the sciatic nerve from the spine to the hamstrings. Potential entrapment sites are beneath the piriformis (not shown, see Fig 7–29) and at the hamstrings.

symptoms and use of assistive devices should also be noted.

The patient's standing posture should then be observed from the side, back, and front. The clinician can obtain information about hip and lumbo–pelvic alignment from the side view. Tight hamstrings can cause a posteriorly rotated pelvis, flattened lumbar lordosis, and an extended hip in standing (Fig 7–8, left). Tight hip flexors can cause an anteriorly rotated pelvis, increased lumbar lordosis, and a flexed hip posture in standing (Fig 7–8, right). The contour of the musculature, including the quadriceps anteriorly and the gluteals posteriorly, should be noted bilaterally.

The back view includes an assessment of pelvic obliquity. This is done by comparing bilateral heights of the iliac crests, posterior superior iliac spine (PSIS), trochanters of the hip, ischial tuberosities, and gluteal folds. Any asymmetries should be noted. The relative alignment of the lumbar spine to the sacrum and pelvis should be observed.

The front view includes soft tissue assessment and a quick comparison of the bilateral heights of the

iliac crests, ASIS's, and trochanters of the hip. The standing alignment should be noted. The patient is told to place his or her feet parallel and facing straight ahead a few inches apart. The angle of the hips to the knees is noted. The position of the patella is also

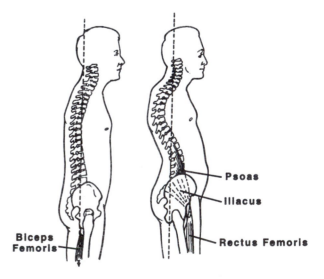

Figure 7–8. Hip muscle length can affect the position of the lumbar spine. Left: tight hamstrings rotate the pelvis posteriorly, extend the hips, and flatten the lumbar lordosis. Right: tight hip flexors rotate the pelvis anteriorly, flex the hips, and increase the lumbar lordosis.

assessed because patellar position will reflect the rotational alignment of the femur (Fig 7–9). "Squinting patellæ" will face inward and reflect anteverted or internally rotated femur alignment. "Frog–eyed" patellæ will face outward, reflecting a retroverted or externally rotated femur alignment.

When inspecting the soft–tissues and bony contours, the color of the skin, any bruises, any incisions or scars, and any edema should be noted. Edema in the hip is difficult to detect unless it results from superficial trauma. Any obvious leg length discrepancy or deformity should also be noted.

Mobility

Physiological Mobility

Physiological mobility refers to the movements of the hip in standard planar and functional combined movements.

Active Mobility

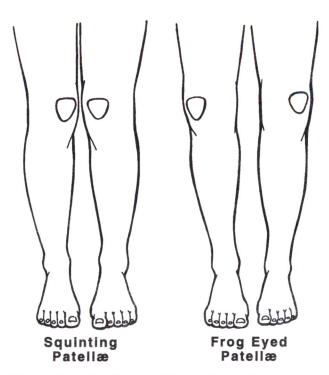

**Squinting   Frog Eyed
Patellæ   Patellæ**

Figure 7–9. Patellar position reflects the rotational alignment of the femur. Left: "Squinting patellæ" reflect femoral anteversion. Right: "Frog-eyed" patellæ reflect femoral retroversion.

Active mobility testing assesses the patient's willingness to move the joint. Overpressure is applied at the end of the available active range of motion to assess the end feel of the joint. The important features to note include: available active range of motion; the symptom complaints during the motion; any crepitus felt or heard (possibly indicating "snapping hip syndrome" or degenerative changes); and the response to overpressure. When performing overpressure, the clinician is assessing whether the range of motion increases or the symptoms change.

The order and number of motions tested will be determined by the subjective clues. For example, motions that by history cause severe symptoms or irritability should be checked last; the clinician may choose to defer testing of motions that will interfere with further examination or cause a non–productive flare–up of complaints. On the other hand, a patient with chronic problems can usually tolerate the full motion testing regime. Comparison should be made to the contralateral limb and to what is expected to be normal. The motions that can be tested at the hip include: flexion, extension, abduction, adduction, internal rotation, and external rotation. Any combination of these motions can be used to further assess function if the subjective clues point to it, or if straight planar motions fail to provoke the symptoms or dysfunction.

Passive Mobility

Passive mobility testing assesses the integrity of the non–contractile components of the hip. Passive mobility should be examined in any movements where active motion is not within normal limits and the clinician is unable to assess the end–feel. Range of motion, symptom response, end–feel, and the pattern of motion restriction should be noted. The clinician should compare results to the opposite limb and to normal responses. The pattern of motion restriction can be capsular or non–capsular. The capsular pattern of the hip is: *internal rotation and abduction more restricted than flexion and extension.*

The symptom response to passive motion can reveal the stage of the problem (see Chapter 2, Principles of Extremity Evaluation). Hip passive range of motion testing is usually performed with the patient supine (Fig 7–10).

Accessory Mobility

Accessory mobility refers to component motions and joint play (see Chapter 2, <u>Principles of Extremity Evaluation</u>). Joint play movements of the hip are usually assessed with the patient supine (see Chapter 11, <u>Mobilization Techniques</u>). The joint play movements of the hip are: distal distraction, lateral distraction, anterior glide, posterior glide, and compression. The clinician should compare findings to the contralateral limb and to normal. These findings include the available range of motion, the end–feel, any crepitus noted, and any symptoms provoked. The results should be consistent with the findings of the physiological mobility examination and will be used to plan treatment. For example, limited lateral distraction and posterior glide is consistent with decreased internal rotation of the hip.

Strength

Manual muscle testing (MMT) assesses the contractile elements of the hip. The tests are performed in the mid–range position to avoid stress on the non–contractile structures. The patient is told to gradually increase effort to a voluntary maximum contraction. This avoids substitution of synergistic muscles. The clinician resists the attempt with an isometric contraction. The muscle strength should be graded and any symptom responses noted. Any muscle acting on, crossing, or influencing the hip should be included. Cyriax's four patterns of response (see Chapter 2, <u>Mobilization Techniques</u>) can help with assessment and the eventual treatment plan. Bilateral comparison should be made.

Functional strength tests at the hip joint can provide additional information about the status of hip musculature. Examples of functional strength tests at the hip include sitting and standing from a chair without use of the arms and placing the foot up on a step (testing hip extensors and flexors, respectively).[43]

Neurological

The neurological examination should be carried out as outlined in Chapter 2, <u>Principles of Extremity Evaluation</u>. Indications for the examination include the patient's complaints of functional weakness, neurological symptoms, or symptoms consistent with neurological involvement. The neurological examination includes motor function, light touch sensation, and deep tendon reflexes (DTR's). Motor function is assessed with resistive muscle tests in lumbosacral myotomes, as performed in the lower quarter screening examination (see Chapter 2,

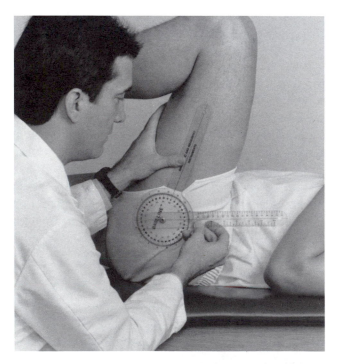

Figure 7–10A. Passive mobility testing at the hip: flexion.

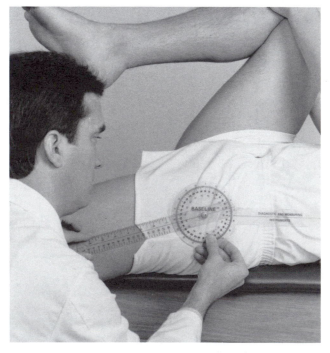

Figure 7–10B. Passive mobility testing at the hip: extension.

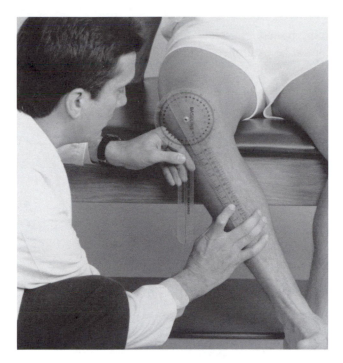

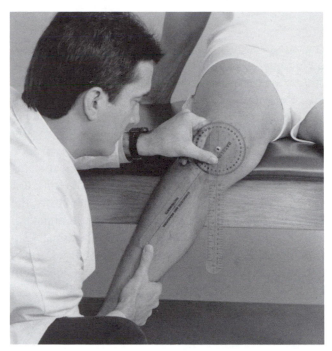

Figure 7-10C. Passive mobility testing at the hip: external rotation.

Figure 7-10D. Passive mobility testing at the hip: internal rotation.

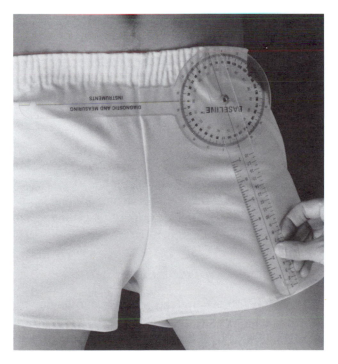

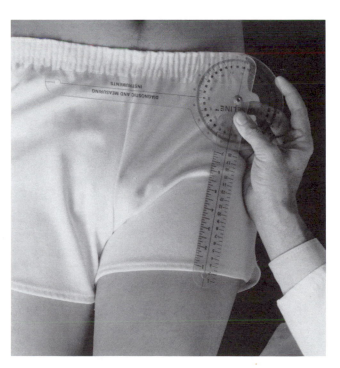

Figure 7-10E. Passive mobility testing at the hip: abduction.

Figure 7-10F. Passive mobility testing at the hip: adduction.

Principles of Extremity Evaluation). Light touch sensation should be tested in the lower limb, including the L1–S4 dermatomes and the regional cutaneous nerve fields (see Fig 2–12 on pages 24 and 25). Relevant DTR's include the knee jerk (L3–L4), the medial hamstring reflex (L5–S1), and the ankle jerk (S1–S2) (see Chapter 2, Principles of Extremity Evaluation). Proprioception of the hip can provide additional information about the neurological status of the hip. Proprioception is tested using the stork test (Fig 7–11). With each of these neurological tests, the involved side should be compared to the contralateral extremity and to normal. Neural tension tests can help implicate the nervous system as a contributor to signs and symptoms at the hip. These tests are more thoroughly described in Chapter 2, Principles of Extremity Evaluation. Internal rotation and adduction of the hip can be added to the SLR and Slump tests to increase their sensitivity.

Palpation

Palpation of the hip should proceed as outlined in Chapter 2, Principles of Extremity Evaluation. The clinician should use the layered palpation technique, gradually proceeding from the surface to deeper tissues. Bilateral comparison should be made. The

skin, bones, muscles, tendons, bursæ, and nerves should be examined. The following structures should be palpated:

Anterior (Fig 7–12)

- anterior superior iliac spines (ASIS's)
- anterior inferior iliac spines (AIIS's)
- lateral femoral cutaneous nerve (LFCN)
- greater trochanters
- trochanteric bursæ
- inguinal ligament
- psoas bursæ
- femoral nerve
- pubic symphysis
- adductor muscles
- flexor muscles

Posterior (Fig 7–13)

- iliac crests
- posterior superior iliac spines (PSIS's)
- ischial tuberosities
- sciatic notches
- gluteal muscles
- piriformis
- hamstring muscles
- abductor muscles

The clinician should try to correlate the palpation findings with the rest of the objective examination findings. Palpation of the sacral and lumbar spine joints should be included if they are thought to contribute to the clinical picture.

Special Tests

Special tests help the clinician rule–out or confirm specific hip pathologies. There are three types of special tests at the hip: musculotendinous, joint and ligamentous, and alignment. These tests are summarized in Table 7–5.

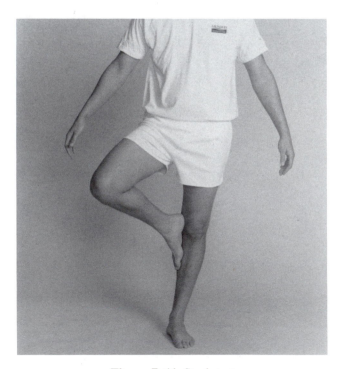

Figure 7–11. Stork test.

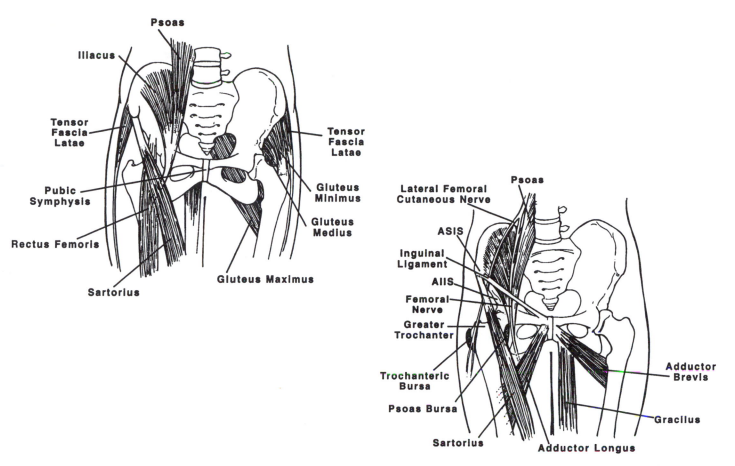

Figure 7–12. Structures to palpate on the anterior hip

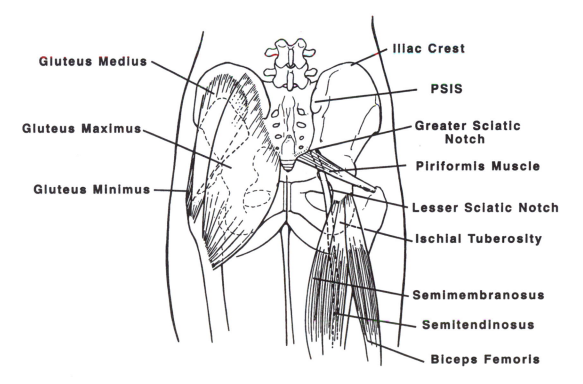

Figure 7–13. Structures to palpate on the posterior hip.

Table 7–5. Special Tests for the Hip

Test Type	Test Name	Purpose
Muscular	Trendelenburg Test	Hip abductor weakness
	Piriformis Test	Piriformis syndrome
	Thomas Test	Tight hip flexors
	Ely's Test	Rectus femoris tightness
	Ober's Test	Iliotibial band tightness
	Noble Compression Test	Iliotibial band friction
	Hamstring Tightness Test	Hamstring tightness
Joint/Ligamentous	Quadrant Test	Articular cartilage Posterolateral joint capsule
	FABERE Test	Hip and pelvic dysfunction
	Torque Test	Capsular stability
Alignment	Craig's Test	Rotational alignment
	Leg Length Tests	Discrepancies in leg length

Musculotendinous Tests

Trendelenburg Test

The Trendelenburg Test is a classic test for weakness in the hip abductor muscles (primarily gluteus medius). The patient is asked to stand on one leg. The test is positive if the pelvis drops on the opposite side, with compensatory lumbar sidebending toward the stance side (Fig 7–14).

Piriformis Test

The piriformis test implicates muscle pain or sciatic nerve impingement.[21,35,51] In sidelying, the clinician places the patient's upside hip in about 60° of flexion and slight internal rotation, then resists abduction and external rotation (Fig 7–15A). A modified version is done in the kneeling position as shown (Fig 7–15B). The test is positive if the patient complains of local muscle symptoms or sciatica.

Thomas Test

The Thomas Test is a classic test for tight hip flexors. The patient assumes the position shown in Figure 7–16A. The test is positive if the extended limb rises from the examination table while the opposite hip is maximally flexed to the chest or if attempts to push the extended thigh to the table result in increased lumbar lordosis. Rectus femoris muscle length is assessed by repeating the Thomas Test with the extended limb off the end of the table; tightness is present when the hip remains slightly flexed and the knee remains extended (Fig 7–16B).

Ely's Test

Ely's Test[26] for rectus femoris tightness is performed with the patient prone. The knee is flexed passively. The test is positive if the same hip flexes as the knee is flexed (Fig 7–17).

Ober's Test

Ober's Test assesses iliotibial band (ITB) tightness (the tendinous extension of the tensor fascia latæ muscle).[42] The test can be performed with the knee flexed or extended; the ITB is most taut in knee extension. In sidelying, the uppermost hip is passively extended and abducted, then relaxed into adduction. The test is positive when the hip does not adduct past midline or when symptoms or complaints of tightness are reproduced (Fig 7–18).

Noble Compression Test

The Noble Compression Test assesses ITB friction syndrome.[41] The patient is supine with hip and knee flexion to 90°. While the clinician palpates the lateral femoral condyle, the patient is asked to extend the knee. The test is positive if the patient complains of pain as the ITB passes over the lateral femoral condyle at ≈30° of flexion (Fig 7–19A). We

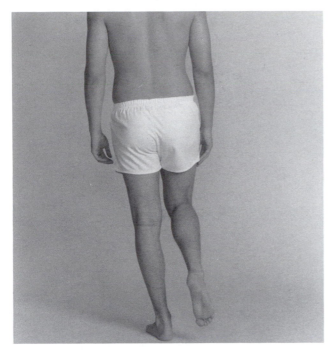

Figure 7–14A. Normal Trendelenberg Test.

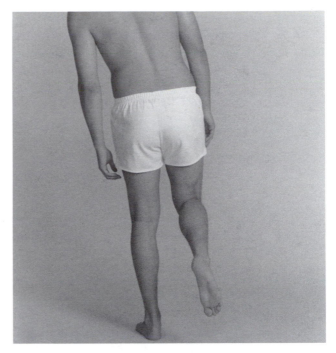

Figure 7–14B. Abnormal Trendelenberg Test.

prefer a modified way to perform the test using the sidelying Ober's Test position (Fig 7–19B).

Hamstring Tightness Tests

Hamstring tightness can be tested in the positions shown in Figure 7–20. These include the long–sitting test, the tripod sign,[1] and the active straight leg raise (SLR).[43] These tests are positive if the pelvis rotates posteriorly as the knee is extended or if the patient is unable to achieve full knee extension. Restriction and symptoms in the hamstring muscle must be differentiated from adverse neural tension and nerve root irritation. If neck flexion or ankle dorsiflexion

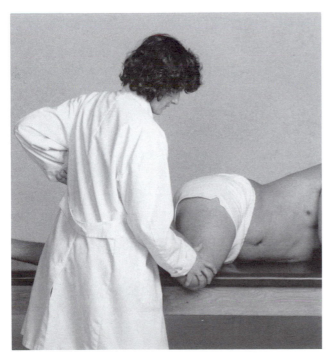

Figure 7–15A. Piriformis test: standard test position.

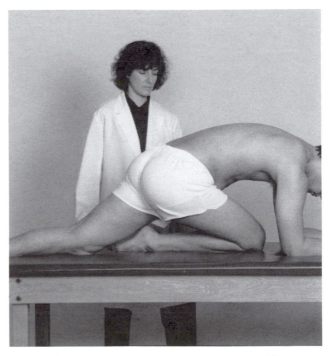

Figure 7–15B. Piriformis test: optional test position.

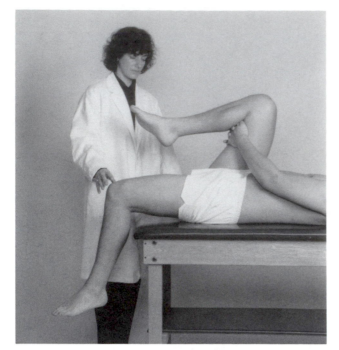

Figure 7–16A. Thomas Test: hip flexor tightness.

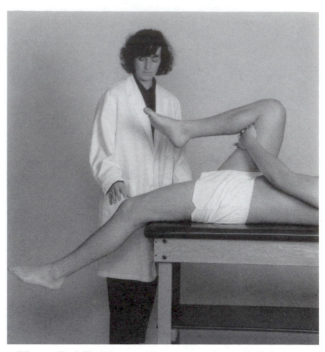

Figure 7–16B. Thomas Test: rectus femoris tightness.

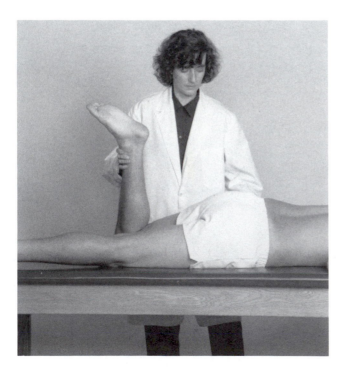

Figure 7–17. Ely's Test.

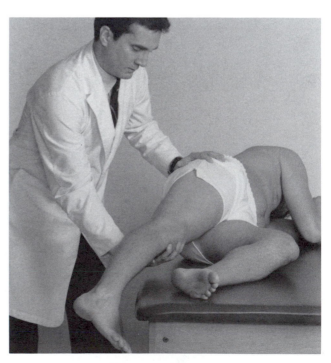

Figure 7–18. Ober's Test.

increase the complaints or cause distal or proximal migration of symptoms, there is probable nerve involvement.

Joint/Ligamentous Tests

Quadrant Test

The quadrant test (scouring) assesses degenerative changes in the articular surfaces of the hip. The hip is positioned passively in adduction and is moved between 90° flexion and full passive flexion (Fig 7–21). This stresses the lateral and posterior joint capsule and compresses the articular cartilage. The test is positive if it provokes apprehension, pain, or crepitus.[38]

FABERE Test

The FABERE test[3] can be used to differentiate between hip and sacroiliac joint pain. The hip is Flexed, ABducted, and Externally Rotated, and the lateral malleolus is allowed to rest on the opposite thigh above the knee (Fig 7–22). Pain located in the groin or anterior thigh is more indicative of hip joint pathology. Pain over the trochanteric region indicates hip capsular problems. Pain in the sacroiliac joint indicates sacroiliac joint involvement.

Torque Test

The torque test assesses the integrity of the capsular ligaments of the hip.[35] The patient's leg is extended over the edge of the examination table, and the clinician applies posterolateral stress to the femoral neck while internally rotating the femur (Fig 7–23). The test is positive if it provokes pain or apprehension.

Alignment Tests

Craig's Test

Craig's Test (or Ryder's Method for measuring femoral rotation) is one way to assess rotational alignment. The patient lies prone with the knee flexed to 90°. The clinician palpates the posterior aspect of the greater trochanter of the femur. The hip is passively rotated (internally and externally) until the greater trochanter is parallel to the examination table or in its most lateral position. The degree of ante– or retroversion can be measured based on the angle of the lower leg to vertical (Fig 7–24). Femoral anteversion results in an internally rotated lower limb and the corollary findings of increased internal rotation of the hip and restricted external rotation. Retroversion results in an externally rotated lower limb, and the corollary findings at the hip of increased

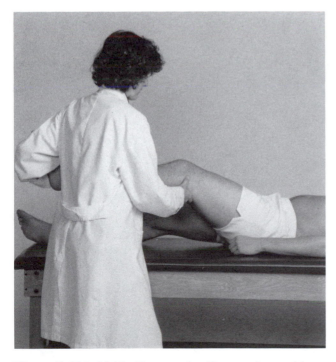

Figure 7–19A. Noble Compression Test, supine position.

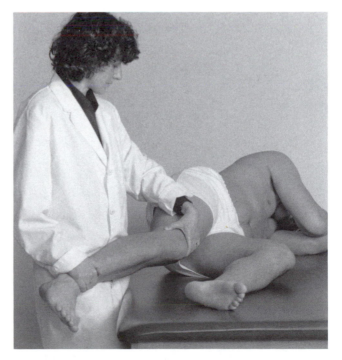

Figure 7–19B. Noble Compression Test, sidelying position.

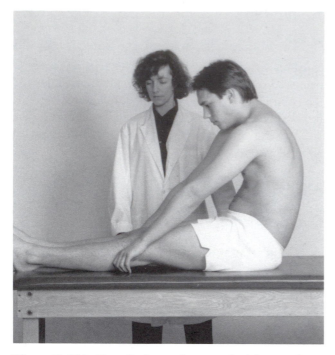

Figure 7–20A. Tests for hamstring muscle tightness: long sitting.

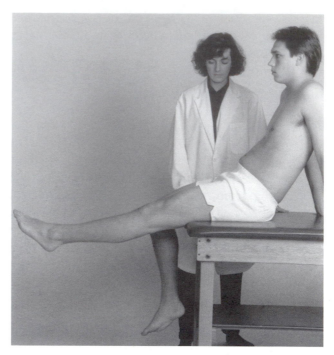

Figure 7–20B. Tests for hamstring muscle tightness: tripod.

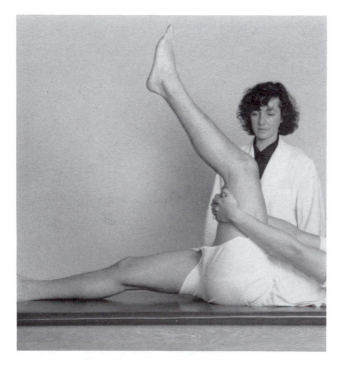

Figure 7–20C. Tests for hamstring muscle tightness: active straight leg raise.

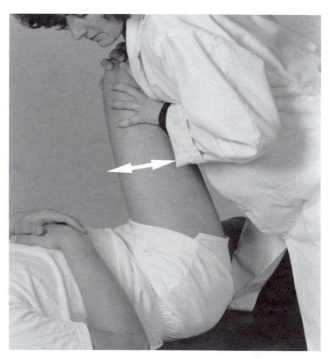

Figure 7–21. Hip quadrant test.

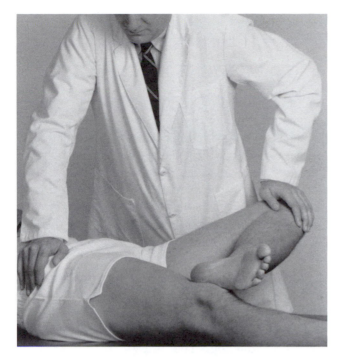

Figure 7–22. FABERE test.

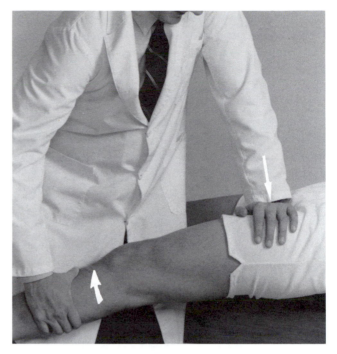

Figure 7–23. Torque test.

external rotation and restricted internal rotation of the hip.[11,54] The test is positive if there is excessive anteversion or retroversion when compared to the uninvolved limb.

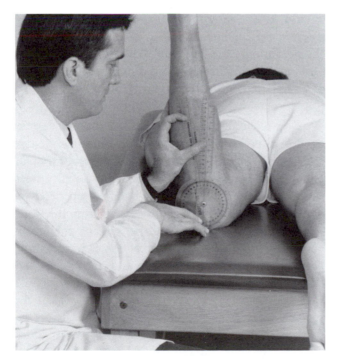

Figure 7-24. Craig's Test.

Leg Length Tests

These tests identify leg length discrepancies. Measuring leg length in supine is not always accurate but is still useful clinically. The patient lies supine and a tape measure is stretched from the ASIS to the ipsilateral lateral malleolus (Fig 7–25).[10,57] The lateral malleolus is preferred to the medial malleolus because the latter is more affected by hip malalignment or obesity. Standing radiographic measurement of leg length inequality is more accurate when precision is needed.[17] The Weber–Barstow Maneuver[58] and simple positioning to check for tibial and femoral limb length differences can also identify leg length inequality (Fig 7–26). The patient lies supine with the hips and knees flexed. The limbs can be viewed from the side (femur length) and front (tibial length) to compare relative limb lengths. The clinician moves to the foot end of the table and palpates the medial malleoli with the thumbs. The patient is asked to lift, or "bridge" the pelvis off the table, hold it for a short time, then rest back on the table. This maneuver levels the pelvis and prevents any misinterpretation of pelvic obliquity. The clinician then passively extends the hips and knees to lie flat on the table, and the malleoli levels are compared for any differences. In standing, the levels of the iliac crests, ASIS's, PSIS's, trochanters, gluteal

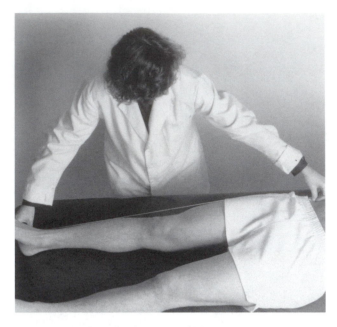

Figure 7–25. Measurement of leg length discrepancy.

folds, and fibular heads can be compared bilaterally. Any of the above tests are positive if there is a difference in leg length from one side to the other.

Any asymmetries should be interpreted carefully.[19] Leg length asymmetries are not always clinically significant. The clinician should correlate findings with the rest of the examination findings to avoid misinterpretation.

Objective Examination Summary

There are many structures that can contribute to the patient's complaints of hip problems. The hip joint itself, the musculotendinous units, and the mechanical interfaces of the nerves as they enter the thigh are the areas most commonly involved. Other structures that can contribute to hip symptoms include the lumbar spine, pelvis, and knee. The initial evaluation must be geared toward screening these joints, and subsequent re–evaluation should include reconsideration of these potential contributing areas, especially if the patient is not benefiting from treatment.

At the conclusion of the evaluation, the clinician determines what problems the patient has and then develops a problem list. The problem list reminds the clinician of the patient's problems so that each is addressed in treatment. The problem list also helps prioritize treatment and set goals.

TREATMENT STRATEGIES

The use of assistive devices to control weightbearing loads should be considered whenever the patient's symptoms are aggravated by weightbearing activities. Using a cane on the opposite side of the involved limb can reduce the weightbearing load transmitted to the involved hip up to 40%.[6] The patient should be weaned from the assistive device as symptoms resolve and the gait pattern becomes symmetrical.

It often helps to review the patient's daily routines to determine which standing, sitting, and sleeping postures are creating symptoms. For example, most people will shift their weight from limb to limb during prolonged standing. The use of a step stool to intermittently take some load off the involved leg will help improve standing tolerance and possibly decrease symptoms. Deep squatting puts the hip joint in flexion, and kneeling on one leg stresses the anterior hip; these positions may need to be avoided until symptoms resolve. Stride length in walking or sport activities should be assessed and shortened initially to decrease stresses on the anterior hip while the symptoms are calming down. Hip wrapping techniques (e.g., hip spica wrap) can often help control stride in gait and decrease stress to the anterior–medial hip joint (Fig 7–27). Stair climbing should initially be kept to a minimum. Avoiding prolonged sitting may prevent the common complaint of a catch in the hip when rising from sit to stand.

New technology has made total joint replacement a viable alternative for patients suffering from severe joint disease or trauma. Because of the temporary lack of hip mobility after surgery, patients usually need assistive devices (such as long handled reachers) for daily activities like picking objects up from the floor. Post–operative weakness of the gluteus medius is very common, and early intervention is important to prevent this problem. Post–surgical hip patients are not always elderly. Professional baseball player Bo Jackson actually returned to play after a total hip replacement. This illustrates the need to consider the patient's potential level of post–operative function when establishing rehabilitation goals.

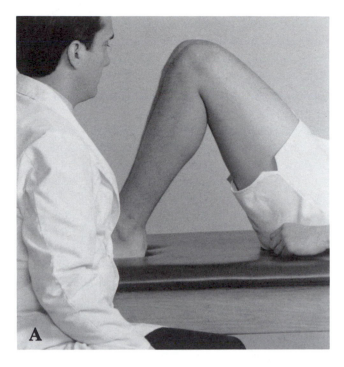

General treatment strategies are discussed in Chapter 3, <u>Pathology and Treatment Principles</u>. See Chapter 11, <u>Mobilization Techniques</u> and Chapter 12, <u>Exercise</u> for further information on mobilization techniques, stretching and strengthening exercises, and proprioceptive training for the hip.

COMMON CLINICAL CONDITIONS

Osteoarthritis

Significant disability can result when progressive osteoarthritis occurs at the hip joint. Unfortunately, it is the most common disorder affecting the hip. Primary osteoarthritis refers to the degenerative process that occurs from aging. Secondary osteoarthritis occurs when degenerative changes are precipitated by disease or mechanical trauma.[30]

Osteoarthritis of the hip begins with the initial asymptomatic changes that occur from inadequate stresses to the cartilage. Intermittent compression is needed to maintain healthy cartilage. When there are decreased compressive forces (e.g., when the patient is non–weightbearing) cartilage begins to degenerate. Older people tend to move around less and in smaller ranges of motion in their daily activities; therefore, some parts of the cartilage are not subjected to normal stresses, and this lack of stress predisposes the joint to osteoarthritis.

However, arthritic changes are not always a result of disuse. The degenerative changes caused by primary osteoarthritis occur in the areas undergoing

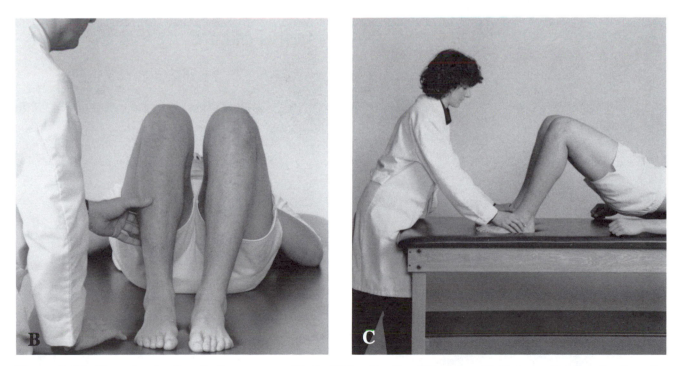

Figure 7–26. Observing leg length discrepancy with the Weber-Barstow Maneuver. A) Compare leg lengths from the side; B) Compare leg lengths from the front; C) Patient bridges to level the pelvis. After bridging the hips and knees are extended on the treatment table, and the relative lengths of the limbs are compared.

the most stress in reaction to abnormal or increased stresses to the joint over time.[18,22,39,45] Four factors contribute to the predisposition of these degenerative joint changes: congenital hip dysplasia,[7,24] leg–length discrepancy,[23] capsular tightness,[7,36,44] and obesity.[30] Disease and mechanical trauma (previous capsular sprain, fracture, etc.) are the predisposing factors in the etiology of secondary arthritis.[30]

History

The patient usually complains of progressive increase in stiffness and symptoms over time. There may be a history of hip problems or trauma that predisposes the hip to changes; a careful history should help identify these factors. Many patients ignore the stiffness and pain until it affects their daily activities. The patient complains of pain that increases after activity; as the problem progresses, the pain may occur even with simple movements.

Signs/Symptoms

The patient typically complains of pain in the anterior hip, groin, and sometimes the lateral hip and buttock. Referred symptoms are eventually felt in the anterior–medial thigh near the knee. Some patients have a primary complaint of knee pain and do not realize the symptoms are related to hip pathology.

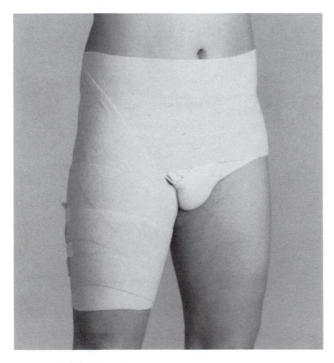

Figure 7–27. Hip spica wrap.

Weightbearing activities aggravate the symptoms. Progressive joint stiffness ensues, and getting dressed can become a problem. Pain and stiffness often occur after activity and accompany getting out of bed, squatting, and getting up from a chair. Pain is eased by rest and decreased weightbearing.

The patient may present with an antalgic gait pattern. A capsular pattern of joint restriction will be seen (loss of flexion, internal rotation and abduction). The quadrant test will be positive, and the Trendelenburg Sign may be seen in moderate to severe cases. Hip flexion contractures are common, and these will limit the patient's stride during gait (Thomas Test and Ely's Test). Joint play mobility of the hip will be restricted to different degrees depending on the duration of the problems. Lumbo–pelvic complaints may accompany the problem because of the change in hip and lumbo–pelvic mechanics.

Diagnostics

Radiographic evidence of osteoarthritis is not conclusive. Some patients present with symptoms but show no radiographic signs while others have radiographic signs but no symptoms; therefore, the degree of degeneration detected on x–ray does not necessarily correlate with the degree of pain or dysfunction (Fig 7–28).

Problem List

Patients with osteoarthritis may present with the following clinical problems:

1. Decreased range of motion and decreased capsular mobility

2. Decreased weightbearing tolerance

3. Gluteus medius weakness

4. Pain with weightbearing

5. Decreased tolerance of functional activities

Treatment

Patients presenting with early signs and symptoms of joint problems will probably gain the most from early therapeutic intervention. Grade I and II oscillatory mobilizations can help decrease pain. Patient's can be shown how to do these mobilization techniques themselves. These techniques can be performed either supine or standing, with the patient putting most of his or her weight on the uninvolved limb to unload the involved hip. Restoring capsular mobility via joint mobilization, ultrasound, and stretching exercises allows progression to strengthening and proprioceptive training. Any predisposing factors should be addressed. For example, a shoe lift on the short limb side may decrease the stresses on the involved joint, which is usually on the long side. A mobility exercise program should also be initiated; modifications in lifestyle, work, and recreational activities should be implemented; and a weight control program should be addressed as needed. The use of an assistive device during weightbearing activities should be firmly recommended. The clinician often meets with patient resistance but must convince him or her that the benefits of unloading the hip outweigh the stigma attached to using a cane or other device.[6] Non–steroidal anti–inflammatory drugs (NSAID's) are often prescribed, and the therapist should encourage the patient to comply with the physician's instructions. Assistive devices such as reachers and raised toilet seats should be considered. Hip abductor strengthening exercises are important. This muscle

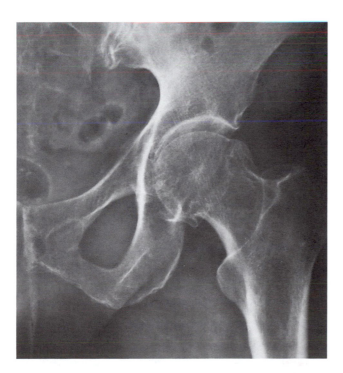

Figure 7–28. Radiographic evidence of degenerative joint disease at the hip.

should be trained in a closed kinematic chain under controlled loads to simulate functional pelvic control demands. Open kinematic chain strengthening does not recreate the demands placed on the gluteus medius in weightbearing activities. In severe cases, the goals are preparation for possible surgical intervention by maintaining or increasing range of motion, controlling weightbearing forces and symptoms, and adequately strengthening the hip musculature. Pool therapy can be quite useful here. Pre–operative intervention of this sort will ensure the optimal post–operative results.

Capsular Sprain

Hip joint pathology is frequently seen without severe trauma (e.g., fracture) or osteoarthritis. Many patients with hip joint pathology may not even be referred to the physical therapist. With a capsular sprain, the injury may have occurred insidiously or with a minor twisting motion during weightbearing. The complaints are similar to those of an arthritic hip: pain on weightbearing, restricted range of motion, and difficulty getting out of bed and up from sitting to standing. The complaints are usually in the anterior hip and groin. These patients may have early osteoarthritis, even when the radiographs are negative. Athletes frequently suffer from capsular sprains at the hip joint. Generally, the acute symptoms from these problems resolve, even without intervention; however, residual capsular tightness may predispose the patient to further hip problems including osteoarthritis,[36] so prompt identification and treatment of this problem is important to prevent recurrence and degenerative changes.

History

The patient may present with or without a history of significant trauma. If there is a traumatic event, the injury usually involves a twisting motion. This occurs in weightbearing activities more often than in non–weightbearing. Pain and stiffness follow, and patients have varying degrees of difficulty resuming weightbearing activities. Often, the acute symptoms resolve quickly and the patient does not seek medical care. In the absence of severe pathology, many patients never seek the help of a physical therapist unless problems continue or progress.

Signs and Symptoms

The patient will complain of problems in daily activities, especially after periods of inactivity such as prolonged sitting. Typical sites of pain are the anterior hip and groin, but some patients will complain of pain in the buttock. Ambulation is painful, especially running. Sometimes the complaints are quite severe for an instant when misstepping or after getting up from bed or a chair. The findings on examination show a capsular pattern of restriction of motion (limited flexion, internal rotation, and abduction). Overpressure is painful, especially in the direction of combined flexion and internal rotation. Muscle guarding can be present with attempts to move into the painful range. Joint play movements are restricted, but they may be limited by pain and have a spongy end–feel. There can be other contributing features on objective examination, including leg length or pelvic asymmetry. The gait pattern is antalgic on the involved limb.

Diagnostics

Radiographs of the hip are negative. There are no signs of osteoarthritis or other pathology. No further tests are performed at this point unless a labrum injury is suspected. A labrum injury is typified by patient complaints of catching, joint instability, and excessive apprehension in weightbearing. An MRI can help determine if there is concurrent damage to the acetabular labrum.

Problem List

Patients with a capsular sprain may present with the following clinical problems:

1. Decreased hip range of motion with decreased capsular mobility

2. Decreased weightbearing tolerance

3. Decreased stride length

4. Pain with weightbearing and transfers

5. Decreased tolerance of functional activities

Treatment

Treatment of capsular sprains is similar to treatment of early osteoarthritis of the hip. The patient should be taught about controlled weightbearing

activities as soon as possible and a cane or crutches issued as needed. A hip spica wrap (Fig 7–27) can decrease stress to the anterior hip structures and functionally shorten stride length. Mobilization techniques for symptom relief include Grade I and II distal distraction, with a progression to higher grades to improve joint lubrication and prevent residual capsular tightness.[8,59] Physical agents can be used as needed to decrease pain and to increase the extensibility of the hip capsule. These are particularly helpful in preparation for higher grades of mobilization to increase joint range. Strengthening exercises should be initiated as soon as tolerated; pillow adductor squeezes and elastic bands (to strengthen other muscle groups) can be used in pain free positions. Functional strengthening exercises, including proprioceptive training on a balance board, complete the rehabilitation program. Pool exercises can help progress the weightbearing tolerance in a more controlled environment and should be considered when appropriate. Range of motion exercises should be initiated early in the rehabilitation process and continued indefinitely to prevent the progression of capsular stiffness to osteoarthritis.[36]

Trochanteric Bursitis

The clinician often sees "trochanteric bursitis" written on the referral form.[27] It is a common misdiagnosis and differentiation of the many other causes of lateral hip symptoms is important. The lateral hip is a common site for referred pain from the lumbar spine, sacroiliac joint, and the deep external rotator muscles of the hip. Tensor fascia latæ syndrome and femoral neck stress fractures can occur in runners and should be ruled out.

History

The patient usually has an insidious onset of complaints, but occasionally a traumatic fall onto the lateral hip predisposes the bursa to mechanical irritation in daily activities.

Signs/Symptoms

The patient usually complains of pain directly over the lateral hip. Pain may refer distally into the iliotibial band or posteriorly into the buttock. Symptoms are most evident when rising from sitting or when climbing stairs. In these activities, the trochanteric bursa is susceptible to mechanical irritation by the overlying iliotibial band. Most patients are unable to lie or sleep on the involved side and often wake when rolling onto the involved side at night. They may also complain of pain with palpation. In some cases, the patient will limp if the symptoms are severe. The mobility examination is usually normal, and no capsular restriction is noted unless there are concurrent joint signs (decreased capsular mobility and complaints consistent with capsular sprain or osteoarthritis). Tenderness to palpation over the posterolateral trochanter is very common, and lateral thigh tenderness may also be present. Stretch to the lateral hip (Ober's Test with overpressure) may show restriction and symptom provocation. Pain with resisted abduction and external rotation of the hip are common findings as an inflamed bursa may be stressed with these maneuvers.

Diagnostics

There are no routine diagnostic tests for this bothersome but benign problem; however, an injection can diagnose the trochanteric bursa as the problem. If the symptoms are dramatically relieved after the injection, then the bursa is probably the site of the complaints. On rare occasions, tomograms or a bone scan can rule out a femoral neck stress fracture that can be the source of the lateral hip pain in runners. Standard radiographs can occasionally show a complication of traumatic bursitis—a calcification of the bursa at the lateral trochanter.[55]

Problem List

Patients with trochanteric bursitis may have the following problems:

1. Tenderness to palpation at the lateral hip

2. Iliotibial band tightness

3. Pain on weightbearing

4. Decreased sleep tolerance

Treatment

Initial treatment should include measures to decrease the inflammation and pain. These could include ice, ultrasound, and iontophoresis. The physician may prescribe NSAID's or elect to treat with a steroid injection. Activity modification is important, with the patient avoiding those factors that aggravate the symptoms. Alternate sleep postures should be reviewed. The treatment of concurrent muscle tightness (i.e., a tight iliotibial band) may be necessary to decrease the stresses on the trochanter and bursa.[48] If present, muscle weakness should be addressed with strengthening exercises.

Piriformis Syndrome

Piriformis syndrome[52] describes the mechanical irritation of the sciatic nerve by the overlying piriformis muscle (Fig 7–29). The sciatic nerve pierces the muscle in 15–20% of the population. The sciatic nerve can be entrapped under the muscle and against the ischium or it may be entrapped within the muscle belly itself. The muscle may be hypertonic due to concurrent lumbo–pelvic pathology, postural factors, or sacral dysfunction. The clinician should carefully identify possible contributing factors that predispose the patient to this problem or mimic piriformis syndrome symptoms.

History

The patient will complain of a gradual onset of buttock, hip, and posterior thigh symptoms. These complaints may occur simultaneously with a lumbo–

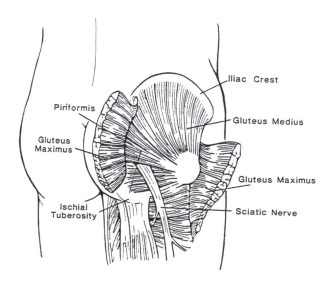

Figure 7–29. The piriformis muscle is a common culprit in sciatic nerve impingement.

pelvic problem (sacral torsion, lumbar disc, etc.) Pain may be felt when first getting out of bed or standing from a chair. The pain usually decreases with mild activity but worsens with prolonged activity or sustained postures. The problem usually presents unilaterally.

Signs/Symptoms

Patients generally complain of pain in the buttock that increases with prolonged weightbearing activities and prolonged sitting. Symptoms can be referred distally down the posterior thigh to the knee and possibly the calf. The legs and feet may "fall asleep" during prolonged sitting. The paresthesia dissipates after getting up and moving around. Findings include a tight piriformis muscle on the involved limb and palpation tenderness over the muscle belly. In a supine position, the foot of the involved side will be externally rotated. Deep palpation or sustained stretching of the piriformis will provoke distal symptoms. Internal rotation of the hip will be restricted and painful. Manual muscle test of the piriformis muscle can provoke local symptoms. The piriformis test (see the "Special Tests" section of this chapter) will be positive. There may be neural tension signs: the SLR test will be provocative, especially with the hip internally rotated and adducted to sensitize the test by tightening the piriformis muscle. The Slump test can also be positive, depending on the degree of compression on the sciatic nerve or if there is lumbar or sacral involvement proximally.

Diagnostics

There are no routine diagnostic procedures for this problem; however, in severe cases, an MRI could implicate the piriformis–sciatic nerve interface as the point of nerve entrapment.

Problem List

Patients with piriformis syndrome may present with the following problems:

1. Decreased sitting and standing tolerance

2. Decreased hip mobility (limited internal rotation and adduction)

3. Radiating pain in the lower extremity

4. Neural tension signs

5. Concurrent lumbo–pelvic joint signs

Treatment

Initial treatment is directed toward symptom relief, with physical agents and soft–tissue mobilization, allowing progression to passive stretching techniques. A combination of ultrasound and stretching or soft tissue mobilization techniques while stretching can be helpful. The patient should be taught passive stretching exercises early in the treatment program. Daily activities and hip postures should be reviewed to decrease stresses on the area. Concurrent treatment for sacral torsions or lumbar problems should be carried out if these factors are thought to be contributing to the problem. Neural mobilization techniques can be incorporated into the treatment regime to treat any AMNT component. This can be done in the SLR or Slump positions as needed.

Maintaining mobility of the piriformis muscle at its interface with the sciatic nerve is essential to prevent recurrence. Surgical release of chronic piriformis syndrome in 12 cases resulted in 10 hips rated as normal or greatly improved after surgery.[56]

Muscle Strains (Hamstring and Rectus Femoris)

The muscles of the hip can easily be strained in work or recreational activities.[20,47,48] The etiology of muscle strains is multifactorial: the muscle tendon unit can be susceptible to overload and injury due to muscle imbalances, poor flexibility, overstretching, violent muscle contraction against heavy resistance, leg length discrepancies, and AMNT.[20,32] Restoration of muscle length is important in reinjury prevention,[20] and addressing the mobility of neural structures may be equally important.[32] Carefully assessing the tissues involved and treating all contributing factors is critical to success of treatment and prevention measures. This section will specifically address two common strains: the hamstring and the rectus femoris.

History

The patient with a hamstring strain usually has a problem at either the origin of the muscle (ischial tuberosity) or the muscle belly. The biceps femoris muscle (short head) is thought to be the most commonly injured hamstring muscle.[20] The onset is acute in most cases. In severe cases, the patient may report feeling a tear or a pop in the muscle. Concurrent complaints of a neurological nature may be present if the neural tissues are involved. For example, the sciatic nerve can be stretched in a hamstring strain, causing lines of pain or paresthesias into the calf and foot.

A patient with strain of the rectus femoris muscle has a very similar history to that of a hamstring strain, except the mechanisms are opposite (i.e., rectus femoris strain with hip extension or knee flexion versus hamstring strain with hip flexion or knee extension). If a Grade I strain occurs, treatment is often as simple as "stretching it out" and gradually resuming activity. Grade II and III injuries to either muscle are usually disabling to the point where the aggravating activity must be discontinued.

Signs/Symptoms

The patient with a hamstring strain may walk with a shortened stride and decreased hip flexion. The patient with a rectus femoris strain will tend to limit hip extension in gait; a limp may be present. The patient may have local pain, swelling, or bruising over the involved muscle. The patient will be tender to palpation and manual muscle testing. The involved muscle may appear weak on examination in more severe cases. Combining the dual functions of the muscles when performing resisted muscle testing can be quite helpful (e.g., symptoms from resisting hip flexion and knee extension will implicate the rectus femoris muscle; symptoms from resisting hip extension and knee flexion will implicate the hamstrings). Passive stretching will also provoke symptoms. Neural tension tests may be positive (Slump test and SLR for hamstrings and prone knee bend (PKB) for rectus femoris).[32,34]

Diagnostics

There are no routine diagnostics for these problems. The degree of pathology can be determined with an MRI scan, but the cost for the test is prohibitive. An adequate clinical examination is usually enough to indict the specific muscles. The hamstring muscle will occasionally avulse at the ischial tuberosity, as will the rectus femoris at the

AIIS or at the superior rim of the acetabulum. These avulsions usually show up on a standard radiograph, but a tomogram may be necessary. Avulsion injuries are usually confined to the adolescent athlete, but an avulsion injury has been reported at the ischium in an adult runner training with retro (backward) running.[50] This was diagnosed with a physical examination and a bone scan.

Problem List

Patients with a muscle strain may present with the following clinical problems:

1. Local muscle pain
2. Decreased muscle length secondary to pain
3. Decreased stride length
4. Decreased tolerance to weightbearing
5. Decreased muscle strength
6. Concurrent neural tension signs

Treatment

The acute phase of treatment involves PRICE and NSAID's to decrease pain, swelling, and local inflammation in the muscle and the surrounding tissues. An elastic wrap should be used for support initially, and crutches are sometimes necessary in the more severe injuries.

Although restoration of muscle length is important, it should not interfere with healing; therefore, the patient should feel a stretching sensation rather than pain when performing mobility exercises and stretching techniques. Pain indicates the muscle is not ready for stretching.[9] Combining hold–relax proprioceptive neuromuscular facilitation (PNF) contractions with intermittent icing is a good alternative if muscle spasm and guarding are present.[31] The patient should ice until the area is numb, then immediately perform the stretch technique; icing can also be performed during stretching. If signs of AMNT are present, it is necessary to stretch the tissue interfaces. Neural tissue stretching has been shown to alter the sympathetic outflow to the lower limbs;[33] thus, there may be a physiological rationale for stretching neural structures to treat and prevent Grade I hamstring injuries.[32]

Muscle strengthening should proceed as tolerated, avoiding pain. Progressive functional exercise should be performed in a manner consistent with the actions of the muscles at the hip and knee, in closed and open kinematic chains.

SUMMARY

The evaluation, treatment, and prevention of problems at the hip has been presented. Many contributing factors can express themselves as "hip" pain. The hip, pelvis, and lumbar spine function as an integrated biomechanical unit, so careful assessment of the contributions from each of these areas is important to identify the proper areas to be treated. The hip is also influenced biomechanically from below by the knee, foot, and ankle. It is susceptible to stress from the large loads it accepts during weightbearing and from the muscles crossing it. Management of hip problems should include all related neuromusculoskeletal structures, and assessment and treatment should be approached in a functional manner.

REFERENCES

1. American Orthopaedic Association: Manual of Orthopaedic Surgery. Chicago IL 1972.
2. Barrett PG: The HS Injury in Footballers. South Australian Institute of Technology, Adelaide 1987. Unpublished thesis.
3. Beetham WP, et al: Physical Examination of the Joints. WB Saunders Co, Philadelphia PA 1965.
4. Bjerkman I: Secondary Dysplasia and Osteoarthritis of the Hip Joint in Functional and Fixed Obliquity of the Pelvis. Acta Orthop Scand 45:873-882, 1974.
5. Bourke A, et al: Hamstring Symptoms and Lumbar Spine Relationship in Sports People. In Proceedings of the Australian Physiotherapy Association National Conference, Hobart 1986.
6. Brand RA, Crownshield RD: The Effect of Cane Use on Hip Contact Force. Clin Orthop and Rel Res 147:181, 1980.
7. Cameron HU, MacNab I: Observations on Osteoarthritis of the Hip Joint. Clin Orthop 108:31-40, 1975.
8. Cibulka MT, DeLitto A: A Comparison of Two Different Methods to Treat Hip Pain in Runners. JOSPT 17(4):172-176, 1993.
9. Cibulka MT: Rehabilitation of the Pelvis, Hip, and Thigh. Clin Sports Med 8:777-803.
10. Clarke GR: Unequal Leg Length: An Accurate Method of Detection and Some Clinical Results. Rheumatology and Physical Medicine 11:385, 1972.
11. Crane L: Femoral Torsion and its Relation to Toeing-In and Toeing-Out. JBJS 41A:421, 1959.
12. DeLitto RS, Sahrmann S: Applied Anatomy of the Low Back Region. Post-Graduate Advances in Evaluation and Treatment of Low-Back Dysfunction. Forum Medicum I-IV:1-22, 1989.
13. Dostal WF, Andrews JG: A Three-Dimensional Biomechanical Model of Hip Musculature. J Biomech 14:803-812, 1981.
14. Echternach JL: Physical Therapy of the Hip. Churchill-Livingstone, New York NY 1990.
15. Edelson EG: Meralgia Paresthetica: An Anatomical Interpretation. JBJS 58A:284, 1986.
16. Favill J: Outline of the Spinal Nerves. Charles C Thomas, Springfield IL 1946.
17. Fisk JW, Balgent ML: Clinical and Radiological Assessment of Leg Length. New Zealand Medical Journal 81:477, 1975.
18. Freeman MAR: The Fatigue of Cartilage in the Pathogenesis of Osteoarthritis. Acta Orthop Scand 46:323-328, 1975.
19. Friberg O: Clinical Symptoms and Biomechanics of Lumbar Spine and Hip Joint in Leg Length Inequality. Spine 8(6):643-651, 1983.
20. Gallaspy JB: Hamstrings, Quadricep, and Groin Rehabilitation. In Physical Rehabilitation of the Injured Athlete. J Andrews, G Harralson, ed. WB Saunders Co, Philadelphia PA 1991.
21. Garrick JG, Webb DR: Sports Injuries: Diagnosis and Treatment. WB Saunders Co, Philadelphia PA 1990.
22. Gofton JP, Trueman GE: Studies in Osteoarthritis of the Hip I: Classification. Can Med Assoc Joul 104:679-683, 1971.
23. Gofton JP, Trueman GE: Studies in Osteoarthritis of the Hip II: Osteoarthritis of the Hip and Leg Length Disparity. Can Med Assoc Joul 104:791-799, 1971.
24. Gofton JP, Trueman GE: Studies in Osteoarthritis of the Hip III: Congenital Subluxation and Osteoarthritis of the Hip Disparity. Can Med Assoc Joul 104:911-915, 1971.
25. Gray's Anatomy. PL Williams PL and R Warwick, ed. 36th ed. WB Saunders Co, Philadelphia PA 1980.
26. Gruebel-Lee DM: Disorders of the Hip. JB Lippincott Co, Philadelphia PA 1983.
27. Gunn CC, Milbrandt WE: Bursitis Around the Hip.

Am J Acupuncture 5:53-60, 1977.

28. Hollingshead H, Jenkins D: Functional Anatomy of the Limbs and Back. WB Saunders, Philadelphia PA 1981.

29. Jefferson D, Eames RA: Subclinical Entrapment of the Lateral Femoral Cutaneous Nerve: An Autopsy Study. Muscle and Nerve 2:145-154, 1979.

30. Kessler R, Hertling D: The Hip-Common Lesions. In Management of Common Musculoskeletal Disorders-Physical Therapy Principles and Methods, 2nd ed. JB Lippincott, Philadelphia PA 1992.

31. Knight KL: Cryotherapy: Theory, Technique, and Physiology. Chattanooga Corporation, Chattanooga TN 1985.

32. Kornberg C and Lew P: The Effect of Stretching Neural Structures on Grade I Hamstring Injuries. JOSPT 10(12):481-487, 1989.

33. Kornberg C, McCarthy T: The Effect of Neural Stretching Technique on Sympathetic Outflow to the Lower Limbs. JOSPT 16(6):269-274, 1992.

34. Kornberg C: The Incidence of Positive Slump Test in Australian Rules Football Player with Grade I HS Strain. Proceedings of 10th International Congress, Sydney Australia 1987.

35. Lee D: The Pelvic Girdle. Churchill-Livingstone, Edinburgh 1989.

36. Lloyd-Roberts GC: The Role of Capsular Changes in Osteoarthritis of the Hip Joint. JBJS 35(B):627-642, 1953.

37. Magee D: Orthopedic Physical Assessment, 2nd ed. WB Saunders, Philadelphia PA 1992.

38. Maitland GD: Peripheral Manipulation, 2nd ed. Butterworth & Co, Stoneham MA 1977.

39. Mankin HJ: Biomechanical and Metabolic Aspects of Osteoarthritis. Orthop Clin North America 2:19-31, 1971.

40. Murphy JP: Menalgia Paresthetica: A Nerve Entrapment Syndrome. Maryland State Medical Journal 23:57-58, 1979.

41. Noble HB, et al: Diagnosis and Treatment of Iliotibial Band Tightness in Runners. Phys Sports Med 10:67, 1982.

42. Ober FB: The Role of the Iliotibial and Fascia Lata As a Factor in the Causation of Low Back Disabilities and Sciatica. JBJS 18:105, 1936.

43. Palmer ML, Epler M: Clinical Assessment Procedures in Physical Therapy. JB Lippincott Co, Philadelphia PA 1990.

44. Paul JP: Forces Transmitted at the Hip and Knee of Normal and Disabled Persons During a Range of Activities. Acta Orthop Belg Suppl 41:78-88, 1975.

45. Radin E, Paul IL: The Mechanics of Joints As It Relates To Their Degeneration. In Symposium on Osteoarthritis. CV Mosby Co, St Louis MO 1976.

46. Radin EL: Biomechanics of the Human Hip. Clin Orthop 152:28-34, 1980.

47. Renstram P, Peterson L: Groin Injuries in Athletes. British Journal of Sports Medicine 14:30-36, 1980.

48. Sammarco G: The Hip in Dancers. Medical Problems of Performing Artists 2:5-14, 1987.

49. Sarala PK, et al: Meralgia Paresthetica: An Electrophysiological Study. Arch Phys Med Rehabil 60:30-31, 1979.

50. Satterfield MJ, et al: Retro Runner With Ischial Tuberosity Enthesopathy. JOSPT 17(4):191-194, 1993.

51. Saudek CE: The Hip. In Orthopaedic and Sports Physical Therapy. CV Mosby Co, St Louis MO 1990.

52. Saunders HD: Pathology and Treatment Concepts-Extremities. In Evaluation, Treatment, and Prevention of Musculoskeletal Problems, 2nd ed. R Saunders, ed. Educational Opportunities, Minneapolis MN 1985.

53. Soggard I: Sciatic Nerve Entrapment. Journal of Neurosurgery 58:275-276, 1983.

54. Staheli LT: Medical Femoral Torsion. Orthop Clin North America 11:39, 1980.

55. Standard Nomenclature of Athletic Injuries. American Medical Association. Monroe WI 1976.

56. Tinel J: Le signe du fourmillent dans les lesions des nerfs peripheriques. La Presse Medicale 47:388-389, 1915.

57. Woerman AL, Binder-MacLeod SA: Leg Length Discrepancy Assessment Accuracy and precision in Five Clinical Methods of Evaluation. JOSPT 5:230, 1984.

58. Woerman AL: Evaluation and Treatment of Dysfunction in the Lumbar-Pelvic-Hip Complex. In Orthopaedic Physical Therapy. R Donatelli and MJ Wooden, ed. Churchill-Livingstone, Edinburgh 1989.

59. Yoder E: Physical Therapy Management of Non-Surgical Hip Problems in Adults. In Physical Therapy of the Hip. JL Echternach, ed. Churchill-Livingstone, New York NY 1990.

CHAPTER 8

THE KNEE

INTRODUCTION

The knee has the unenviable position of being between the body's two longest lever segments. It must withstand considerable loads and externally applied forces in daily activities, especially in work and sports. The knee receives little stability from bony structures; thus, the soft tissues must withstand these forces, and injury results when they are overloaded.

There are actually two joints at the knee: the tibiofemoral and patellofemoral. The patellofemoral joint is unique because it has the largest sesamoid bone in the body—the patella. The patella acts as a pulley and gives a mechanical advantage to the quadriceps. The patellofemoral joint is very susceptible to cumulative trauma from repetitive stresses and is a major source of pain and dysfunction at the knee.[49]

The tibiofemoral joint receives its stability from static and dynamic restraints. Injury to the static restraints, which includes the ligaments and meniscus, can lead to significant disability. Advances in reconstructive surgery and rehabilitation have decreased the risk of permanent disability from injuring these structures.

Symptoms felt at the knee can be referred from the hip, ankle, and lumbar spine; therefore, effective management of knee problems must include the related neuromusculoskeletal structures.

FUNCTIONAL ANATOMY

Osseous and Capsuloligamentous Components

The joints and ligaments of the knee are shown in Figure 8–1. The proximal tibiofibular joint will be considered as part of the knee.

Tibiofemoral Joint

The tibiofemoral joint is a modified hinge joint between the distal end of the femur and proximal end of the tibia. The joint capsule of the knee surrounds the femoral condyles and tibial plateaus and contains the largest synovial joint in the body.[42] The joint capsule provides stability to the knee by blending with the collateral ligaments. During knee movement, it helps lubricate the articulating surfaces by distributing synovial fluid. The joint capsule blends with many bursæ around the joint, which are often a source of pain and inflammation.

The medial and lateral femoral condyles are located at the distal femur (Fig 8–2). These condyles are convex in the frontal and sagittal planes, and covered with hyaline cartilage. The trochlear groove, which lies between the condyles, cradles the patella and is also covered with cartilage. In the frontal plane, the height of the lateral condyle is usually greater than the medial condyle. This added height helps prevent lateral patellar subluxation. The medial condyle extends farther distally than the lateral condyle. This

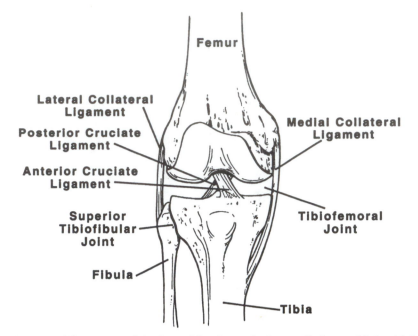

Figure 8-1. The joints, bones and ligaments of the knee. Not shown is the patellofemoral joint (right knee, anterior view).

added length makes the tibia spiral around the femur during flexion and extension.[45] The tibial plateaus are concave in the frontal planes to fit congruently with the femoral condyles; however, the lateral tibial plateau is convex in the sagittal plane, creating an incongruity that allows increased joint play at the knee. The movement of tibial external rotation during knee extension is called the screw–home mechanism. This provides more stability to the knee than would the simple hinge configuration of the tibiofemoral joint.[42]

Menisci

A unique feature of the tibiofemoral joint is two semi–lunar shaped fibrocartilage discs called menisci. These structures deepen the tibial fossa, make the joint surfaces more congruent and increase

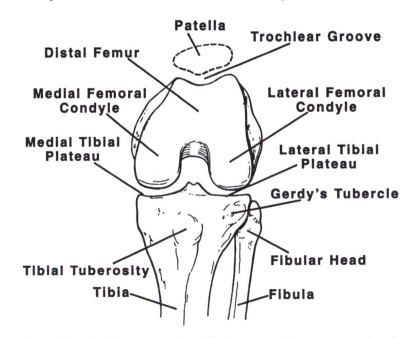

Figure 8-2. The distal femoral and tibial plateaus (left knee, anterior view)

knee stability. The menisci also act as shock attenuators, spreading the load over the articular cartilage and preventing displacement of the menisci (Fig 8–3).[84] They are stabilized by the intermeniscal, meniscofemoral, and meniscotibial ligaments (Fig 8–4). The menisci move posteriorly during knee flexion and anteriorly during knee extension. The lateral meniscus moves more than the medial meniscus. The menisci transmit 50% of the compressive forces across the knee in full extension and 85% of the compressive forces at 90° of flexion in weightbearing.[1] The menisci resist tension in a circumferential direction, consistent with the orientation of the majority of their fibers.[14] Compressive forces develop tension in these fibers, which helps transmit forces to the tibial plateau and prevent peripheral displacement of the menisci. Rotational weightbearing motions at the knee are stressful and are more difficult for the menisci to resist than sagittal plane motions.[42] The anterior aspects of the menisci buffer knee hyperextension and dampen the pendulum effect of the leg during the swing phase of gait.[28]

The mechanical movement of the menisci helps distribute synovial fluid over the articular cartilage. The menisci are avascular in their cartilaginous inner 2/3 and partly vascular in their outer fibrous 1/3.[6] Tears in the avascular meniscus have limited potential for healing.

Ligaments

The ligamentous structures of the knee are the main static restraints that provide knee stability. There are four main stabilizers: the medial collateral ligament (MCL), the lateral collateral ligament (LCL), the anterior cruciate ligament (ACL), and the posterior cruciate ligament (PCL).

The collateral ligaments are the primary restraints to varus and valgus stresses at the knee, especially when the knee is between full extension and 30° of flexion. They become more lax as flexion increases. The collateral ligaments also resist rotation at the knee; the LCL is more taut in internal rotation, and the MCL is more taut in external rotation.[42] The MCL has an attachment to the medial meniscus, but the LCL does not attach to the lateral meniscus.

The cruciate ligaments stabilize the knee in the anterior–posterior and rotational planes of movement. Due to different fiber lengths, some portion of both cruciate ligaments is taut throughout knee range of motion.[60]

The PCL is the strongest ligament in the knee.[60] It consists of two bundles—a posteromedial band that is taut in extension and an anterolateral band that is taut in flexion. This arrangement makes it difficult to reconstruct the PCL surgically because anatomical placement of the graft would require two grafts to maintain some ligament tension throughout the range of motion.[117] The primary function of the PCL is to resist hyperextension of the knee and posterior displacement of the tibia relative to the femur.[36]

The ACL is the most commonly injured ligament in the knee. The ACL is actually a continuum of fibers with different portions taut throughout the range of motion. The posterolateral fibers are more taut in

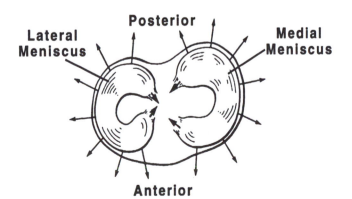

Figure 8–3. The menisci spread out forces and transmit forces to the cartilage.

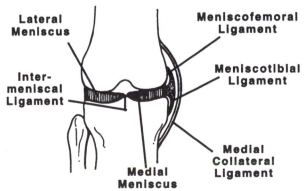

Figure 8–4. The intermeniscal, meniscofemoral, and meniscotibial ligaments.

extension; the anteromedial fibers are more taut in flexion. These bundles are less distinct than in the PCL.[127]

The primary function of the ACL is to resist anterior translation of the tibia on the femur.[11] Both of the cruciate ligaments also restrain rotational movements at the knee. Internal rotation of the tibia on the femur causes the cruciates to tighten and intertwine as the articular surfaces approximate. To some degree, the opposite occurs in external rotation of the tibia on the femur.[42]

The cruciates are covered by a synovial membrane with a rich vascular supply from the middle geniculate artery. This synovial membrane is the main blood supply to the cruciates. This blood supply can be interrupted with a partial tear of the cruciates, rendering the residual ligaments avascular.

The tibial nerve innervates the cruciate ligaments. Some of the terminal branches of the nerve lie along the ligament fascicles. These branches may supply proprioception.[85]

Two types of instability can occur at the knee: straight and combined. Straight instability occurs when there is excessive joint laxity in a single plane of motion. Straight instabilities at the knee can occur in an anterior, posterior, medial, or lateral direction. Combined instability occurs when there is excessive joint laxity in more than one plane of motion at one time. These are referred to as rotational instabilities. The possible rotational instabilities at the knee are: anteromedial rotational instability (AMRI), anterolateral rotational instability (ALRI), posteromedial rotational instability (PMRI), and posterolateral rotational instability (PLRI). These are presented schematically in Figure 8–5. The incidence of PMRI is low, and some clinicians question whether the condition actually exists.

Two types of restraints counter excessive joint laxity: primary and secondary (Fig 8–6). A primary restraint is the structure most responsible for resisting excessive joint laxity in a particular direction. A secondary restraint is a back–up structure that resists excessive joint movement when the primary structure is injured. For example, the ACL is the primary restraint to straight anterior laxity at the knee joint. Injury to the ACL puts more stress on the secondary

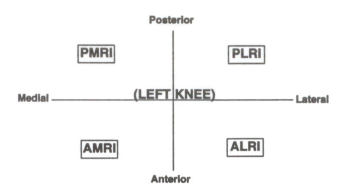

Figure 8–5. Schematic representation of the potential types of knee instability. PMRI is very rare.

restraints: the remaining ligaments, the joint capsule, and the hamstrings.

Patellofemoral Joint

The patellofemoral joint is formed by the articulation of the patella and the femoral condyles in the trochlear groove. This joint has little bony stability. The height of the lateral femoral condyle helps prevent lateral subluxation of the patella. Soft tissue surrounds the joint to increase stability (Fig 8–7). Superiorly, the quadricep tendon attaches to the patella, and inferiorly, the patellar tendon continues distally to the tibial tubercle. The tendon expansions of the vastus medialis and vastus lateralis muscles form the medial and lateral retinaculum. The joint capsule and patellofemoral ligaments attach to the medial and lateral patellar borders. The lateral border also has an attachment from the iliotibial band (ITB) expansion—the iliopatellar band—that blends with the lateral retinaculum.[116] Tightness of this lateral structure can cause decreased medial patellar glide and subsequent patellofemoral dysfunction.[101]

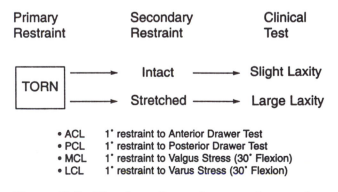

Figure 8–6. The knee has primary and secondary restraints to joint laxity.

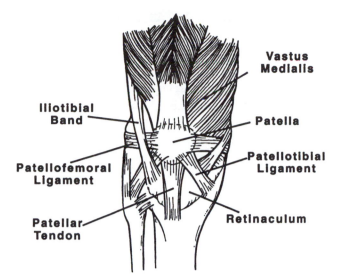

Figure 8–7. Soft tissue surrounds the patellofemoral joint to provide stability.

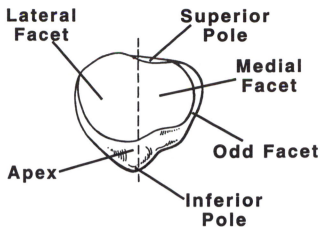

Figure 8–8. The posterior surface of the patella (left knee).

The patellofemoral joint increases the mechanical advantage of the quadricep muscles and resists mechanical loading (Fig 8–2). This is particularly important during weightbearing, when the patella may be subjected to compressive loads of up to 10 times body weight.[13]

The underside of the patella is completely covered with hyaline cartilage, except for the inferior portion or apex.[1] There are three facets on the underside of the patella: the medial, the lateral, and the odd (Fig 8–8).[14] The facets increase the stability of the patellofemoral joint and help transmit forces across the joint.

The underside surface of the patella undergoes a particular pattern of contact through the knee range of motion (Fig 8–9).[44] In patellofemoral dysfunction, this pattern of contact is disrupted, leading to excessive compression at the joint.

Superior Tibiofibular Joint

The superior tibiofibular joint is a plane synovial joint formed where the proximal ends of the tibia and fibula meet on the lateral side of the knee (Fig 8–1). No physiological movements occur at this joint. The only movement here is accessory motion caused by ankle motion. Dysfunction at this superior tibiofibular joint can lead to symptoms felt at the lateral knee.

Table 8–1 summarizes the movements and range of motion at the knee.

Neuromuscular Components

The neuromuscular components of the knee interact with the static stabilizers to provide a balance of intrinsic and extrinsic forces that contribute to functional knee stability.[90] The functional capabilities

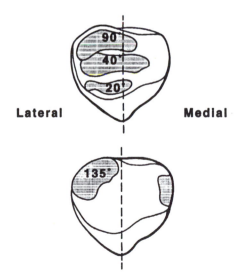

Figure 8–9. The patellofemoral contact pattern during knee flexion. Shaded areas represent areas of contact between the patella and femur at different ranges of knee flexion (adapted from Goodfellow, Hungerford and Zindel).[44]

Table 8–1. Movements and Range of Motion at the Knee

Physiological Movements	
Flexion	125-135°
Extension	5-10°
Tibial Rotation	
Internal rotation	20-30°
External rotation	30-40°

of the knee muscles form the basis for appropriate and successful rehabilitation.

There are two functional muscle groups: extensors and flexors (Fig 8–10). Many of the muscles that act on the knee also act proximally at the hip or distally at the ankle. These combined functions allow effective muscle interactions to produce smooth lower limb movements.[109]

Muscular Structures

Extensors

The quadriceps muscles are the rectus femoris; vastus medialis, including the vastus medialis obliquus (VMO); vastus lateralis; and vastus intermedius. In a closed kinematic chain, these muscles contract eccentrically to control knee flexion, absorb compressive forces, and decelerate the lower extremity. They are antagonistic to the force of gravity and the hamstring muscles.[42]

The quadriceps play a large role in knee stability. Quadriceps contractions increase tension in the anteromedial and anterolateral joint capsules through their retinacular attachments. They stabilize the menisci through the meniscopatellar ligaments. Medial quadriceps contraction decreases strain on the MCL.[20] The quadriceps help the cruciates prevent posterior tibial displacement from 90–75° of knee

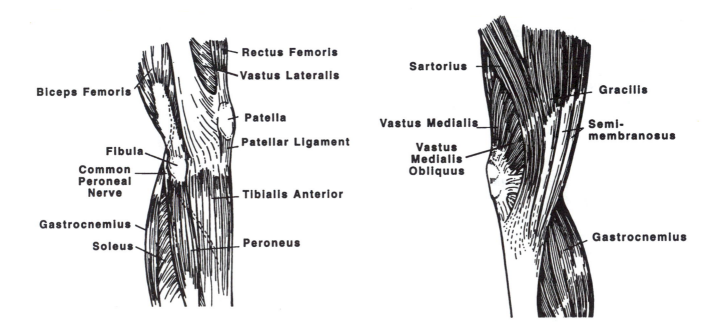

Figure 8–10. The muscles of the knee. The vastus intermedius lies beneath the rectus femoris.

extension.[4] From 75–0° of extension, the quadriceps pull the tibia anteriorly, antagonistic to the ACL.[4,20] The most stress on the ACL from a quadriceps contraction occurs from 45–0° of extension.[68]

The oblique orientation of the VMO's fibers stabilizes the patella during knee motion and during loading by controlling patellar tracking and resisting lateral displacement of the patella out of the trochlear groove. The VMO's primary function is to resist lateral forces that act on the patella in a closed kinematic chain.[12,72,81,111] It is unclear whether the VMO is responsible for terminal extension of the knee in the open kinematic chain.

Flexors

The hamstring muscles are the primary flexors of the knee joint in an open kinematic chain. They help the ACL restrain anterior displacement of the tibia on the femur; thus, hamstring muscles have an important role in rehabilitating the ACL deficient knee.[123] Collectively, the hamstrings also influence the rotation of the tibia on the femur, analogous to using reins to control a horse. The semimembranosus muscle attaches to the medial tibial condyle, the medial and posteromedial capsules, and the medial meniscus by an expansion in the tendon.[42] It helps internally rotate the tibia and retract the medial meniscus[42] and resists external rotation of the tibia, especially with the knee flexed. The pes anserine group (semitendinosus, gracilis, and sartorius) attach to the anteromedial tibia at the distal insertion of the MCL. These muscles flex the knee, internally rotate the tibia, and resist external rotation of the tibia when the knee is flexed. The biceps femoris attaches to the fibular head at the distal insertion of the LCL. It also attaches to the posterolateral capsule and the iliotibial tract.[78] The biceps femoris externally rotates the tibia on the femur and resists internal rotation. During flexion, this muscle retracts the joint capsule and pulls the iliotibial tract posteriorly, keeping it taut throughout the range.[42] The iliotibial tract inserts distally at Gerdy's Tubercle on the lateral tibia; thus, the iliotibial tract flexes the knee beyond 30° but helps in terminal knee extension (final 30°).[78] It also externally rotates the tibia after 30° of flexion.

The popliteus muscle stabilizes the lateral compartment of the knee through its attachment to the lateral meniscus and posterolateral capsule.[110] It retracts the lateral meniscus during knee flexion and helps the PCL prevent forward displacement of the femur on the tibia in a closed kinematic chain.[10] This muscle helps "unlock" the fully extended, weightbearing knee by internally rotating the tibia. Gait studies have shown the popliteus maintains the internally rotated position of the tibia during stance.[77]

The medial and lateral heads of the gastrocnemius muscle originate at the posterior femur and at the joint capsule of the knee. In addition to flexing the knee, the gastrocnemius helps the quadriceps resist posterior translation of the tibia in the closed kinematic chain.[42] At the midstance phase of gait, the gastrocnemius maintains knee flexion tension to control knee extension. It also decelerates internal rotation of the femur and flexes the knee, lifting the heel to initiate swing.[42]

The hamstrings and rectus femoris muscles have combined functions because they cross the hip and knee joints. In an open kinematic chain, the rectus femoris extends the knee and flexes the hip. It helps control knee flexion and hip extension in the closed kinematic chain. In an open kinematic chain, the hamstrings extend the hip and flex the knee. They control hip flexion and knee extension in the closed kinematic chain. These muscles balance each other and control the appropriate length–tension relationships of each other in gait.[109]

In summary, the muscles of the knee have dual roles—controlling motion and providing stability for a joint that has little inherent bony stability. The muscles, their actions, and their peripheral and segmental nerve innervations are shown in Table 8–2.

Neural Structures

The neural structures at the knee are continuations of the proximal nerves—the sciatic nerve (posteriorly) and the femoral nerve (anteriorly).

Posteriorly, the sciatic nerve courses distally from the sciatic notch of the pelvis through the hamstring compartment, between the biceps femoris and the underlying adductor magnus. At the superior apex of the popliteal fossa, the sciatic nerve divides into its tibial and peroneal branches. The tibial nerve runs down the middle of the popliteal fossa and passes deep between the heads of the gastrocnemius. Some

Table 8–2. Muscles of the Knee: Their Actions, Peripheral Nerve Supplies, and Nerve Roots

Muscles	Actions	Peripheral Nerve Supply	Spinal Segment
Biceps femoris	knee flexion tibia external rotation	sciatic	L5, S1, S2
Gastrocnemius	knee flexion	tibial	S1, S2
Gracilis	knee flexion tibia internal rotation	obdurator	L2, L3
Plantaris	knee flexion	tibial	S1, S2
Popliteus	knee flexion tibia internal rotation	tibial	L4, L5, S1
Rectus femoris	knee extension	femoral	L2, L3, L4
Sartorius	knee flexion tibia internal rotation	femoral	L2, L3
Semimembranosus	knee flexion tibia internal rotation	sciatic	L5, S1, S2
Semitendinosus	knee flexion tibia internal rotation	sciatic	L5, S1, S2
Tensor fascia latæ (in 0-30° flexion)	knee extension	superior gluteal	L4, L5
Tensor fascia latæ (in 45-145° flexion)	knee flexion	superior gluteal	L4, L5
Vastus intermedius	knee extension	femoral	L2, L3, L4
Vastus lateralis	knee extension	femoral	L2, L3, L4
Vastus medialis	knee extension	femoral	L2, L3, L4

people have a fibrous arch in the origin of the soleus muscle. The tibial nerve may be trapped or compressed here.[70]

The common peroneal nerve courses medially to the biceps femoris tendon and passes into the peroneus longus muscle, wrapping around the neck of the proximal fibula. The peroneal nerve may be compressed here by direct trauma to the lateral knee or by prolonged postures (such as cross–leg sitting). In the peroneus longus muscle, the nerve bifurcates, forming the deep peroneal (motor) and superficial peroneal (sensory) nerves.

Anteriorly, the femoral nerve courses distally from the femoral triangle in the anterior proximal thigh and divides into many cutaneous and motor branches. The saphenous nerve is the largest division, branching off just distal to the femoral triangle and coursing down the medial thigh to cross the knee. The infrapatellar branch originates from the saphenous nerve here and innervates the medial tibial subcutaneous periosteum and the overlying skin. This infrapatellar branch pierces the sartorius muscle and joins the cutaneous branches of the femoral nerve to supply cutaneous sensation at the patellofemoral joint. The saphenous nerve can be subject to intermittent compression as it pierces the sartorius muscle near the pes anserine insertion.

The following nerves can be compressed or entrapped: A) the tibial nerve as it enters the fibrous arch at the origin of the soleus muscle; B) the common peroneal nerve at the neck of the fibula; and C) the infrapatellar branch of the saphenous nerve as it pierces the sartorius muscle (Fig 8–11).

EVALUATION

Subjective Examination

The subjective examination should proceed as in Chapter 2, Principles of Extremity Evaluation. The patient's main complaints should give the clinician

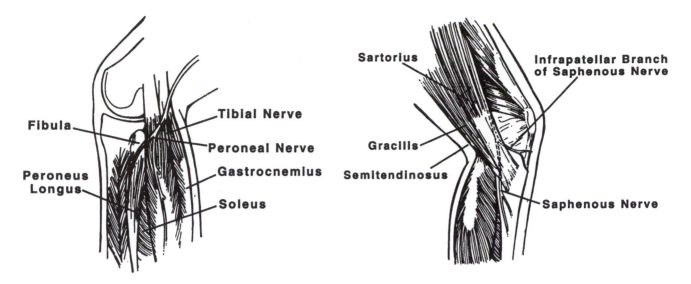

Figure 8–11. Potential sites of nerve entrapment around the knee. Left: the tibial nerve at the soleus muscle, and the common peroneal nerve at the neck of the fibula (posterior-lateral view). Right: the infrapatellar branch of the saphenous nerve at the sartorius muscle (medial view).

valuable clues about the patient's problems and help plan the objective examination. The mechanism of injury can help determine the structures that may be injured, especially in cases of acute trauma. Acute knee injuries can range from patellofemoral dislocation to ligamentous ruptures or meniscal tears. If the patient felt or heard a "pop" and subsequently developed a hemarthrosis with a moderate to large amount of effusion, there is up to a 70% chance the ACL is involved.[24] Repetitive trauma can affect the ligaments, tendons, and bursæ around the knee. Patellofemoral dysfunction is a common problem, often caused by repetitive trauma. The patterns of symptoms and mechanism of injury will help guide the objective examination of the knee.

Planning the Objective Examination

The objective examination of the knee is based on the subjective clues found during the patient interview. A well–planned examination will limit the possibility of inadvertently aggravating the problem. Tests should be prioritized to avoid excessive symptom provocation, which may interfere with a complete and accurate assessment. Suspected contributing areas such as the hip, ankle, and lumbar spine should be evaluated as needed to implicate or rule out their involvement.

The severity, irritability, and nature (SIN) of problems at the knee should be considered when planning the objective examination. If the knee problem is severe, the patient will have difficulty maintaining a position, especially in weightbearing. In such a case, the mobility examination should be limited to pain free points in the range, perhaps only in non–weightbearing.

If the knee problem is irritable, the problems will be provoked easily but will not settle down easily. For patients with irritable conditions, the number of motions tested should be limited to avoid exacerbating symptoms. The nature of the problem can limit the objective examination. For example, patients with a recent fracture or joint replacement should not be subjected to the full complement of objective tests.

Objective Examination

The objective examination should be performed as in outlined in Chapter 2, <u>Principles of Extremity Evaluation</u>. The areas that may contribute to symptoms felt at the knee should be checked first. This should include the lumbar spine, especially if movement of the low back provokes pain in the knee area. The hip, pelvis, and ankle should be considered in a thorough examination if these structures are thought to contribute to the clinical picture.

Structural Observation

Structural observation of the knee includes looking for alignment problems at the spine, pelvis, hips, and entire lower extremity.

ANTERIOR

The patient should first be observed from the front. The patient should stand comfortably, with the feet no farther than shoulder width apart and pointed straight ahead. This posture allows comparison from side to side and from patient to patient. Any asymmetries should be noted. The normal angle between the femur and the tibia is ≈7° of valgus in adults (Fig 8–12). The relative position of the patellæ should be noted.

The patient should then be asked to put the feet together. Any genu varus or "bow–legged" deformity will stand out. If the knees hit each other and prevent a normal stance, excessive genu valgus, or "knock–knee," is present. The position of the patellæ reflects the rotational alignment of the hip. Squinting patellæ reflect internally rotated or anteverted hips, while "frog–eye" patellæ reflect externally rotated or retroverted hips (Fig 8–13).

The relative position of the thigh and patella to the tibial tubercle should be noted. The clinician should look for tibial torsions while the patient stands with the patellæ pointing straight ahead.

Lastly, the patient should be asked to stand in a normal, relaxed posture. Patients will usually stand in a posture of ease to keep stress off stiff or painful tissues. This may provide valuable clues, especially when comparing the standard "toes straight ahead" alignment to the patient's habitual stance.

In addition to observing bony structure, the clinician should look for any soft tissue changes or asymmetries. Edema should be measured and all incisions inspected. Muscle wasting or atrophy is common at the knee after surgery or in chronic problems. Particular attention should be paid to the VMO, as it is usually the first portion of the quadriceps to be affected. The quadriceps angle (Q–angle) is the angle between a line running from the ASIS to the middle of the patella and a line from the middle of the patella to the tibial tuberosity. This is traditionally measured with the patient supine and the knee fully extended and relaxed; however, the position of the feet and hips can alter the Q–angle, especially in weightbearing;[96] therefore, the Q–angle should be measured with the patient standing so it represents normal weightbearing function (Fig 8–14). Normal Q–angles measure ≤10° for men, and ≤15° for women.[64] The Q–angle should be measured and compared bilaterally.

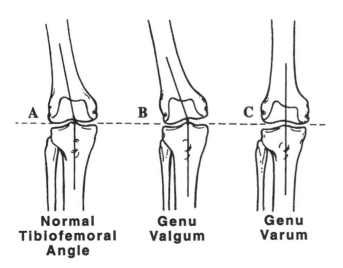

Figure 8–12. The angle between the femur-tibia. A) normal; B) genu valgum; C) genu varum.

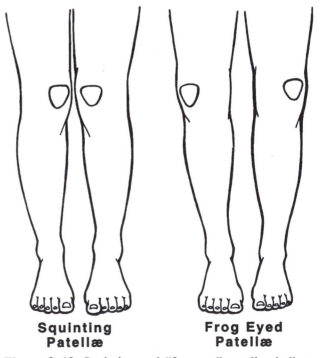

Figure 8–13. Squinting and "frog-eye" patellae indicate hip rotational alignment.

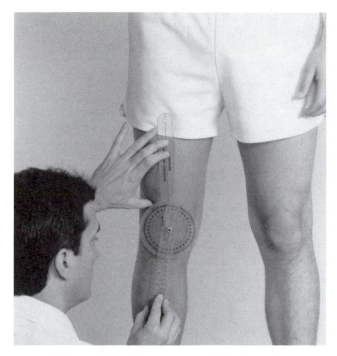

Figure 8–14. Measurement of the Q-angle.

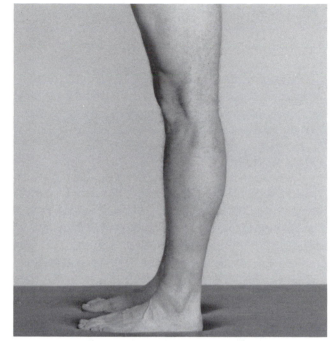

Figure 8–15. Genu recurvatum.

LATERAL

The patient's alignment should be noted from the sides and compared bilaterally. Any relative hyperextension at the knee—called genu recurvatum—should be noted (Fig 8–15). Recurvatum can be caused by the structure of the knee or by a postural compensation from tight hip flexors or an increased lumbar lordosis. If the knees are positioned in flexion, there may be intra–articular swelling or recent injury. Although some research suggests abnormal patellar positions can be seen from the side, these are only significant if correlated with radiographic findings. A high riding patella is called *patella alta* (Fig 8–16). A low riding patella is called *patella baja*. Patella baja is sometimes a complication of prolonged edema and inflammation in the post–operative ACL reconstructed knee, referred to as patellofemoral entrapment syndrome. Any differences in the size of the tibial tubercle should be noted. This area is commonly hypertrophied in Osgood–Schlatter's Disease (tibial tubercle epiphysitis).

POSTERIOR

The posterior structures and alignment of the knee are observed next. The popliteal crease and fibular head heights should be compared. Any

asymmetry in the calf musculature should be noted. There may be an abnormal finding such as swelling from a popliteal cyst (Baker's Cyst). These findings should be correlated to the symptoms since these are not always problematic.

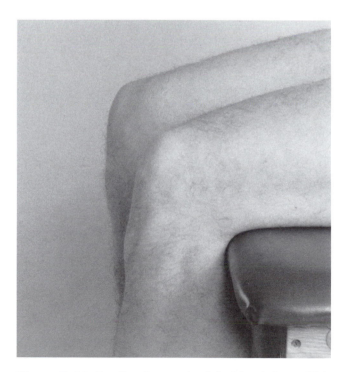

Figure 8–16. Patella alta on the left (close) knee. This condition can also be observed in standing.

Mobility

Physiological Mobility

Physiological mobility refers to the movement of the knee in standard planar movements and functional combined motions. Physiological mobility is tested actively and passively.

Active Mobility

Active mobility of the knee is examined to assess the patient's ability and willingness to move the knee. The important features include: the available range of motion, the complaints during motion, and any crepitus felt or heard. Abnormal joint sounds may indicate patellofemoral dysfunction, possibly chondromalacia (softening of the underside of the patella). Depending upon the severity and irritability of the joint, overpressure may be applied at end range. The response to overpressure should be noted: *Did the range of motion increase? Was there a symptom response?* The clinician can also get an initial impression of the joint's end–feel. Comparison should be made bilaterally and to normal. Testing is usually performed with the patient sitting, but it may be useful to check active mobility in a functional position such as standing. Weightbearing may affect symptoms and the available range of motion at the knee. The motions that can be actively tested at the knee include flexion and extension.

Passive Mobility

Passive mobility should be examined in any active motion of the knee that was not within normal limits or where the clinician was unable to test the end–feel. The following should be noted: range of motion, symptom response, end–feel, and the pattern of motion restriction. Passive motion should be compared bilaterally and to normal. The capsular pattern of the knee is *flexion limited greater than extension.* Passive mobility is usually tested in a supine position (Fig 8–17). In addition to knee flexion and extension, internal and external rotation of the tibia should be tested passively (Fig 8–18).

Accessory Mobility

Accessory mobility refers to joint play and component motions. Accessory mobility should be tested at any joint in which physiological mobility is limited or where abnormal responses to physiological mobility tests are found (see Chapter 11).

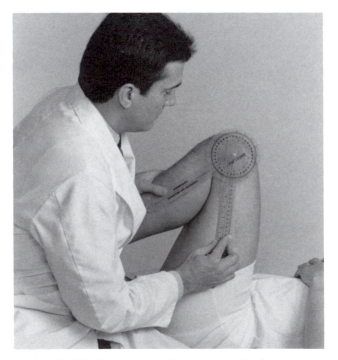

Figure 8–17A. Passive mobility testing at the knee: flexion.

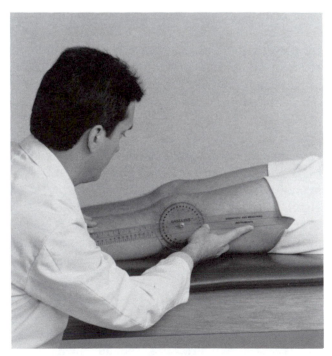

Figure 8–17B. Passive mobility testing at the knee: extension

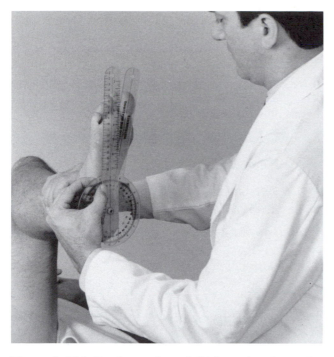

Figure 8–18A. Passive testing of tibial rotation: internal rotation.

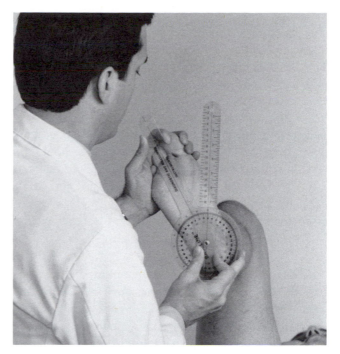

Figure 8–18B. Passive testing of tibial rotation: external rotation.

By joint, the following glides should be tested:

Tibiofemoral joint

- anterior
- posterior
- medial
- lateral

Patellofemoral joint

- superior
- inferior
- medial
- lateral

Superior tibiofibular joint

- anterior
- posterior

Pertinent findings include the available range of motion, the end–feel, any crepitus noted, and any symptoms provoked. All findings should be compared to the contralateral limb and to normal accessory mobility. The results should be consistent with the findings of the physiological mobility examination. For example, a common finding after immobilization is limited posterior glide of the tibia, which coincides with a restriction in knee flexion.

Strength

Specific manual muscle testing (MMT) assesses the status of the contractile elements of the knee. The tests are performed in the mid–range of motion to avoid stress on the noncontractile structures. The patient is told to gradually increase effort to a voluntary maximum contraction. The clinician resists the contraction isometrically. The muscle strength should be graded and any symptom response noted. Any muscle acting on, acting across, or influencing the knee should be included. Cyriax's four patterns of response (see Chapter 2, Principles of Extremity Evaluation) can help interpret the results of muscle tests. The result should be compared bilaterally and to normal strength.

Neurological

The neurological examination should be performed as outlined in Chapter 2, Principles of Extremity Evaluation. Indications for the examination include complaints of functional weakness; paresthesia or anesthesia; or other complaints that may indicate neurological impairment (e.g., balance or coordination problems). The basic neurological examination includes motor function, light touch sensation, and deep tendon reflexes (DTR's). Motor function is assessed per the lower quarter screening examination, assessing gross strength in the L1–S2 myotomes. The lumbosacral dermatomes and cutaneous nerve fields should be tested for light touch sensation (see Fig 2–12 on page 24). The relevant DTR's include the knee jerk (L3–L4), the medial hamstring reflex (L5–S1), and the ankle jerk (S1–S2). All neurological tests should be performed bilaterally for comparison.

Other neurological tests that may be relevant include proprioception testing and neural tension tests. Proprioception should be assessed, especially when there has been damage to ligament structures.[123] If adverse mechanical neural tension (AMNT) is suspected to contribute to the patient's complaints, the straight leg raise (SLR), prone knee bend (PKB), and the Slump tests should be performed. These tests are described in Chapter 2, Principles of Extremity Evaluation.

Palpation

The palpation examination should be consistent with layered palpation, as described in Chapter 2, Principles of Extremity Evaluation. Comparisons should be made bilaterally. The anterior structures are palpated with the patient supine or sitting. Posterior structures are best palpated with the patient prone. The medial and lateral structures can be palpated in sidelying, sitting, supine or prone. The following structures should be palpated:

Anterior (Fig 8–19)

- patella
- prepatellar bursa
- patellar retinaculum
- suprapatellar pouch
- quadricep tendon
- patellar tendon
- infrapatellar fat pad
- synovial plicæ (if present)

- quadriceps
- sartorius

Anterior, with knee flexed (Fig 8–20)

- joint lines (anteromedial and anterolateral)
- tibial plateau and tibial tubercle
- femoral condyles
- anteromedial and anterolateral borders of the menisci

Posterior (Fig 8–21)

- posterior capsule
- tibial nerve
- arcuate ligament
- posterior oblique ligament
- biceps femoris tendon
- semimembranosus tendon
- semitendinosus tendon
- hamstrings
- gastrocnemius
- popliteus muscle

Lateral (Fig 8–22)

- ITB
- lateral patellar facet
- fibular head
- common peroneal nerve
- LCL

Medial (Fig 8–23)

- Medial patellar facet
- MCL
- pes anserine
- saphenous nerve

It is important to correlate palpation findings to the rest of the objective examination findings. The clinician may need to palpate other sites that may contribute to the patient's problems.

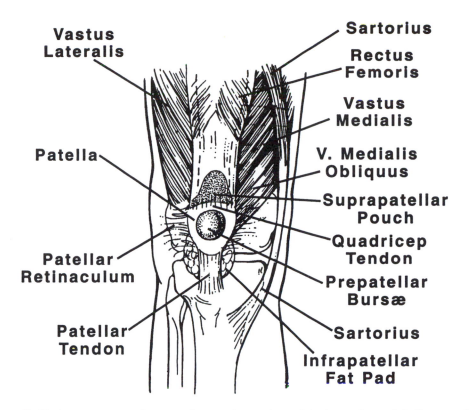

Figure 8–19. Structures to palpate on the anterior surface of the knee. Synovial plica not shown.

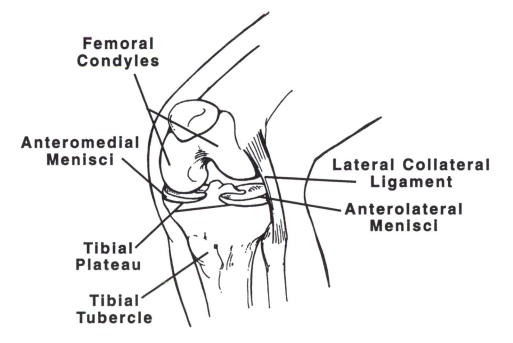

Figure 8–20. Structures to palpate on the anterior surface, with the knee flexed.

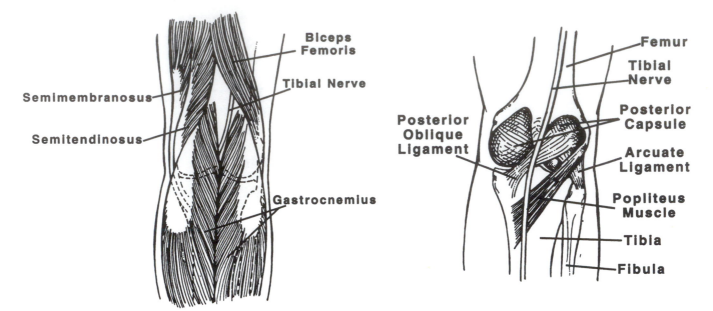

Figure 8–21. Structures to palpate on the posterior surface. Left: Superficial structures. Right: Deep structures.

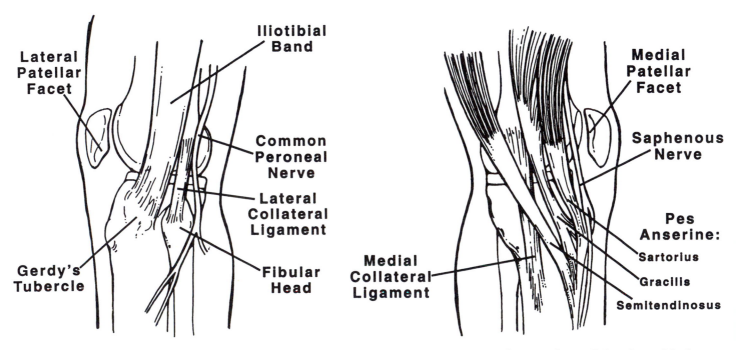

Figure 8–22. Structures to palpate on the lateral surface of the knee.

Figure 8–23. Structures to palpate on the medial surface of the knee.

Special Tests

Special tests gather more information about the knee problem and identify the contributing factors of the patient's problem. Special tests of the knee are classified as musculotendinous, effusion, joint and ligamentous, and functional. These tests are summarized in Table 8–3.

Musculotendinous Tests

Hamstring Tightness

Hamstring tightness can be tested in the positions shown in Fig 8–24. These include the long–sitting test, the tripod sign,[2] and the active SLR.[98] The test is positive if the patient's pelvis rotates posteriorly to

Table 8–3. Special Tests for the Knee

Test Type	Test Name	Purpose
Musculotendinous	Hamstring length	Hamstring Tightness
	Ely's	Rectus femorus tightness
	Ober's	Iliotibial band tightness
	Noble's Compression	Iliotibial band syndrome
Effusion	Stroke	Minimal joint effusion
	Fluctuation	Moderate to severe effusion
	Patellar tap	Moderate to severe effusion
Joint/Ligamentous	Patellar tilt	Tight lateral retinaculum/lateral patellar instability
	Lateral pull	Balance of quadriceps pull lateral patellar instability
	McConnell	Lateral patellofemoral instability
	Apprehension	Lateral patellofemoral instability
	Varus stress	Straight lateral instability
	Valgus stress	Straight medial instability
	Lachman's	Straight anterior instability
	Posterior sag	Straight posterior instability
	Posterior drawer	Straight posterior instability
	Quad active	Straight posterior instability
	AMRI	Anteromedial rotational instability
	ALRI	Anterolateral rotational instability
	Flexion rotation Drawer	Anterolateral rotational instability
	Slocum's ALRI	Anterolateral rotational instability
	McIntosh	Anterolateral instability
	External rotation	Posterolateral rotational instability
	Reverse pivot shift	Posterolateral rotational instability
	Squat	Meniscal injury
	Steinman's	Meniscal injury
	Hyperflexion-hyperextension	Meniscal injury
	McMurray-Anderson	Meniscal injury
	Plica	Synovial plica irritation
Functional Tests		Functional knee status

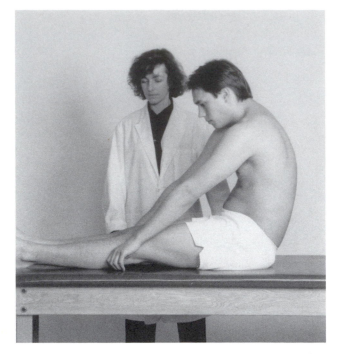

Figure 8–24A. Tests for hamstring tightness: long-sitting.

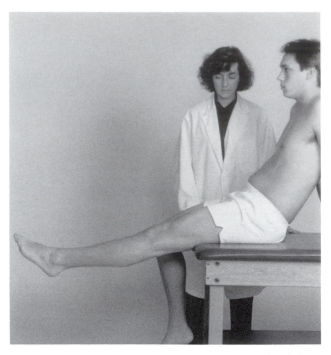

Figure 8–24B. Tests for hamstring tightness: tripod sign.

allow increased range or if the patient is unable to attain straight knee position. Restriction and symptoms in the hamstring muscle must be differentiated from AMNT and nerve root irritation. If neck flexion or ankle dorsiflexion can increase the complaints or cause distal or proximal migration of symptoms, then there is probable nerve involvement.

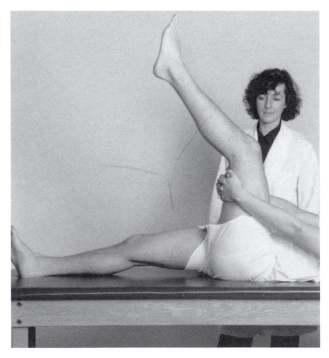

Figure 8–24C. Tests for hamstring tightness: active SLR.

Ely's Test

Ely's Test[47] for rectus femoris tightness is performed with the patient prone. The knee is flexed passively. The test is positive if the same hip flexes simultaneously (Fig 8–25).

Ober's Test

Ober's Test assesses tightness of the ITB.[94] The test can be performed with the knee flexed or extended; the ITB is most taut in knee extension. In sidelying, the uppermost hip is passively extended and abducted, then relaxed into adduction. The test is positive when the hip does not adduct past midline or when symptoms or complaints of tightness are reproduced (Fig 8–26).

Noble's Compression Test

Noble's Compression Test identifies ITB friction syndrome.[97] The clinician palpates the lateral femoral condyle while the knee is passively extended as shown (Fig 8–27, left). The test is positive if the patient's pain is reproduced as the ITB passes over the lateral femoral condyle. The test position we prefer is also shown (Fig 8–27, right). This is Noble's Compression Test performed in the Ober's Test position.

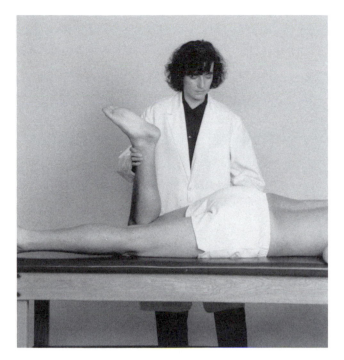

Figure 8–25. Ely's Test.

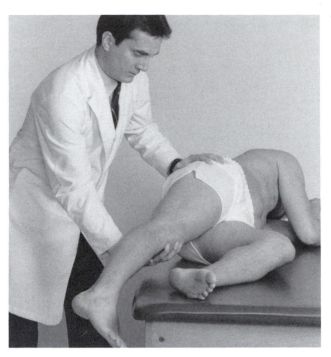

Figure 8–26. Ober's Test

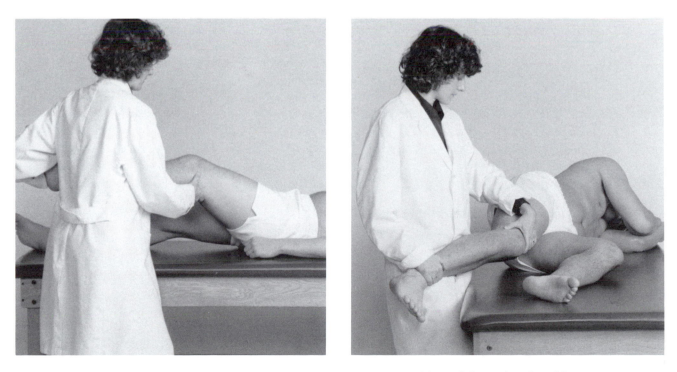

Figure 8–27. Noble's Compression Test. Left: standard position. Right: optional position.

Effusion Tests

Swelling can be assessed with circumferential measurements at and around the joint line; however, since many factors contribute to asymmetrical measurements (e.g., swelling, muscle atrophy, hypertrophy), other tests are needed to determine the cause of differences. There are three common ways to assess swelling at the patellofemoral joint: the stroke test, the fluctuation test, and the patellar tap test.

Stroke Test

The stroke test detects minimal effusion. The patient is supine with the knee relaxed. Beginning on the medial side of the patella, just distal to the joint line, the clinician strokes proximally. On the lateral side, the clinician begins above the joint line, stroking downward (Fig 8–28). These strokes are alternated several times. The test is positive if there is a palpable "wave" of fluid passing toward the medial patellofemoral joint.

Fluctuation Test

The fluctuation test detects moderate to severe effusion.[75] The patient is supine with the knee relaxed. The clinician places one hand proximal to the patella and the other distal to the patella (Fig 8–29). Pressure is applied by pushing down with each hand alternately. The test is positive if there is palpable movement of fluid beneath the skin.

Patellar Tap Test

The patellar tap test assesses moderate to severe joint effusion. The clinician pushes the patella inferiorly and taps the patella (Fig 8–30). The test is positive if the patella seems to "float" or bounce.

Joint/Ligamentous Tests

Joint and ligamentous tests assess the stability of the patellofemoral and tibiofemoral joints. Ligament testing guidelines are as follows:

- Make sure patient is as relaxed as possible
- Test contralateral limb first for comparison
- Apply firm stress
- Note amount of excessive joint motion
- Note end-feel during test

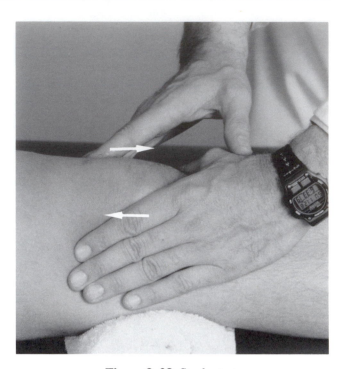

Figure 8–28. Stroke test.

A positive test indicates a significant deficit in the primary ligamentous restraint. A negative test does not necessarily mean the primary restraint is intact; the secondary restraints may be preventing excessive motion.

Patellar Tilt Test

The patellar tilt test assesses patellofemoral stability. The clinician lifts the lateral edge of the patella up away from the femur (Fig 8–31). The patella should remain in the trochlear groove. The test is positive if the patella moves less than 15° upward from a line parallel to the table while the patient is supine.[69] This lack of mobility indicates a tight lateral retinaculum, which predisposes the patella to lateral instability.

Lateral Pull Test

The lateral pull test assesses patellofemoral stability. The patient is seated or supine. The clinician evaluates the amount of superior and lateral pull of the patella by having the patient perform a voluntary quadricep contraction with the knee in full extension (Fig 8–32). Normally, there will be equal superior and lateral pull. The test is positive if there is excessive lateral pull.[69]

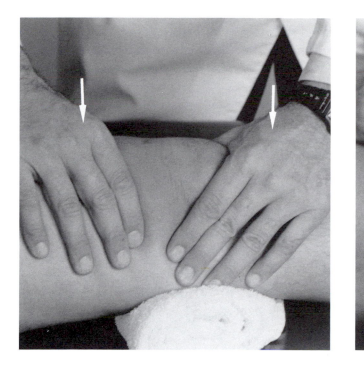

Figure 8–29. Fluctuation test.

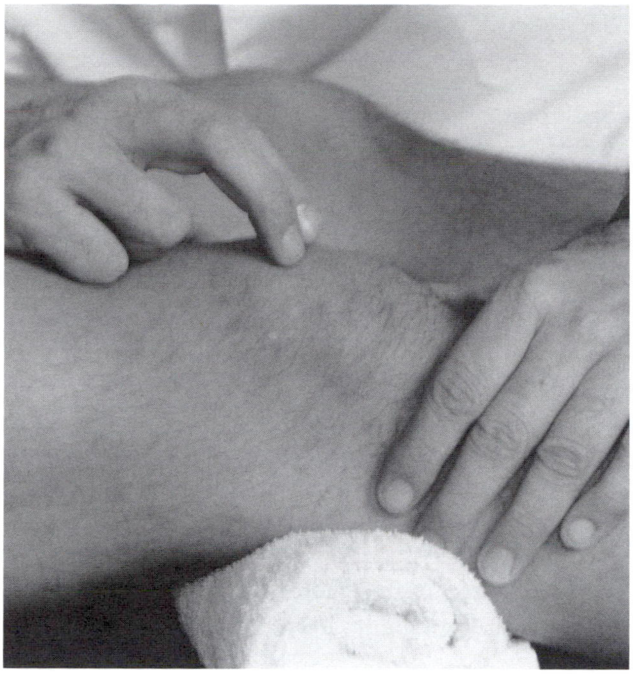

Figure 8–30. Patellar tap test.

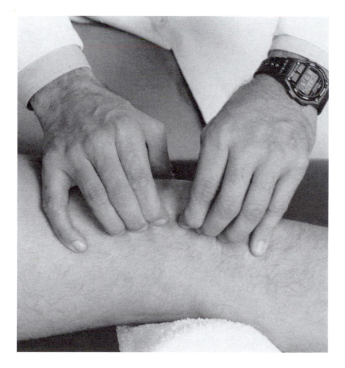

Figure 8–31. Patellar tilt test.

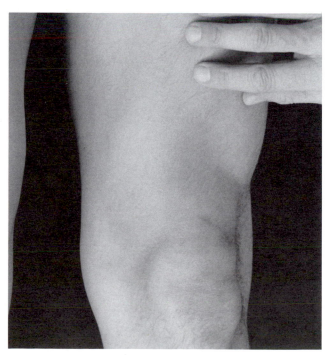

Figure 8–32. Lateral pull test.

McConnell Test

The McConnell Test assesses lateral patellofemoral instability. This test consists of repeated isometric testing of the quadriceps at 0°, 30°, 60°, 90°, and 120° of knee flexion with the patient sitting. If the patient complains of pain, the clinician repeats the tests at the painful angles while stabilizing the patella laterally (Fig 8–33). The test is positive if lateral stabilization eliminates the pain.[81]

Apprehension Test

This is another common test for lateral patellofemoral instability. The clinician glides the patella to its maximum lateral position (Fig 8–34). The test is positive if there is pain and apprehension. The test can be performed in the opposite direction; however medial patellar instability is rare.

Varus Stress Test

The varus stress test assesses straight lateral knee stability. Testing is performed with the knee in full extension and in 30° of flexion (Fig 8–35). Testing in slight flexion primarily stresses the LCL, while tests in full extension also stress the joint capsule. The test is positive if there is excessive mobility and pain. If the LCL is torn, the cruciates become secondary restraints to varus stress. Marked joint laxity in 0° of extension implicates cruciate ligament involvement. This should be confirmed with other ligament tests.

Valgus Stress Test

The valgus stress test assesses straight medial knee stability. Pressure is applied medially with the knee in full extension and at 30° of knee flexion (Figure 8–36). Testing in slight flexion primarily stresses the MCL, while tests in full extension also stress the joint capsule. The test is positive if there is excessive laxity and pain. If the MCL is torn, the cruciates act as secondary restraints to valgus stress. Marked joint laxity in 0° of knee extension implicates cruciate involvement. This should be confirmed with other ligament tests.

Lachman's Test

This test is the classic test for ACL instability (straight anterior instability). The patient is positioned with the knee in 20–35° of flexion. The patient's femur is stabilized with one hand, while the proximal tibia is stressed in an anterior direction (Fig 8–37). The test is positive if there is excessive joint laxity when compared to normal.

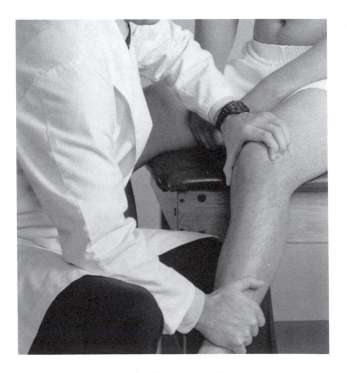

Figure 8–33. McConnell Test.

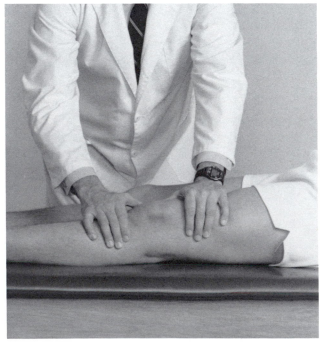

Figure 8–34. Apprehension test.

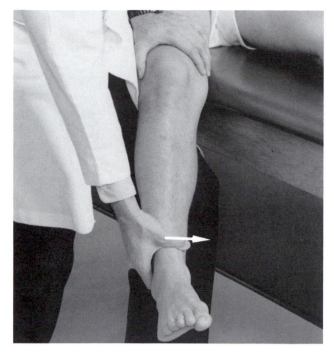

Figure 8–35. Varus stress test shown in ≈30° of flexion

Anterior Drawer Test

The anterior drawer test detects straight anterior stability. The patient's knee is positioned in 90° of knee flexion (Fig 8–38). The clinician applies a straight anterior force on the proximal tibia. The test is positive if there is excessive joint laxity.

Posterior Sag Sign

The posterior sag sign is a positional test to help the clinician implicate PCL involvement by determining if posterior instability is present. The patient is in 90° of knee flexion (Fig 8–39). The test is positive if there is a posterior sag of the tibia on the femur. The anterior drawer test may seem positive if the posterior sag is present because the tibia started in a relatively posterior position.

Posterior Drawer Test

The posterior drawer test detects PCL injury. The patient is in 90° of knee flexion. The clinician applies a straight posterior force to the proximal tibia (Fig 8–40). The test is positive if there is excessive joint laxity.

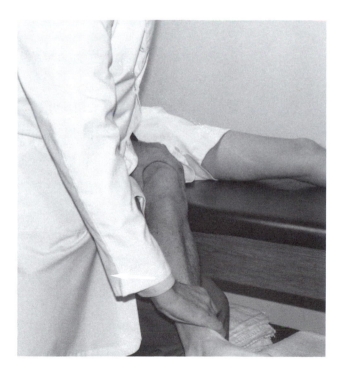

Figure 8–36. Valgus stress test shown in ≈30° of flexion

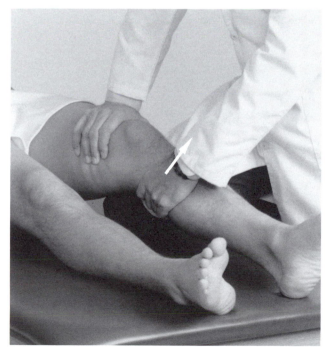

Figure 8–37. Lachman's Test.

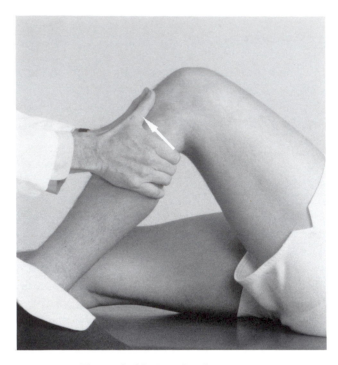

Figure 8–38. Anterior drawer test.

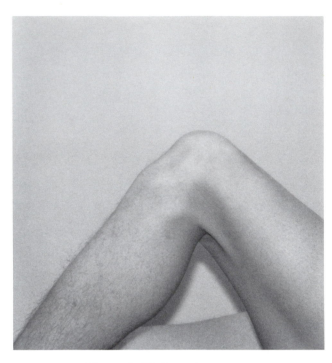

Figure 8–39. Posterior sag test

Quadricep Active Test

The quadricep active test detects posterior instability. The patient is supine with the knee flexed to 90°. The patient is asked to actively contract the quadriceps while knee flexion is maintained (Fig 8–41). The test is positive if the tibia moves anteriorly.[22]

Anterior Medial Rotational Instability (AMRI) Test

Although the clinician could infer AMRI is present if a Lachman's Test and a valgus stress test are positive, an easy modification of the drawer test can confirm this condition. The tibia is externally rotated ≈15°, and the anterior drawer test is performed (Fig 8–42). The test is positive if the medial aspect of the tibial plateau moves anteriorly relative to the lateral aspect.

Anterior Lateral Rotational Instability (ALRI) Test

The drawer position detects this instability. The clinician places the tibia in about 15–30° of internal rotation. Too much rotation may tighten the ITB and the PCL, giving a false negative test result. The anterior drawer test is performed. The test is positive

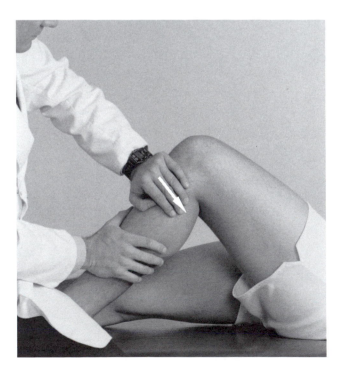

Figure 8–40. Posterior drawer

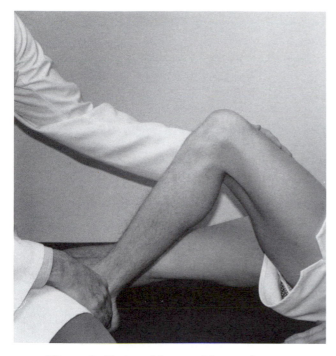

Figure 8–41. A positive quadricep active test.

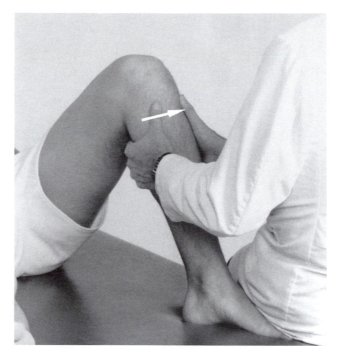

Figure 8–42. Anterior medial rotational instability (AMRI) test

if the lateral tibial plateau moves more anteriorly than the medial side (Fig 8–43).

Pivot Shift Tests

The pivot shift tests detect ALRI. These tests try to re–create the tibial subluxation that can occur with this instability. The surface of the lateral tibial plateau is convex in the sagittal plane. Injury to the lateral structures creates a pivot point that the lateral femoral condyle can roll back and forth over.[82] The aim is to prove instability is present by subluxing and reducing the tibia on the femur. This usually occurs between 20°–40° of knee flexion. The test is positive if a shift or clunk can be seen or felt; however, in cases of excessive swelling, muscle guarding, or even subtle instability, re–creation of the patient's complaint of apprehension or "giving way" is enough to indicate a positive test. There are three pivot shift tests for ALRI: the flexion rotation drawer test, Slocum's ALRI Test, and the McIntosh Test.

Flexion Rotation Drawer Test

The flexion rotation drawer test is performed with the tibia held in neutral rotation and the knee flexed to ≈20° (Fig 8–44).[88] The weight of the thigh causes the femur to drop relatively posterior and into external

rotation. The test is positive if the tibia is relatively anteriorly subluxed and internally rotated. This subluxed position is reduced with a combined movement of slight flexion (10–20°) and a posterior drawer.

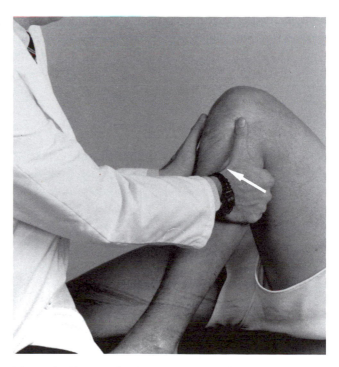

Figure 8–43. Anterior lateral rotational instability (ALRI) test.

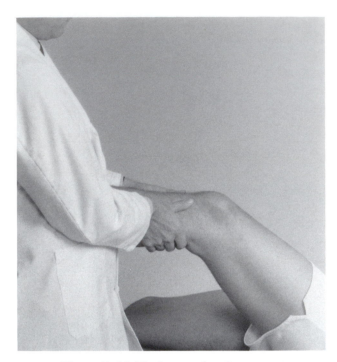

Figure 8–44. Flexion rotation drawer test.

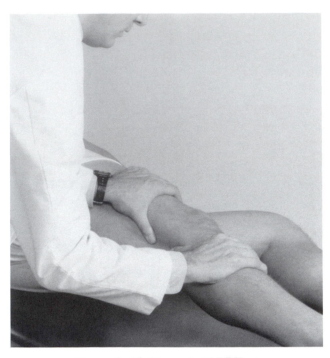

Figure 8–45. Slocum's ALRI Test.

Slocum's ALRI Test

This test is performed with the patient in sidelying, with the involved leg up. The heel of the involved leg rests on the examination table, with the knee in about 20° of flexion (Fig 8–45).[40] This positions the knee in relative internal tibial rotation. In this position, the clinician applies a valgus stress by pressing down toward the table, while flexing the knee to 30–40°. The test is positive if the clinician feels a clunk or shift as the tibia reduces on the femur.

The McIntosh Test

This test is performed with the patient in supine and the knee comfortably extended. The clinician internally rotates the tibia, and a valgus stress is added. This recreates the anterolateral subluxed position of the tibia on the femur. The knee is then flexed to about 20–40° (Fig 8–46). The test is positive if the clinician feels a clunk or shift as the tibia is moved into flexion.[113]

External Rotation Test

This test assesses PLRI. There are two positions from which it may be performed:

1. The patient is positioned in a modified drawer position, with the knee flexed to 90° and the tibia

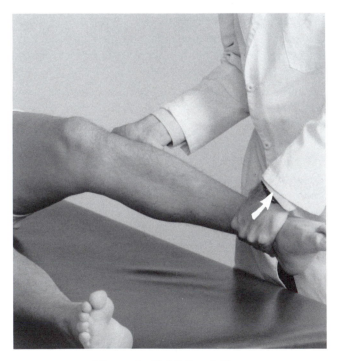

Figure 8–46. McIntosh Test.

externally rotated ≈15–20°. A posterior force is applied to the proximal tibia (Fig 8–47A). The test is positive if there is excessive joint laxity in the posterior lateral knee.

2. The patient positions the knee in mild flexion (20–35°) and is asked to bend the knee further while the clinician holds it in external rotation (Fig 8–47B).[30] The clinician palpates the posterolateral joint line for any excessive motion. The test is positive if there is excessive joint laxity.

Instrumented Ligament Testing

There are now knee arthrometers that measure joint laxity. These instruments can help make the initial diagnosis of knee instability and help reassess ligamentous stability after reconstructive knee surgery. Instrumented testing has advanced ligamentous injury management at the knee, but further research is needed to examine the validity and reliability of these methods. A recent text provides an excellent review of instrumented examination of the knee.[15]

Meniscal Tests

Clinical experience and review of the literature suggest none of the available meniscal tests are definitive. The diagnosis of meniscus impairment is often made by history alone; however, meniscal tests can help clarify the patient's problem. Comparison to the uninvolved limb is critical. Four meniscal tests are presented here: the squat walk test, Steinman's Sign, the hyperflexion/hyperextension test, and the McMurray–Anderson Test.

Squat Walk Test

The patient is asked to walk in the full squat position—a "duck walk" (Fig 8–48). The test is positive if there is guarding, clicking, or pain, especially if there is a difference between the involved and uninvolved sides.[113]

Steinman's Sign

For this test, the clinician observes the patient for tenderness that seems to move when the knee is moved.[83] The joint line is palpated with the knee flexed and extended. The test is positive if joint line pain is more anterior with knee extension and more posterior with knee flexion.

Hyperflexion–Hyperextension Test

The patient is positioned in full knee flexion and the clinician applies overpressure with internal tibial rotation. Then the patient is positioned in full knee

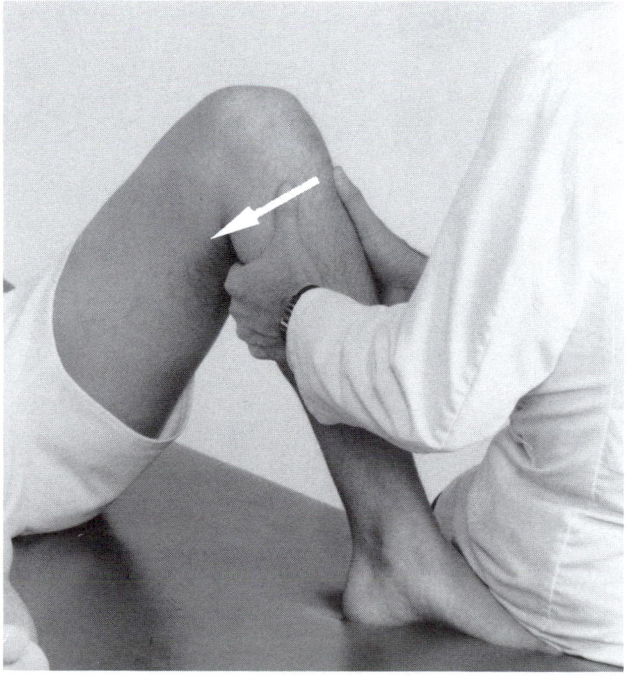

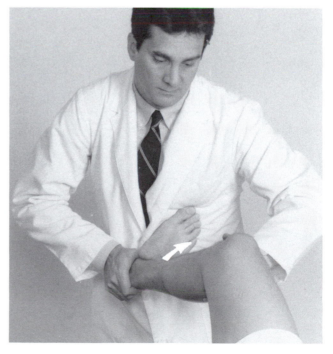

Figure 8–47A. External rotation test in 90° flexion.

Figure 8–47B. External rotation test in slight flexion.

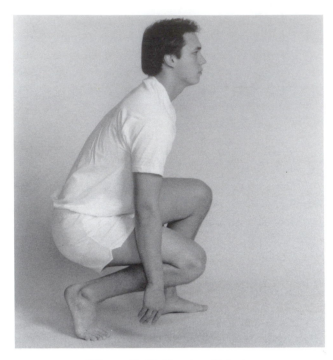

Figure 8–48. Squat walk test.

extension, and the clinician applies overpressure with external tibial rotation (Fig 8–49). The test is positive if there is guarding, clicking, or pain.

McMurray–Anderson Test

This test is a combination of the McMurray Test[3] and Anderson's Medial–Lateral Grinding Test.[53] The patient's tibia is held in internal rotation while the knee is flexed from 0–45°. A valgus stress is applied with this movement. Then the knee is extended from 45–0° while varus stress is applied and the tibia is externally rotated (Fig 8–50). The test is positive if it reproduces clicking, grinding or possibly pain.

If the clinician suspects the menisci are internally deranged, the patient should be referred to an orthopædic surgeon for examination and diagnostic tests.

Plica Test

This test detects a symptomatic synovial plica. The patient is supine as the clinician palpates the medial patella and applies a mild medial stress. The tibia is held in internal rotation as the knee is repeatedly moved from flexion to extension (Fig 8–51). The test is positive if the plical band pops with

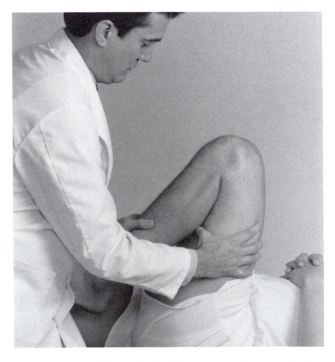

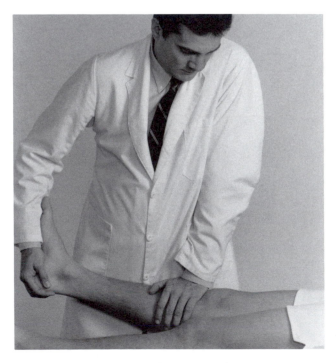

Figure 8–49. Hyperflexion-hyperextension test. Left: hyperflexion. Right: hyperextension.

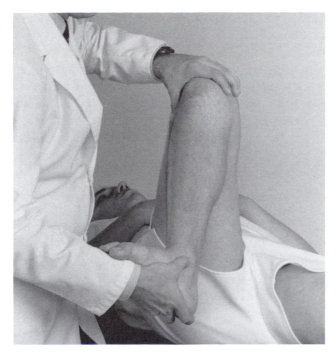

Figure 8–50. McMurray-Anderson Test.

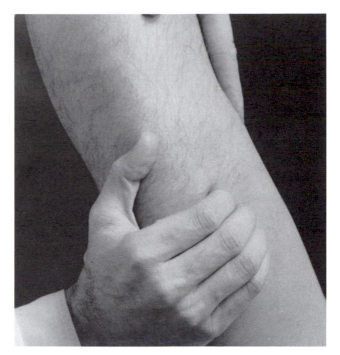

Figure 8–51. Plica test.

palpation. This may occur anywhere in the range of motion, but most commonly occurs at 45–60°.[87]

FUNCTIONAL TESTS

There have been many attempts to appropriately assess knee function. Two of the common rating scales used are the Cincinnati Rating System[89] and the Knee Society Rating Scale.[56,93,98] A simple group of functional tests can be performed to help the clinician gain valuable information. These are: two–legged full squat; one–legged half squat; and circular one–leg hopping in a clockwise and counterclockwise direction. Research on the validity of using the one–leg hopping test as a predictor of function has shown inconclusive results.[8,76,93,118]

The results should be compared bilaterally and to normal. The following responses should be noted: the patient's willingness to perform the test; the symptom response; and signs of apprehension.

Objective Evaluation Summary

The objective and subjective examination findings should be reviewed and correlated. Many structures can contribute to knee symptoms. The contribution of all knee tissues (including the ligaments, menisci, tendons, muscles, bursæ, nerves,

and the joints themselves) should be considered. Other sources of knee complaints include the hip, the foot and ankle, and the lumbar spine. The initial evaluation must be geared toward screening these joints. Re–assessments should include reconsideration of these areas, especially if the patient is not benefiting from treatment.

At the conclusion of the evaluation, the clinician determines what problems the patient has and develops a problem list. This list helps the clinician set goals and plan treatments.

TREATMENT STRATEGIES

If the problem is not caused by acute injury to the knee, the proximal contributing structures should be treated first. This will help determine the extent to which problems in these areas relate to symptoms and dysfunction at the knee. Their contribution can be measured after treatment by reassessing any change in knee symptoms or range of motion.

The clinician should consider the use of assistive devices to control weightbearing for any patient whose knee problems are aggravated by weightbearing activities. The assistive device should be used until the symptoms resolve and the gait pattern is symmetrical. Immobilizers and knee braces that limit range of motion can help protect the joint after acute injury. Their prolonged use should be avoided to prevent the deleterious effects of immobilization (see Chapter 3, Pathology and Treatment Principles).

The patient should avoid pivoting if the knee is unstable. The patient should be taught to turn on the ball of the foot and to avoid twisting at the knee. This should continue until joint proprioception is restored. Work and sport activities should be modified as needed.

Open kinematic chain exercises can be used at the knee, but closed kinematic chain exercises should be included in the treatment program because they more closely mimic function. Proprioceptive exercises should also be included in the treatment of any knee disorder. This is especially important when instability is present. Pool exercises are an excellent means of functional progression, especially when controlled weightbearing is needed.

The reader should refer to Chapter 11, Mobilization Techniques, and Chapter 12, Exercise, for mobilization techniques, stretching, strengthening, and proprioceptive exercises for the knee.

COMMON CLINICAL CONDITIONS

Patellofemoral Instability

Patients with pain at the patellofemoral joint are often referred to physical therapy. The causes of the pain have been attributed to abnormal stresses to the subchondral bone of the patella, abnormal stresses to the retinaculum, and even to venous engorgement that intermittently compresses nerves.[38,39,57,122] There are numerous medical articles referring to patellofemoral problems as "chondromalacia patellæ." In fact, this term describes only the pathological changes that occur with cartilage degeneration, and it is not an appropriate diagnosis for all patients with patellofemoral problems.[39,43,54] Most authors agree the underlying cause of patellofemoral problems is poor patellofemoral mechanics. In this condition, the normal path of the patella in the trochlear groove of the femur is altered. This is referred to as altered patellofemoral tracking or "instability."

Very high forces are transmitted across this joint, as shown in Table 8–4. The greater the flexion in weightbearing, the greater the force across the patellofemoral joint.[111] These forces are offset by an increase in the area of patellar contact during closed kinematic chain movements. This increased contact transmits the forces over a wider area, diminishing the effects at any one point in the joint. This increased contact does not occur in resisted open kinematic chain exercises.[41]

Most patellar instability occurs in the first 30° of knee flexion as the patella moves medially in the trochlear groove. Beyond this point the patella has greater bony stability in the groove.[23] Minor instability of the patella in the trochlear groove can lead to mild symptoms. Moderate instability can require changes in the patient's lifestyle, and severe instability can result in subluxation or dislocation of the patella.

Patellofemoral problem management requires thorough examination and treatment of all contributing factors. Recurrence is very common, therefore teaching patients the importance of continuous self–management is necessary for lasting results.

History

Patients usually describe a gradual onset with activity, but there may be a history of trauma that resulted in subluxation or dislocation. Patellofemoral subluxation sometimes occurs with a valgus–external rotation stress when pivoting. Repetitive trauma is the most common cause of patellofemoral problems.

Signs/Symptoms

Patients usually complain of peripatellar pain. If the problem is precipitated by traumatic subluxation or dislocation, there may be swelling around the joint. Pain is usually worst in weightbearing, but sitting can also irritate the problem. Patients who have pain when standing after prolonged sitting have what is termed "movie–goer's sign."[43]

The complaints can be activity specific. Stair climbing, squatting, running, pivoting, and jumping may cause pain. Many patients also report crepitus or noise in this joint. Some complain of pain "behind the

Table 8–4. Forces at the Patellofemoral Joint[75]

Position	Force
Standing	0.0 x BW
Walking	0.5 x BW
Stairs	3.3 x BW
Deep knee bend (130° knee flexion)	7.8 x BW
Sitting (90° knee flexion)	0.0 x BW
Sitting (36° knee flexion)	1.4 x BW
Sitting (0° Knee Flexion)	0.5 x BW
Sitting (isokinetic exercise 60-180°/sec, <20° knee flexion)	<1.0 x BW
Sitting (isokinetic exercise 60-180°/sec, <70-75° knee flexion)	5.0 x BW

kneecap." In the objective examination the clinician should look for the static and dynamic contributors noted above. The apprehension test may be positive in cases of marked instability. The McConnell Test may be positive. The clinician should observe the patient's gait pattern to get a complete picture of the lower kinematic chain and its effect on patellofemoral mechanics.

Diagnostics

There are no routine diagnostic tests for patellofemoral dysfunction. Radiographs may be used if a fracture is suspected after subluxation, dislocation, or blunt trauma. Radiographs can also help identify any predisposing bony factors contributing to the patellar instability (Fig 8–52). A lateral x–ray may show a patella alta or high–riding patella, which may contribute to excessive lateral tracking, patellar subluxation, and dislocation.[58,101] MRI can pick up retropatellar cartilage defects.

Problem List

Patients with patellofemoral instability may have any of the following problems:

1. Anterior knee pain with closed kinematic chain activities

2. Crepitus with open kinematic chain resisted exercise

3. Episodes of knee cap "going out"

4. Poor VMO activation

5. Lateral patellar tracking

6. Intolerance of weightbearing or prolonged sitting

Treatment

PRICE and anti–inflammatory drugs can help decrease symptoms associated with patellar

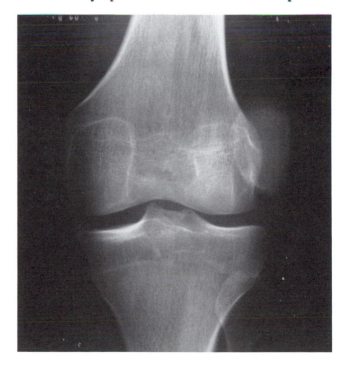

Figure 8–52. Radiograph of a right patellar lateral dislocation.

instability. Immobilization for 3–7 days after dislocation may be needed to control symptoms and promote healing. Any exercises performed in a closed kinematic chain should be done in a pain free range. It is essential to control any edema, since joint effusion can inhibit VMO activation.

If muscle tightness contributes to the problem the patient should be taught stretching exercises. These may include stretching the piriformis, hamstrings, ITB, and gastrocsoleus muscles. ITB tightness is particularly problematic as it can limit medial patellar glide.[86]

The VMO pulls the patella medially and resists lateral tracking, so it is essential for this muscle to work effectively. VMO reeducation may include electrical stimulation, biofeedback, and patellofemoral taping.

Since the biomechanics of the foot and ankle can contribute to knee pain, any problems in this area should be addressed with appropriate footwear or orthoses.[108] This is particularly important if there is abnormal pronation at the subtalar joint.[41,108]

Closed kinematic chain exercises are critical to lasting results. These may include biking, squats, stair climbing, and balance board exercises.[29,55,81] Proprioceptive training in weightbearing can also aid functional rehabilitation. A recent study casts doubt on the use of short–arc quadricep strengthening in the open kinematic chain to increase strength of the VMO. Subjects using this method to strengthen their quadriceps showed abnormal patellar tracking despite an increase in quadricep muscle strength. Open kinematic chain strengthening exercises do not seem to help the patella relocate medially and may predispose the patella to lateral subluxation.[29] Other research has shown that performing quad sets and SLR with the hip in adduction does not preferentially strengthen the VMO;[66] however, contraction of the adductors in a weightbearing position has been shown to preferentially increase VMO activity relative to the vastus lateralis.[52]

Taping can help control lateral glide, lateral tilt, anterior–posterior tilt, and rotation of the patella (Fig 8–53). When used with closed kinematic chain strengthening of the VMO, taping has shown promising clinical results.[55,81] Recent research supports the use of a functional approach to retraining the quadriceps with help from biofeedback and patellofemoral taping.[29,55,67,81] Minimizing symptoms while promoting patellar stability is crucial to long term management of these problems.

Iliotibial Band (ITB) Syndrome

ITB syndrome is most commonly seen in competitive athletes,[27] but may occur in workers and recreational athletes. The onset of the symptoms can be gradual. The symptoms are initially subtle and brought on by activity, but pain can become quite severe in some cases.

The ITB has two components at the lateral knee: the iliopatellar band and the iliotibial tract. The iliopatellar band reinforces the lateral retinaculum and adds stability to the lateral knee. The iliotibial tract courses distally to its insertion at Gerdy's Tubercle at the lateral proximal tibia. The patellotibial ligament connects the iliopatellar band to the iliotibial tract. Iliotibial tract attachments include the lateral intermuscular septum; the lateral femoral condyle; the lateral capsular ligament; biceps femoris tendon; and the fibula.[101]

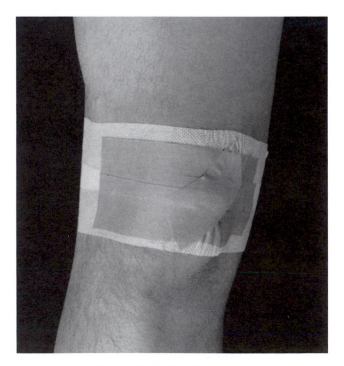

Figure 8–53. Patellar taping.

The mechanics of the ITB are affected by the gluteus maximus and the tensor fascia lata, from which it arises.[74,102] The iliotibial tract is pulled posteriorly by the biceps femoris tendon, keeping it taut throughout knee flexion. Because of its angle of insertion, the ITB is a knee extensor from 0–30° of extension and a knee flexor when the knee is flexed 30° or more.[78]

The ITB is most taut when the knee is in a varus position.[34,62] ITB syndrome is caused by excessive friction between the ITB and the underlying lateral femoral condyle; therefore, individuals with ITB tightness are more prone to this problem.

ITB syndrome occurs most frequently in runners who have pes cavus (high arches) and genu varus (bow legs).[114]

History

The patient usually has a gradual onset of lateral knee pain. The mechanism of injury is usually overuse at the knee. Occasionally, the onset is sudden after the knee is subjected to an unaccustomed stress. Symptoms at the lateral knee will increase if the repeated stresses are not modified. ITB syndrome often recurs. Many of these patients also have a history of patellofemoral problems.

Signs/Symptoms

The patient complains of an aching pain in the lateral knee. This can become sharp at a certain level of activity (e.g., at a specific mileage threshold in a runner). Climbing stairs or running on inclines aggravates pain. The condition is irritated on the downhill side when running on a sidehill (Fig 8–54).

The patient can usually point to a specific spot on the lateral knee when asked to identify the painful site. The pain is usually felt near the lateral femoral condyle, but it may refer proximally or distally. The area will be tender to palpation. There may be palpable crepitus on repeated flexion and extension of the knee. Ober's Test for iliotibial tightness will be positive, as will Noble's Compression Test. Because of its attachment to the ITB, the lateral retinaculum may also be tender to palpation.

Diagnostics

There are no standard diagnostic tests for this problem. Diagnosis is usually made by history and objective examination only; however, a cortisone injection at the ITB may prove diagnostic if the symptoms are relieved.

Problem List

Patients with ITB syndrome may have any of the following problems.

1. Lateral knee pain with activity

2. Tight ITB

3. Pain on palpation at lateral femoral condyle

4. Inability to run due to pain

5. Decreased tolerance to stair climbing

Treatment

ITB syndrome management should address all contributing factors. Symptomatic relief measures such as ice, ultrasound, and iontophoresis can help control pain and inflammation and speed healing. The

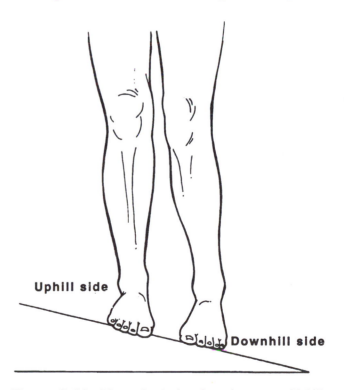

Figure 8–54. Biomechanical adaptations to sidehill running.

physician may prescribe anti–inflammatory drugs. A tight ITB should be stretched to decrease the stresses on this area. Friction massage and soft tissue mobilization may help lengthen the ITB and stimulate healing. Patients should avoid activities that increase mechanical stress on the ITB.

Abnormal foot mechanics should be addressed. Orthoses may decrease the lateral knee stresses by controlling foot position.

Patients should be gradually progressed back to a normal routine. Runners should avoid excessive sidehill running and all patients with this problem should avoid excessive use of stairs. ITB syndrome can resist therapeutic intervention. Clinical studies have shown pes cavus–related ITB syndrome can take up to twice as long to resolve as pronation–related patellofemoral problems.[114]

Meniscal Tears

The menisci are frequently involved in knee pain and dysfunction. For a long time total meniscectomy was the treatment of choice for any injury to these structures; however, as early as 1948, some clinicians were already discovering patients who underwent total meniscectomy showed degenerative joint changes as soon as three months after surgery.[115] More recent studies have shown similar findings.[1,63,84] When the menisci are removed, several mechanical functions are lost:

1. The menisci act as mechanical spacers and prevent contact between the femoral condyles and tibial plateaus in non–weightbearing situations. After a total meniscectomy, there is a small amount of joint space narrowing.[71]

2. The menisci normally distribute greater than 50% of the total forces across the knee in weightbearing situations.[27] The force distribution capabilities of the menisci are lost with total meniscectomy (Fig 8–3).

3. The menisci normally help the ligaments limit joint translation. After a meniscectomy, this extra translation limitation is lost. Meniscectomy performed after ACL disruption can allow up to 6 mm of additional anteroposterior tibial translation.[26]

The menisci also participate in joint lubrication, nutrition, and shock absorption.[71] Arthroscopic partial meniscectomy has been the primary alternative to total meniscectomy and is one of the more common surgical procedures of the knee;[71] however, there is increasing evidence partial meniscectomies also lead to unsatisfactory results. Partial meniscectomies result in degenerative joint changes directly related to the amount of meniscus removed.[28,73]

A newer surgical alternative is meniscal repair. Clinical studies have shown symptom relief, high healing rates, and low reinjury rates after surgical repair of an injured meniscus.[26,48,105] These studies show healing rates as high as 90% in the peripheral meniscus.[25] Other surgical techniques for repairing damaged menisci are being researched. These include introducing fibrin clots and fascial patches as scaffolding to the avascular areas of meniscal injury.[5,50] Future surgery may even place collagen–based scaffolds as superstructures for meniscal regeneration. Early results using this procedure are encouraging.[112]

Certainly, non–operative treatment is an option. There is some evidence of meniscal healing with conservative care.[126]

History

Non–contact stresses to the knee are the most frequent mechanisms of injury to the menisci.[25] Patients usually report a mechanism of injury related to a sudden change of direction (e.g., an abrupt start, stop, pivot, or twist). Meniscal injuries often occur when the knee is twisted or when landing from a jump with the knee in hyperflexion or hyperextension. Degenerative meniscal tears are common in active older patients, and may occur with minimal stresses.[18] Sixty–five percent of patients with an acute ACL injury have concurrent injury to the menisci.[24] Up to 98% of patients with chronic ACL insufficiency also have meniscal damage.[125]

Signs/Symptoms

The patient has a variety of complaints, including joint line pain, joint locking, and giving way of the knee. All these symptoms occur during weightbearing. The patient may also be unable to fully straighten or extend the knee. There may be swelling around the joint, and there is frequently concurrent injury to the ligamentous structures and the patellofemoral joint. The special tests for meniscal injury may be positive (see the "Special Tests" section of this chapter). The end–feel is usually spongy and the patient may have joint line or posterior knee pain with overpressure. Occasionally, a patient's knee may lock during examination. If the clinician cannot manually unlock the joint, the patient should be referred to an orthopædic surgeon.

Diagnostics

MRI examination is the test of choice for diagnosing meniscal pathology (Fig 8–55).[61] The use of an arthrogram, which is invasive, is not as common as it once was. Standard radiographs are sometimes used when the patient is an adolescent. These can rule out a growth plate fracture in an acute injury, but do not provide information about the menisci.

Problem List

Patients with meniscal tears may present with any of the following problems:

1. Knee joint line pain

2. Catching or locking of the knee

3. Painful, limited knee flexion or extension

4. Intolerance of weightbearing activities

5. Antalgic gait pattern

Treatment

Treatment of injury to the menisci may vary from non–operative to partial meniscectomy to meniscal repair. Rehabilitation guidelines for meniscus injury are based on multiple factors, including: the location and extent of the lesion; weightbearing surface degeneration; duration of injury; and joint stability. The patient's fitness also affects predicted recovery time. A professional athlete with a partial meniscectomy usually returns to the sport more quickly than the middle aged weekend athlete with a similar injury. Generally, rehabilitation of non–operative meniscal injury and partial meniscectomy patients requires 6–12 weeks. Rehabilitation after meniscal repair can take up to six months.

Short term treatment for both the non–operative and post–operative patient includes symptom relief measures and joint effusion control. The patient should use assistive devices to decrease weightbearing loads and facilitate a normal gait pattern. Partial meniscectomy patients can begin full weightbearing as early as 4–7 days after surgery. Meniscal repair patients are usually non–weightbearing for 3–6 weeks after surgery.

Open kinematic chain exercises should be used early in rehabilitation. These exercises help build strength and increase range of motion while controlling weightbearing forces. The exercise program should be gradually progressed to closed kinematic chain exercises. These exercises should be carefully controlled, avoiding unnecessary joint pain, effusion, and reinjury. The patient should be gradually returned to full weightbearing status. Pool therapy or underwater treadmills are useful for gradually increasing weightbearing forces. Proprioceptive training should be gradually introduced, especially when the patient has a history of recurrent ligamentous injuries. Recent texts outline

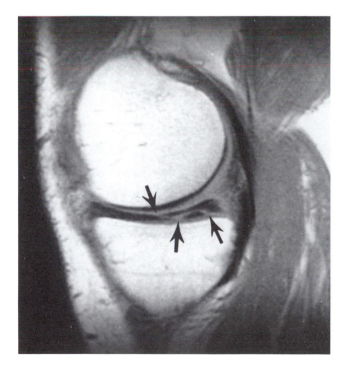

Figure 8–55. MRI showing a complex tear of the posterior horn of the medial meniscus. Note the linear increased signal intensity seen extending through several areas of inferior and superior surface (arrows) of the normally low signal intensity meniscus.

protocols for rehabilitating the knee with a meniscal injury.[14,18,49] The clinician should work closely with the patient's surgeon to establish acceptable guidelines for the rehabilitation.

Conservative Management of ACL Tears

Many physicians and patients decide to rehabilitate the ACL–injured knee through non–operative means. The issue of non–operative treatment for the ACL–injured knee has been widely discussed in the literature.[32,37,65,91,92,100,124] Many complications have been documented in patients with chronic ACL insufficiency, including: chronic synovitis, recurrent meniscal tears, progressive joint laxity, and advanced joint surface erosion.[37,91,92,124] These changes can be accelerated in the ACL deficient knee that has undergone medial meniscectomy.[26] There is a decrease in proprioception and an increased threshold for movement detection in the ACL deficient knee.[9,19] The goal of rehabilitation is to maintain the functional stability of the knee by compensating for the ligament injury with neuromuscular mechanisms.[33,123] Successful treatment appears to be related to the level of proprioception loss; hamstring function; the use of braces; and activity modification after injury.[8,46,91,92,119]

History

There is usually a history of acute trauma. Patients often report a "snap" or "pop" at the time of injury, with the rapid onset of a large effusion and hemarthrosis. In acute injuries, the patient will be unable to bear weight normally, and range of motion will be limited. Seventy percent of patients with this history have injury to the ACL.[24] The patient may also have a history of the knee giving way. The patient with chronic ACL instability usually has a history of episodic giving way, effusion, and pain. Many times, specific activities that irritate the condition will give clues to the mechanical instability present. An example is a patient who complains of a giving way sensation while pivoting on the right foot toward the left when the knee is flexed. This external rotation/valgus stress is consistent with AMRI.

Signs/Symptoms

The patient with acute ACL sprain complains of pain, swelling, and limited weightbearing use of the knee after injury. Patients with chronic ACL sprain complain of positional apprehension and intermittent pain and effusion with specific activities. Examination reveals positive Lachman's test, anterior drawer test, and pivot shift tests. These tests may be difficult to perform in the acutely injured knee due to swelling and muscle guarding. Instrumented testing using a knee arthrometer will be positive. Acute ACL disruptions show a difference ≥3mm of anterior laxity when compared to the uninjured side.[21] Functional knee testing may reveal positional or activity related apprehension or instability in weightbearing. Isokinetic testing may reveal a specific ACL deficient curve consistent with a distinct decrease in strength. This decreased strength on isokinetic testing may be caused by an anterior shift of the tibia on the femur in the open kinematic chain.

Diagnostics

Physical examination and history are often sufficient to confirm an ACL injury. MRI is the definitive diagnostic test for evaluating ACL integrity (Fig 8–56).[61] It can pick up subtle changes in the ligamentous response to injury that may not even be evident to a surgeon probing an apparently intact ACL during diagnostic arthroscopic surgery.

Problem List

Patients who have an ACL tear may present with any of the following clinical problems:

1. Knee instability with weightbearing activity

2. Recurrent episodes of pain and swelling at the knee

3. Decreased proprioception

4. Pain on active movement of the knee

5. Altered gait pattern

Treatment

Conservative treatment of the acute injury should address any pain, effusion, limited weightbearing, and decreased range of motion. Treatment initially consists of PRICE and controlled weightbearing using assistive devices. Knee immobilizers are often used briefly. Patellofemoral mobilization may be required after immobilization to restore normal mobility. Electrical muscle stimulation may help the patient regain muscular control and may help decrease joint effusion. The exercise program should initially emphasize hamstring control of excessive anterior tibial translation.[33,123] This will stabilize the joint and counteract the inherent loss of joint proprioception.[9,33,104] Some authors suggest using closed chain exercises including proprioceptive neuromuscular facilitation (PNF).[31] Joint proprioception and stability can be increased by teaching the patient to pull the tibia into place as an anterior drawer stress is applied to the joint. The patient should be able to resist any anterior translation at this joint (Fig 8–57). Co–contractions of the hamstring and quadriceps can be accomplished initially in a sitting position. Eventually, co–contractions should be performed in full weightbearing.

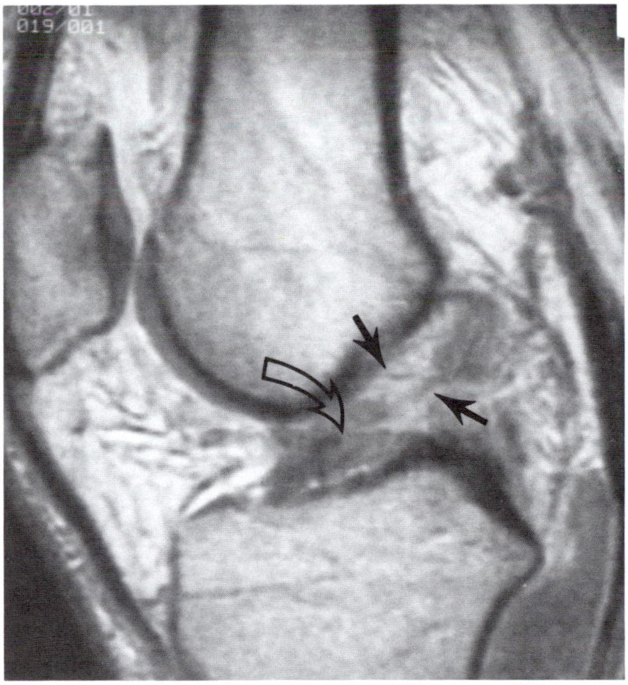

Further exercise progression may include proprioceptive training on a balance board and running. The running program should begin with forward running, progressing to running with gradual changes in direction ("S" running), and eventually to sharp change in direction ("Z" running). Research supports the use of closed kinematic chain strengthening exercises because there is less anterior tibial translation in the closed chain.[51,99,121,129] There are many ways to accomplish this, including using a reclined squat, stair climber machine, stationary bike, surgical tubing.

Functional knee braces have been widely used for ACL injuries despite the lack of strong evidence to support their use.[33] Many patients feel more confident when using braces, and this may be reason enough to use them. Activity modification, especially avoiding positions that lead to giving way, pain, and effusion, is essential to long term success in conservative management of these problems.

ACL Tear (Surgical)

The surgical treatment and rehabilitation of the ACL–injured knee has undergone dramatic change in

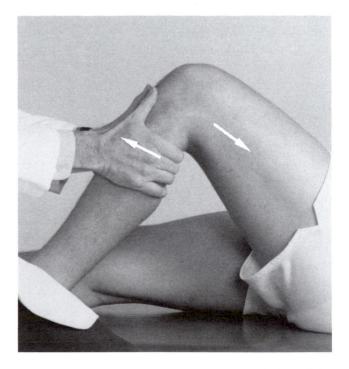

Figure 8–56. MRI showing a complete tear of the proximal aspect of the anterior cruciate ligament. Shown is a full-thickness interruption of the proximal anterior cruciate ligament (straight arrows) with the distal stump seen horizontally-oriented in the intercondylar notch (curved arrow).

Figure 8–57. Patient resisting anterior translation of the tibiofemoral joint. This exercise helps improve joint proprioception.

the last 50 years. The original procedure was described in 1939 using the patellar tendon as a graft.[17] For many years, primary repair of the torn ligament with or without augmentation was advocated,[16,79,80] but there was limited success with this technique.[7,35,95] Non–operative treatment became popular and is still very common; however, patients whose functional goal is to continue a stressful work or sport are prime candidates for a reconstructive procedure.[128] Extra–articular procedures using the ITB as a graft have had discouraging long term results. Intra–articular ACL reconstruction has been advocated by many authors.[128] Recent advances in instrumentation and graft fixation have facilitated more accurate graft placement and stronger graft fixation. Arthroscopically assisted surgery has allowed earlier and more aggressive rehabilitation.[128]

Traditionally, the rehabilitation of ACL reconstructed knees was quite conservative. It was common to have knees immobilized for 6–8 weeks and patient's using crutches for 3–4 months, with a return to vigorous activities at 9–12 months after surgery.[128] Common complications with this post–operative management included: quadriceps weakness; chronic knee effusion; donor site pain; extensor mechanism disruption; and arthrofibrosis (joint stiffening). Aggressive rehabilitation now emphasizes immediate motion; full passive extension; immediate weightbearing; and early muscle strengthening.[128] These accelerated programs have shown much better results.[106,107] With accelerated rehabilitation, there is improved muscle strength; greater range of motion; improved knee stability; less joint stiffness; and fewer complaints.

The most common intra–articular graft is the vascularized patellar tendon graft (bone–tendon–bone). Other grafts are sometimes used. These include the Gore–Tex™ graft, frozen cadaver allografts, and combined techniques such as the ligament augmentation device (LAD), which combines an autograft with polyethylene.

History

The patients have a history as outlined in the "Conservative Management of ACL Tears" section of this chapter. Surgical patients may be more active or have more functional instability than patients managed conservatively. They may also have already failed a conservative approach.

Signs/Symptoms

The patients have the same signs and symptoms as listed in the "Conservative Management of ACL Tears" section of this chapter.

Diagnostics

MRI and diagnostic arthroscopy are the diagnostic tools used to confirm an ACL disruption.

Problem List

Patients with post–operative ACL repairs present with some of the following problems:

1. Moderate joint effusion
2. Poor quadriceps contractions
3. Healing (unstable) ACL graft
4. Poor weightbearing tolerance
5. Decreased knee proprioception

Treatment

There are several good references describing the surgical procedures and post–operative management for ACL reconstructions.[14,49,59,103] The treatment program described here summarizes an accelerated rehabilitation approach to ACL reconstruction using a patellar tendon graft.[128]

Several basic guidelines should be kept in mind during post–operative period:[120]

1. Rehabilitation should be adaptable to patients and their problems.

2. Deleterious immobilization must be prevented.

3. Healing constraints should never be violated.

4. Progression to the next level of rehabilitation depends on success at the previous stage.

5. Communication between the patient, the clinician and the physician is critical to the success of the entire process. Surgery is only the beginning, and

no surgery will be successful without a comprehensive rehabilitation program.

There are six stages in the rehabilitation process: [128]

1. Immediate post–operative phase (day 1–7)—The goals of this phase are to prevent an infection of the surgical wound, prevent deleterious immobilization, gain full passive knee extension, activate the quadricep and hamstring muscles, and safely ambulate with crutches and an immobilizer (brace).

2. Maximum protection phase (week 2–6)—The goals are to improve muscle strength and endurance, gradually increase motion, ambulate independently without an assistive device, and control external forces to protect the graft. Proprioception exercises can be initiated in this phase.

3. Controlled ambulation phase (week 6–9)—The knee brace is discontinued for ambulation and proper gait mechanics are encouraged. It is our experience that using the brace in full extension weightbearing for up to six weeks can cause an infrapatellar catching problem near the graft site. Other protocols do not use the brace for this long in weightbearing. [107]

4. Moderate protection phase (week 9–14)—During this phase there is continued activity modification to protect the knee. The exercises are accelerated in this phase. Isokinetic testing can be considered, with certain limitations. The arc of motion should be limited to 45–90° and an anti–shear device should be used. The anti–shear device helps decrease the anterior shear forces generated with open kinematic chain quad contractions.

5. Light activity phase (12–16 weeks)—Running, cutting (changing directions while running), and agility drills may begin. Strengthening exercises should continue.

6. Return to activity phase (5–6 months)—The patient is progressed through a gradual return to normal vigorous activities. Functional strengthening and proprioception exercises should continue.

Strengthening in a closed kinematic chain is emphasized throughout this post–operative progression. This type of exercise decreases the stresses on the graft and mimics function. Persistent pain or effusion should not be ignored, as they will inhibit muscle function. Proprioceptive training is important and should be initiated as soon as tolerated. Pool therapy or underwater treadmills are useful for gradually increasing weightbearing forces.

There are many different post–operative protocols for ACL reconstructions. The protocol described above is just one example. Another example is found in Table 8–5. The clinician should work closely with the referring surgeon to develop guidelines for patients with these problems.

SUMMARY

Placed between the body's two longest bony segments, the knee must withstand considerable loads in daily activities. Its stability is balanced by an intricate relationship of ligamentous restraints and muscular control. Patients with knee disorders are commonly seen by physical therapists for a variety of problems, from simple patellofemoral irritation to complex reconstructive surgery with meniscal repairs. Recent advances in technology are lessening the disability caused by injury to the bony, cartilaginous, and ligamentous structures of the joint. Rehabilitation continues to play an important role in the successful implementation of these advances.

The evaluation, treatment, and prevention of problems at the knee has been presented. Symptoms at the knee can be referred from the hip, ankle, and lumbar spine. All potential contributing factors should be considered in a comprehensive treatment program.

Table 8-5. Accelerated Rehabilitation for Anterior Cruciate Ligament Reconstruction

POST-OPERATIVE Time	Exercise/Activity
0-1 days	• start physical therapy for gait training and pain control
1-7 days	• inspect wound daily • cryo-cuff and frequent PRICE • immobilizer in full extension for sleeping and weightbearing • weightbearing as tolerated with crutches • patellofemoral mobilizations as tolerated • wall slide exercise for flexion (≤120° as tolerated) • full terminal knee extension ASAP
7-14 days	• closed kinematic chain strengthening • stationary bike for ROM and strengthening • pool exercise if wound healed • start incisional mobilization ASAP • progressive weightbearing to tolerance • PRICE as needed • electrical muscle stimulation as needed • proprioceptive balance board activities
2-6 weeks	• progress flexion to full as tolerated • continue weightbearing to full as tolerated • progressive closed kinematic chain strengthening • prevent excessive inflammation/edema with PRICE post-exercise
6-12 weeks	• progress to jumping rope, sliding board, lateral shuffles • pool running as tolerated • light jogging permitted • continue closed kinematic chain strengthening
12-24 weeks	• increase closed kinematic chain exercise, agility, and functional activities as tolerated (running, jumping, cutting) as needed depending upon goal • functional brace optional for sports or work

REFERENCES

1. Ahmed AM, Burke DL: In-Vitro Measurements of Static Pressure Distributions in Synovial Joints. Part I. Tibial Surface of the Knee. Journal of Biomechanical Engineering, 105:216, 1983.

2. American Orthopaedic Association: Manual of Orthopaedic Surgery. Chicago IL 1972.

3. Anderson AF, Lipscomb AB: Clinical Diagnosis of Mensical Tears-Description of a New Manipulative Test. Am J Sports Med 14:291, 1988.

4. Arms SW, Pope MH, Johnson RJ, et al: The Biomechanics of ACL Rehabilitation and Reconstructions. Am J Sports Med 12:8, 1984.

5. Arnoczky SP, et al: Meniscal Repair Using an Exogenous Fibris Clot. JBJS 70A:1209, 1988.

6. Arnoczky SP, Warren RF: Microvasculature of The Human Meniscus. Am J Sports Med 10:90, 1982.

7. Balkfors B: The Course of Knee Ligament Injuries. Acta Orthop Scand 198:1-99, 1982.

8. Barber SD, Noyes FR, Mangine RR, et al: Quantitative Assessment of Functional Limitations In Nor-

mal and ACL Deficient Knees. Clin Orthop 255:204-214, 1990.

9. Barrack RL, et al: Proprioception in the ACL-Deficient Knee. AM J Sports Med 17:1-6, 1989.

10. Basmajian JV, Lovejoy JF: Function of the Popliteus Muscle in Man. JBJS 53B:557, 1971.

11. Blackburn TA, Craig E: Knee Anatomy: A Brief Review. Phys Ther 60:8, 1981.

12. Bose K, et al: Vastus Medialis Oblique: An Anatomical and Physiological Study. Orthopaedics 3:880-883, 1980.

13. Brownstein B, Mangine RE, Noyes FR, and Kryger S: Anatomy and Biomechanics. In Physical Therapy of the Knee. RE Mangine, ed. Churchill-Livingstone, New York NY 1988.

14. Bullough PG, Munver AL, Murphy J, Weinsteing AM: The Strength of the Menisci as it Relates to their Fine Structure. JBJS 52B: 564, 1970.

15. Butler DS: Mobilisation of the Nervous System. Chicago IL May 1993. Seminar.

16. Cabaud HE, et al: Experimental Studies of Acute ACL Injury and Repair. Am J Sports Med 7:18-22, 1979.

17. Campbell WC: Reconstruction of the Ligament of the Knee. Am J Surg 43:473-480, 1939.

18. Cavanaugh JT: Rehabilitation Following Meniscal Surgery. In Knee Ligament Rehabilitation. RP Engle, ed. Churchill-Livingstone, New York NY 1991.

19. Corrigan JP, Cashman WF, Brady MP: Proprioception of the Cruciate Deficient Knee. British Editorial Society of Bone and Joint Surgery. 74(2):247-250, 1992.

20. Daniel D, et al: The Quadriceps-ACL Interaction. Orthop Trans 6:199, 1982.

21. Daniel DM, et al: Instrumented Measurement of Anterior Knee Laxity in Patients with ACL Disruption. Am J Sports Med 13:401, 1985.

22. Daniel DM, et al: Use of the Quadriceps Active Test to Diagnose Posterior Cruciate Ligament Disruption and Measure Posterior Laxity of the Knee. JBJS 70A:386, 1988.

23. DeCarlo MS, Shelbourne KD, et al: Traditional Versus Accelerated Rehabilitation Following ACL Reconstruction: A One Year Follow-up. JOSPT 15(6):309-316, 1992.

24. DeHaven KE: Diagnosis of Acute Knee Injuries With Hemarthrosis. Am J Sports Med 8(1):9-14, 1980.

25. DeHaven KE: Injuries to the Menisci of the Knee. In The Lower Extremity and Spine in Sports Medicine. JA Nichols, EB Hershmann, ed. CV Mosby, St Louis MO 1986.

26. DeHaven KE: Peripheral Meniscus Repair – An Alternative to Meniscectomy. JBJS 63B:463, 1981.

27. DePalma AF: Diseases of the Knee. JB Lippincott,

Philadelphia PA 1954.

28. DiStefano VJ: Function Post Traumatic Sequelæ and Current Concepts of Management of Knee Meniscus Injuries. Clin Orthop 151:143, 1980.

29. Doucette and Goble: Exercise For Patellofemoral Pain and Tracking. Am J Sports Med 20:434-440, 1992.

30. Engle RP, Canner GC: Posterolateral Instability: Diagnosis and Treatment. In Knee Ligament Rehabilitation. RP Engle, ed. Churchill-Livingstone, New York NY 1991.

31. Engle RP, Canner GC: Proprioceptive Neuromuscular Fasciation (PNF) and Modified Procedures For ACL Instability. JOSPT 11:230, 1989.

32. Engle RP, Canner GC: Rehabilitation of Symptomatic Anterolateral Knee Instability. JOSPT 11:237, 1989.

33. Engle RP: Non-Operative ACL Rehabilitation. In Knee Ligament Rehabilitation. RP Engle, ed. Churchill-Livingstone, New York NY 1991.

34. Fairbank TJ: Knee Joint Changes After Menisectomy. JBJS 30B:664, 1948.

35. Feagin JA, Curl WW: Isolated Tear of the ACL: Five Year Follow-up Study. Am J Sports Med 4:95-100, 1976.

36. Finerman G: American Academy of Orthopaedic Surgeons Symposium on Sports Medicine of the Knee. CV Mosby, Denver CO 1982, St Louis MO 1985.

37. Fowler PJ, Regan WD: The Patient With Symptomatic Chronic ACL Insufficiency. Results of Minimal Arthroscopic Surgery and Rehabilitation. Am J Sports Med 15:321, 1987.

38. Fulkerson J, et al: Histological Evidence of Retinacular Nerve Injury Associated with Patellofemoral Malalignment. Clin Orthop 197:196-205, 1985.

39. Fulkerson J, Hungerford D: Disorders of the Patellofemoral Joint, 2nd ed. Williams & Wilkins, Baltimore MD 1990.

40. Galway HR, MacIntosh DL: The Lateral Pivot Shift: A Symptom and Sign of ACL Insufficiency. Clin Orthop and Rel Res 147:45, 1980.

41. Gerrard B: The Patellofemoral Pain Syndrome. A Clinical Trial of the McConnell Programme. Australian Journal of Physiotherapy, 35:70-80, 1989.

42. Gill DM, et al: Anatomy of the Knee. Knee Ligament Rehabilitation. RP Engle, ed. Churchill-Livingstone, New York NY 1991.

43. Goodfellow J, Hungerford D, Woods C: Patellofemoral Joint Mechanics and Pathology. JBJS 58:291-299, 1976.

44. Goodfellow J, Hungerford DS, Zindel M: Patellofemoral Joint Mechanics and Pathology: I. Functional Anatomy of the Patellofemoral Joint. JBJS 58:287-290, 1976.

45. Grood ES, Suntay WJ: A Joint Coordinate System For the Clinical Description of Three-Dimensional Motion. Application to the Knee. Journal of Biomechanical Engineering 105:136, 1983.

46. Grove TP, et al: Non-operative Treatment of the Torn ACL. JBJS 65A:184, 1983.

47. Gruebel-Lee DM: Disorders of the Hip. JB Lippincott Co, Philadelphia PA 1983.

48. Hamberg P, et al: Suture of the New and Old Peripheral Meniscus Tears. JBJS 65A:193, 1983.

49. Harrelson GL: Knee Rehabilitation. In Physical Rehabilitation of the Injured Athlete. J Andrews and GL Harrelson, ed. WB Saunders, Philadelphia PA 1991.

50. Henning CE, et al: Arthroscopic Meniscal Repair Using an Exogenous Fibris Clot. Clin Orthop 252:64, 1990.

51. Henning CE, Lynch MA, Glick KR: An In Vivo Strain Gauge Study of the ACL. Am J Sports Med 13:22-26, 1985.

52. Hodges P, Richardson C: An Investigation into the Effectiveness of Hip Adduction in the Optimization of the Vastus Medialis Oblique Contraction. Scand J. Rehabil Med. In press.

53. Hughston JC: Patellar Subluxation and Dislocation. WB Saunders, Philadelphia PA 1984

54. Hunter H: Patellofemoral Arthralgia. J Am Osteopath Assoc 85:581-585, 1985.

55. Ingersoll C, Knight K: Patellar Location Changes Following EMG Biofeedback or Progressive Resistance Exercises. Med Sci Sports Exercise 23:1122-1127, 1991.

56. Insal JN, et al: Rationale of the Knee Society Clinical Rating System. Clin Orthop Rel Res 248:13, 1989.

57. Insall J, Salvati E: Patellar Position in The Normal Knee Joint. Radiology 101:101-109, 1971.

58. Insall J: "Chondromalacia Patella": Patellar Malalignment Syndrome. Orthop Clin N America 10:117-127, 1979.

59. Insall J: Current Concepts Review: Patellar Pain. JBJS 64:147-151, 1982.

60. Insall JN: Anatomy of the Knee. Surgery of the Knee. JN Insall, ed. Churchill-Livingstone, New York NY 1984.

61. Jackson DW, et al: Magnetic Resonance Imaging of the Knee. Am J Sports Med 16:29, 1988.

62. Jackson JP: Degenerative Changes in The Knee After Meniscectomy. JBJS 49B:584, 1967.

63. Jackson RJ, et al: Factors Affecting Late Results After Meniscectomy. JBJS 56A:719, 1974.

64. James SL: Chondromalacia of the Patellae in the Adolescent. In The Injured Adolescent Knee, JC Kennedy, ed. Williams & Wilkins, Baltimore MD 1979.

65. Kannua P, Jarvinen M: Conservatively Treated Tears of the ACL. JBJS 69A:1007, 1987.

66. Karst GM, Jewett PD: EMG Analysis of Exercise Proposed for Differential Activation of Medial and Lateral Quadricep Femoris Muscle Components. Physical Therapy 73(5):286-299, 1993.

67. Kennedy J, et al: Nerve Supply of the Human Knee and Its Functional Importance. Am J Sports Med 10:329-335, 1982.

68. Kennedy JC, et al: The Anatomy and Function of the ACL as Determined by Clinical and Morphological Studies. JBJS 56A:223, 1974.

69. Kolowich PA, Paulos LE, et al: Lateral Release of the Patella: Indications and Contraindications. Am J Sports Med 18:359, 1990.

70. Last RJ: Anatomy: Regional and Applied, 7th edition. Churchill-Livingstone, New York NY 1984.

71. Levy M, Torzilli PA, and Warren RF: The Effect of Medial Meniscectomy on Anterior-Posterior Motion of the Knee. JBJS 64A:883, 1982.

72. Lieb F, Perry J: Quadriceps Function: An Anatomical and Mechanical Study Using Amputated Limbs. JBJS 50A:1535-1548, 1968.

73. Lindenfield TN: Arthroscopically Aided Meniscal Repair. Orthopedics 10:1293, 1987.

74. Lutter LD: Foot Related Knee Problems in the Long Distance Runner. Foot, Ankle 1:112-116, 1980.

75. Magee D: Knee. Orthopaedic Physical Assessment. WB Saunders, Philadelphia PA 1992.

76. Mangine R: Rules For Management. Functional Testing, Braces. 1990 Advances on the Knee and Shoulder. Cincinnati Sports Medicine and Deaconess Hospital, Cincinnati OH 1990.

77. Mann RA, Hagy JL: The Popliteus Muscle. JBJS 59:924-927, 1977.

78. Marshall JL, et al: The Biceps Femoris Tendon and Its Functional Significance. JBJS 54:1444, 1972.

79. Marshall JL, Warren RJ, et al: Primary Surgical Treatment of ACL Lesions. Am J Sports Med 10:103-107, 1982.

80. Marshall JL, Warren RJ, et al: The ACL: A Technique of Repair and Reconstruction. Clin Orthop 143:97-106, 1979.

81. McConnell J: The Management of Chondromalacia Patellae: A Long-Term Solution. Austr J Physiother 32:215-223, 1986.

82. McLeod WD, et al: Tibial Plateau Topography. Am J Sports Med 5(1):13-18, 1977.

83. McMurray TP: The Semilunar Cartilages. Br J Surg 29:407, 1942.

84. Meade TD: Meniscus Tears: Diagnosis and Treatment. In Knee Ligament Rehabilitation. RP Engle, ed. Churchill-Livingstone, New York NY 1991.

85. Nicholas JA, Hirshman EB: The Lower Extremity and Spine in Sports Medicine. CV Mosby, St Louis

MO 1986.

86. Noble CA: Iliotibial Band Friction Syndrome in Runners. Am J Sports Med 8:232-234, 1980.

87. Noble HB, et al: Diagnosis and Treatment of Iliotibial Band Tightness in Runners. Physician and Sports Medicine. 10:67, 1982.

88. Noyes FR, Butler DL, Grood ES, et al: Clinical Paradoxes of ACL Instability and a New Test to Detect Its Instability. Orthop Trans 2:36, 1978.

89. Noyes FR, et al: Functional Disability in the ACL Deficient Knee Syndrome-Review of Knee Rating Systems and Projected Risk Factors in Deterring Treatment. Sports Med 1:278, 1984.

90. Noyes FR, et al: Intra-articular Cruicate Reconstruction, Part I: Perspectives on Graft Strength, Vascularization, and Immediate Motion After Replacement. Clin Orthop 172:71, 1983.

91. Noyes FR, et al: The Symptomatic ACL Deficient Knee, Part I The Long-Term Functional Disability in Athletically Active Individuals. Part II: The Results of Rehabilitation, Activity Modification, and Counseling. JBJS 65A:154, 163, 1983.

92. Noyes FR, et al: The Variable Functional Disability of the ACL Deficient Knee. Orthop Clin N Am 16:47, 1985.

93. Noyes FR: Objective Functional Testing. The Noyes Knee Rating System. FR Noyes, ed. Cincinnati Sports Medicine Research and Education Foundation, Cincinnati OH 1990.

94. Ober FB: The Role of the Iliotibial and Fascia Lata as a Factor in the Causation of Low Back Disabilities and Sciatica. JBJS 18:105, 1936.

95. Odensten M:, et al: The Course of Partial ACL Ruptures. Am J Sports Med 13:183-186, 1985.

96. Olerud C, Berg P: The Variation of Q-Angle with Different Positions of the Foot. Clin Orthop Rel Res 191:162, 1984.

97. Paine RM: Instrumented Examination of the Knee. Knee Ligament Rehabilitation. RP Engle, ed. Churchill-Livingstone, New York NY 1991.

98. Palmer ML, Epler M: Clinical Assessment Procedures in Physical Therapy. JB Lippincott, Philadelphia PA 1990.

99. Palmitier RA, et al: Kinetic Chain Exercise in Knee Rehabilitation. Sports Medicine 11:402-413, 1991.

100. Patier GA, et al: 4-10 Year Follow-Up of Unreconstructed ACL Tears. Am J Sports Med. 17:430, 1989.

101. Puniello MS: Iliotibial Band Tightness and Medial Patellar Glide in Patients With Patellofemoral Dysfunction. JOSPT 17(3):144-148, 1993.

102. Renne J: The Iliotibial Band Friction Syndrome. JBJS 57:1110-1111, 1975.

103. Schmidt G: Latest Technique in ACL Surgery and Rehabilitation. JOSPT 15(6):256-322, 1992.

104. Schultz RA, et al: Mechanoreceptors in Human Cruciate Ligaments. JBJS 66:1072-1076, 1984.

105. Scott GA, Jolly BL, Henning CE: Combined Posterior Incision and Arthroscopic Intra-articular Repair of the Meniscus. JBJS 68A:847, 1986.

106. Shelbourne KD, et al: Update on Accelerated Rehabilitation after ACL Reconstruction. JOSPT 15(6):303-308, 1992.

107. Shelbourne KD, Nitz PA: Accelerated Rehabilitation after ACL Reconstruction. Am J Sports Med 18:292-299, 1990.

108. Slocum DB, Larson RL: Rotary Instability of the Knee. JBJS 50:241, 1968.

109. Soderberg G: Knee. Kinesiology: Application to Pathological Motion. Williams & Wilkins, Baltimore MD 1986.

110. Southmayd W, Quigley TB: The Forgotten Popliteus Muscle. Clin Orthop Rel Res 130:218, 1978.

111. Souza DR: Anatomy and Pathomechanics of Patellofemoral Pain Syndrome. Post-Graduate Studies in Sports Physical Therapy. Forum Medicum I-IX:1-13, 1991.

112. Stone KR, et al: Future Directions: Collagen-Based Prosthesis for Meniscal Regeneration. Clin Orthop 252:129, 1990.

113. Stroberl M, Stedtfelt HW: Diagnostic Evaluation of the Knee. Springer-Verlag, Berlin 1990.

114. Sutker AV, et al: Iliotibial Band Syndrome in Distance Runners. Phys Sportsmed 9:69-73, 1981.

115. Tapper EM, Hoover NW: Late Results After Menisectomy. JBJS 51A:517, 1969.

116. Terry GC, Hughston JC, and Norwood LA: The Anatomy of the Iliopatellar Band and Iliotibial Tract. Am J Sports Med 14(1):39-45, 1986.

117. Tewes D: Functional Anatomy of the PCL. Lecture at the Sports Medicine Center, Minneapolis MN 1993.

118. Teynor Y, et al: A Performance Test to Monitor Rehabilitation and Evaluate ACL Injuries. Am J Sports Med 14:156-159, 1986.

119. Tibone JE, et al: Functional Analysis of ACL Instability. Am J Sports Med 14:276, 1986.

120. Tovin BJ, et al: Surgical and Biomechanical Considerations in Rehabilitation of Patients with Intra-articular ACL Reconstructions. JOSPT 15(6):317-322, 1992.

121. Voight M, et al: Instrumented Testing of Tibial Translation During a Lachman's Test and Selected Close Chair Activities in ACL Deficient Knees. JOSPT 15:49, 1992.

122. Waisbrod H, Treiman N: Intra-osseous Venography in Patellofemoral Disorders: A Preliminary Report. JBJS 62:454-456, 1980.

123. Walla DJ, et al: Hamstrings Control and the Unstable ACL Deficient Knee. Am J Sports Med 13:34-

39, 1985.

124. Warren RF, Levy IM: Meniscal Lesions Associated With ACL Injury. Clin Orthop 172:32, 1983.

125. Warren RF, Marshall J: Injuries of the ACL and MCL of the Knee. Clin Orthop 136:191, 1978.

126. Weiss CB, Lundberg M, Hamberg P, et al: Non-Operative Treatment of Meniscal Tears. JBJS 71A:811, 1989.

127. Welsh PR: Knee Joint Structure and Function. Clin Orthop 147:7, 1980.

128. Wilk KE, Andrews JR: Current Concepts in the Treatment of ACL Disruption. JOSPT 15(6):279-293, 1992.

129. Yack, et al: Open Versus Closed Chain Exercises for the ACL Deficient Knee. Am J Sports Med 21:49-54, 1993.

CHAPTER 9

THE FOOT AND ANKLE

INTRODUCTION

Located at the terminal end of the lower kinematic chain, the foot and ankle have an intricate arrangement of joints. The foot's importance as a functional unit is most apparent during gait; the structure and function of the foot and ankle let humans move about upright. The foot and ankle effectively distribute weightbearing forces during standing and the stance phase of gait. In addition, the structures of the foot and ankle must generate adequate forces for propulsion; thus there must be a balance between the *mobility* needed to absorb large forces and adapt to uneven surfaces and the *stability* required to control these forces and propel the body. This balance requires dynamic muscular control and static ligamentous restraint to prevent abnormal stresses from damaging tissues and causing pain and dysfunction.

Many pathologies can disrupt the normal mechanics of the foot and ankle. A patient's gait pattern will often reflect a specific problem that can be easily observed. Abnormal foot and ankle mechanics can have disabling consequences since the entire lower kinematic chain, including the lumbo–pelvic complex, depends on the terminal end to adequately oppose external forces. Footwear can cause many problems and often mirrors the stresses put on it, as seen by wear patterns on the soles of shoes.

Symptoms at the foot and ankle can be referred from the lumbo–pelvic area, the hip, the knee, and the lower leg. Problem management at the foot, ankle, and lower leg needs to include the related neuromusculoskeletal structures.

FUNCTIONAL ANATOMY

Osseous and Capsuloligamentous Components

There are 26 bones in the foot and ankle. These structures form four functional regions: the ankle, the rearfoot, the midfoot, and the forefoot (Fig 9–1).[60,82] The integrity of these regions is maintained by an expansive ligamentous network (Fig 9–2). The joints of the foot and ankle are intricately dependent on each other to provide normal mechanical function; changes in one joint influence changes in the others. Collectively, they influence the entire lower kinematic chain.

The Ankle

The ankle is composed of the talocrural and distal tibiofibular joints. The talocrural joint also functions with the subtalar joint as part of the rearfoot.

The distal tibiofibular joint is a syndesmosis joint between the distal tibia and fibula (Fig 9–1). This joint is stabilized by the inferior transverse ligaments, the interosseus ligament, and the anterior and posterior tibiofibular ligaments. Movements at this joint are small but provide accessory motion to allow greater freedom of movement at the ankle. During pronation, the fibula slides proximally and anteriorly. It rotates laterally with dorsiflexion to accommodate the wider portion of the talus engaging the mortise. During supination, the fibula slides distally and posteriorly. It rotates medially with plantar flexion, narrowing the mortise as the talus disengages.[43,65] Injuries to the distal tibiofibular joint are often overlooked but can adversely affect ankle function.

The Foot

The foot is divided into three functional areas: the rearfoot, the midfoot, and the forefoot. The arches of the foot span these three areas. The medial and lateral longitudinal arches run the length of the foot. The transverse arch runs across the width of the foot. These arches are shown schematically in Figure 9–3.

The medial and lateral longitudinal arches of the foot are maintained statically.[2,36] The medial arch is dynamically stabilized and maintained via the action of the peroneus longus, the posterior tibialis, and the intrinsic muscles (Fig 9–4, top).

The transverse arch of the foot is formed by the cuneiform and cuboid bones. This arch is supported by the metatarsal heads and a musculoligamentous complex, which prevent the metatarsals from splaying or spreading out (Fig 9–4, bottom). The transverse arch gets dynamic stabilization from contractions of the intrinsic muscles.[54]

Rearfoot

The rearfoot consists of the talocrural and subtalar joints. The talocrural joint is sometimes considered part of the ankle and was discussed in "The Ankle" section of this chapter.

The talocrural joint is formed between three bones—the tibia, the fibula, and the talus. The tibiotalar and fibulotalar articulations form a single uniaxial modified hinge joint. The superior concave surface of this joint is shaped like a mortise (Fig 9–1).[86] The mortise is formed between the medial malleolus, the distal tibial plafond, and the lateral malleolus. The convex surface of the talus fits within this mortise. The lateral malleolus extends more distally and sits more posteriorly than the medial malleolus. This makes the axis of motion at the ankle run from anteromedial superior to posterolateral inferior (Fig 9–5). This oblique orientation allows triplanar motion.[65]

Dorsiflexion and plantar flexion are the primary motions at this joint; a mild amount of abduction coupled with dorsiflexion and adduction coupled with plantar flexion also occur. Negligible amounts of inversion and eversion occur at this joint.[65]

The ankle has strong ligamentous support (Fig 9–2). On the medial aspect, support comes from the deltoid ligament. Lateral stability is derived from

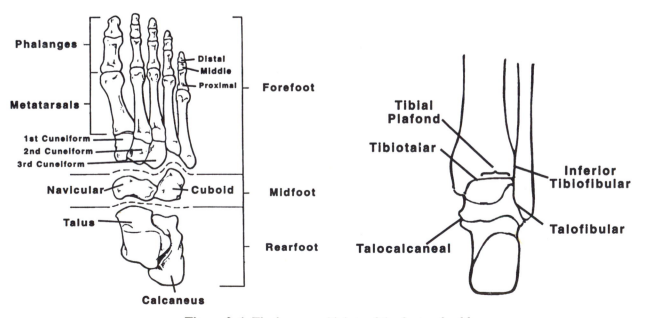

Figure 9–1. The bones and joints of the foot and ankle.

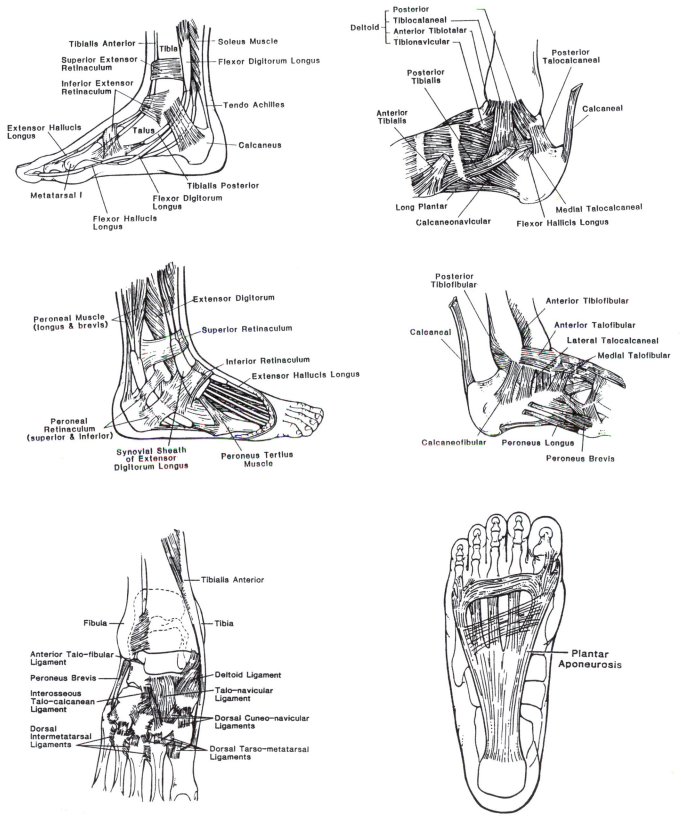

Figure 9–2. The ligaments of the foot and ankle.

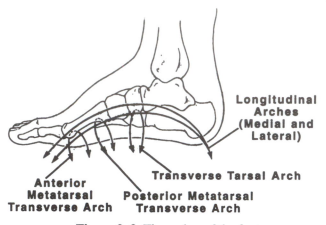

Figure 9–3. The arches of the foot

calcaneofibular, anterior talofibular, and posterior talofibular ligaments. The most common injury at this joint is a sprain of the lateral ligamentous structures.

The talus is wedge shaped and is wider anteriorly than posteriorly.[39,52] This shape and the small amount of anterior–posterior accessory motion present[47] affect the stability of this joint. During dorsiflexion, the talus slides posteriorly on the tibia, wedging into the mortise. This adds stability at the expense of mobility. During plantar flexion, the talus slides anteriorly on the tibia and disengages from the mortise, adding mobility to the joint at the expense of stability.

The subtalar joint is formed between the talus superiorly and the calcaneus inferiorly. The subtalar joint is a synovial joint with an oblique axis that allows triplanar motion. The medial and lateral collateral ligaments, the posterior and lateral talocalcaneal ligaments, the interosseous talocalcaneal ligament, and the cervical ligament support the rearfoot. The interosseous talocalcaneal ligament plays a critical role in stabilizing this joint during static and dynamic activities, becoming taut during eversion.[28,43] The cervical ligament becomes taut during inversion.[28,43]

The oblique axis at the subtalar joint is ≈16° from the midline from a bird's eye view; and inclined 42° from the bottom of the foot when viewed from the side (Fig 9–6). This orientation allows triplanar motion, described as pronation and supination. These motions are composed of three components. In the open kinematic chain, pronation consists of eversion, dorsiflexion, and abduction of the calcaneus.

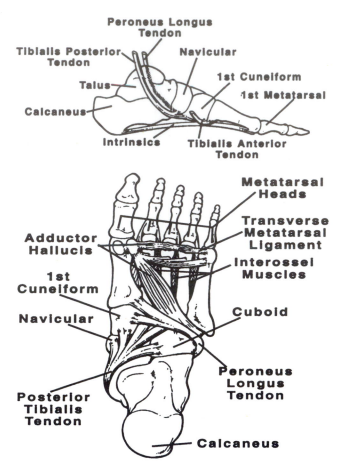

Figure 9–4. Anatomical structures that support the arches of the foot. Top: the peroneus longus, posterior tibialis, and intrinsic muscles support the medial arch. Bottom: the transverse arch is stabilized by the metatarsal heads, the intrinsic muscles of the foot, and the transverse metatarsal ligament.

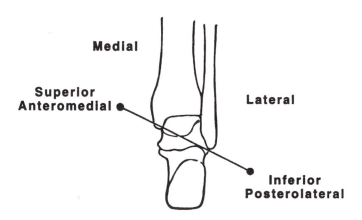

Figure 9–5. The axis of motion of the talocrural joint.

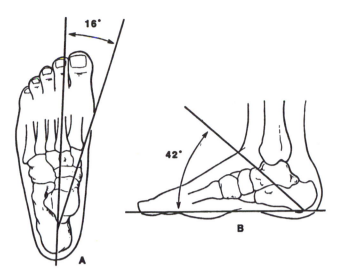

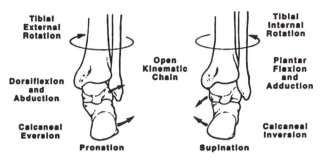

Figure 9-7. Rearfoot pronation and supination in the open kinematic chain (right foot).

Figure 9-6. The axis of motion of the subtalar joint.

Midfoot

Supination consists of inversion, plantar flexion, and adduction of the calcaneus (Fig 9-7).

The components of triplanar motion change in the closed kinematic chain. In the closed chain, pronation consists of calcaneal eversion, with plantar flexion and adduction of the talus on the calcaneus (Fig 9-8). Supination in weightbearing consists of calcaneal inversion, with dorsiflexion and abduction of the talus on the calcaneus. The direction of calcaneal movement is unaffected by the type of motion, whether open or closed kinematic chain.

The subtalar joint plays two roles during gait. In pronation, the joint is a mobile adapter, allowing the foot to conform to irregular surfaces. In supination, the subtalar joint acts as a rigid lever that allows the propulsion required to move the body forward.[72] These two functions are repeated over and over during the gait cycle (see Chapter 10, Gait Evaluation).

The subtalar joint allows tibial rotation during gait. This tibial rotation affects the entire lower kinematic chain. During the gait cycle, pronation causes tibial internal rotation and supination causes tibial external rotation (Fig 9-8).

The accessory motion at the subtalar joint includes lateral glide of the convex portion of the calcaneus during inversion and medial glide during eversion.[65]

The midfoot consists of the calcaneocuboid, talonavicular, naviculocuboid, naviculocuneiform, and intercuneiform joints. The calcaneocuboid joint is a sellar or saddle-shaped joint, and the talonavicular joint is considered a ball and socket joint. Ligamentous support for these joints comes from the deltoid, dorsal talonavicular, calcaneonavicular, and calcaneocuboid ligaments. The articulation between the cuboid and navicular bones is fibrous. The joints between the cuneiform bones and their articulation with the cuboid and navicular bones are plane synovial joints.

All midfoot joints allow gliding and rotation. Two axes of motion allow triplanar motion at the mid tarsal joints so the forefoot can twist on the rearfoot (Fig 9-9). The motions of inversion and eversion occur around a longitudinal axis, observed as the rise and fall of the medial arch during gait.[16,62,72] The motions of plantar flexion-adduction and dorsiflexion-abduction occur around an oblique axis. When the subtalar joint pronates in a closed kinematic chain, the mid tarsal joints "unlock" and adapt to the weightbearing forces. As the subtalar joint supinates in weightbearing, the mid tarsal joints "lock" and

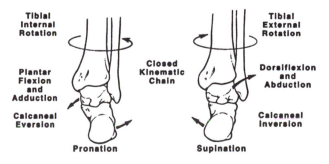

Figure 9-8. Rearfoot pronation and supination in the closed kinematic chain (right foot)

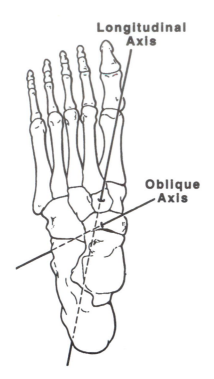

Figure 9–9. The axes of motion in the midfoot.

become more rigid in preparation for propulsion during gait; thus, the mid tarsal joints are quite dependent on the action of the subtalar joint. Every degree of subtalar overpronation produces an increase in mid tarsal joint instability.[71]

Mid tarsal joint position during gait is dictated by muscle contractions during the propulsive phase of gait and by ground reaction forces during the contact and midstance phases of gait.[77]

Forefoot

The forefoot consists of the structures distal to the midfoot. This includes the tarsometatarsal (TMT), intermetatarsal (IMT), the metatarsophalangeal (MTP), and the interphalangeal (IP) joints. The TMT and IMT joints are plane synovial joints. The MTP joints are condyloid synovial joints, and the IP joints are uniaxial synovial hinge joints. The metatarsals provide forefoot stability, and the MTP and IP joints provide forefoot mobility. The metatarsal heads tolerate weightbearing forces, and the toes help stabilize the forefoot dynamically.[16]

Two "rays" of the foot rotate around longitudinal axes: the first ray is composed of the first metatarsal

and the medial cuneiform; the fifth ray is the fifth metatarsal.[75] The first and fifth rays can flex and extend in the sagittal plane. When the subtalar and mid tarsal joints supinate or pronate, the forefoot is twisted into pronation or supination[34] by the reciprocal motion of the first and fifth rays. A pronation twist is a result of first ray plantar flexion and fifth ray dorsiflexion. A supination twist is caused by first ray dorsiflexion and fifth ray plantar flexion (Fig 9–10).[16]

Abnormal alignment of the forefoot can affect the weightbearing position of the subtalar joint (Fig 9–11).[16,17,72] Forefoot varus is a position of forefoot inversion in relation to the rearfoot, with the subtalar joint in neutral. During weightbearing, in a foot with forefoot varus, the medial aspect of the foot is brought in contact with the ground by subtalar joint pronation, causing the calcaneus to evert.[92] Forefoot valgus is a position of eversion of the forefoot relative to the rearfoot, with the subtalar joint in neutral. With a

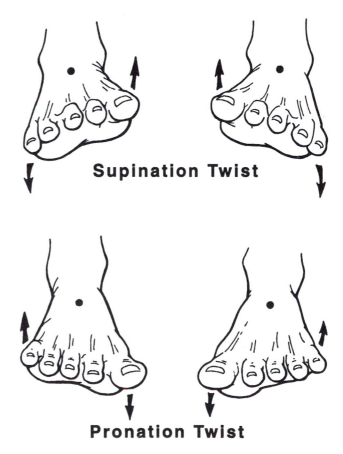

Figure 9–10. Forefoot pronation and supination.

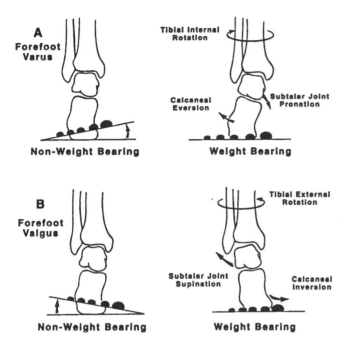

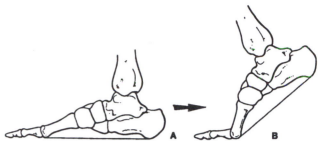

Figure 9–12. Tension in the plantar fascia increases during pushoff in gait, creating the "windlass effect."

Figure 9–11. Forefoot alignment does not affect the position of the subtalar joint in non-weightbearing, but changes subtalar alignment in weightbearing. A) Forefoot varus, B) Forefoot valgus.

valgus forefoot, weight is shifted to the lateral aspect of the foot through subtalar joint supination, causing calcaneal inversion.[92] Excessive forefoot pronation or supination can be detrimental to the foot and ankle and to the entire lower kinematic chain.

Metatarsals

The metatarsals act as beams to support the longitudinal arches of the feet[34,35] and are held together by the plantar fascial aponeurosis. During weightbearing, tension develops within the plantar fascial aponeurosis and is increased by MTP dorsiflexion during the push–off phase of gait as the tension in the aponeurosis pulls the calcaneus and metatarsals closer together. Because of its medial attachment on the calcaneus, tension on the plantar aponeurosis causes calcaneal inversion and subtalar joint supination, helping establish a rigid lever for propulsion in push–off. This is called the "windlass effect" (Fig 9–12).[27,35,70]

The metatarsals are weightbearing structures. In the normal population during static standing, the metatarsals carry about 2.5 times less force than the rearfoot.[10] The forces on the metatarsal bones are about 3 times higher in walking and 5 times higher in running[10] than in static standing.

The first metatarsal is twice as wide and four times as strong as the second metatarsal.[38] It has three muscle attachments (peroneus longus, posterior tibialis, and anterior tibialis) that dynamically stabilize it during propulsion. The head of the first metatarsal has a large joint surface and sesamoid bones on the plantar surface. These bones give the flexor hallucis longus muscle a mechanical advantage, decreasing the forces on the MTP.[16,85]

Toes

The toes play an important role during ambulation. The toes maintain contact with the ground until the final stage of push–off in gait, bearing up to 40% of body weight during this stage.[53,85] Pressures on the toes are minimal in standing and increase with activity. Tension in the toe flexor tendons and sheaths decreases the pressures on the bones themselves and helps stabilize the longitudinal arch. The greatest amount of force transmitted through tendons occurs at the first MTP joint during the stance phase of gait.[10,53,85] Extension of the first MTP joint is crucial to the windlass effect. Adequate first MTP joint extension (60–70°) is needed to develop adequate tension within the plantar aponeurosis.[16] Normal mechanics at the first MTP are also dependent on the mobility of the sesamoid bones. Many foot disorders cause or are the result of altered mechanics at this joint.

The movements and range of motion at the foot and ankle are shown in Table 9–1.[4,16,65]

Table 9–1. Movements and ROM at the Foot and Ankle

ANKLE	Plantar flexion		50°
	Dorsiflexion		20°
	Eversion	Rearfoot	10°
		Forefoot	25°
	Inversion	Rearfoot	20°
		Forefoot	25°
	Abduction	Forefoot	15°
	Adduction	Forefoot	30°
TOE EXTENSION	Great toe	MTP	70°
		IP	0°
	Lateral 4 toes	MTP	40°
		PIP	0°
		DIP	30°
TOE FLEXION	Great toe	MTP	45°
		IP	90°
	Lateral 4 toes	MTP	40°
		PIP	35°
		DIP	60°

Neuromuscular Components

Muscular Structures

The function of the muscles of the lower leg, ankle, and foot depends on whether the foot is fixed in a closed kinematic chain or free in an open kinematic chain. Many of these muscles also have diverse actions because of their multiple joint crossings. The muscles of the foot and ankle are shown in Figure 9–13A and B.

Posterior Muscles

Superficial Group

The superficial group consists of the gastrocnemius and soleus muscles (gastroc–soleus). These muscles share a common insertion on the calcaneus through the Achilles tendon. The gastrocnemius crosses the knee and ankle; the soleus crosses only the ankle. In an open kinematic chain the gastrocnemius causes knee flexion, and the gastrocnemius and soleus together cause ankle plantar flexion and subtalar joint supination.

These muscles are active throughout the stance phase of gait. The gastroc–soleus eccentrically decelerates tibial internal rotation and anterior glide of the tibia during midstance; concentrically supinates the subtalar joint; externally rotates the tibia; and plantar flexes the ankle during late midstance into push–off (see Chapter 10, Gait Evaluation).

Deep Group

The deep posterior muscles are the posterior tibialis, flexor digitorum longus, and flexor hallucis longus. In the open kinematic chain, the posterior tibialis is a plantar flexor and an ankle invertor. In a closed kinematic chain, its main function is to eccentrically decelerate subtalar pronation and internal tibial rotation at heel strike and to decelerate the forward motion of the tibia on the ankle during midstance. It then reverses to concentrically supinate the subtalar joint and externally rotate the tibia during late stance and early push–off.

The flexor digitorum longus and flexor hallucis longus help the posterior tibialis eccentrically decelerate the forward motion of the tibia during midstance. The flexor hallucis longus also concentrically stabilizes the first MTP joint; the flexor digitorum longus stabilizes the other toes. These actions support the medial arch. The flexor hallucis longus and flexor digitorum longus flex the toes concentrically in the open kinematic chain. The flexor digitorum longus also helps supinate the subtalar joint.

Lateral Muscles

The lateral muscles are the peroneus longus and peroneus brevis. In the open kinematic chain, both muscles contract concentrically to evert the foot and ankle. The longus also pronates the subtalar joint and causes first ray plantar flexion and eversion. In the closed kinematic chain, the peroneus longus supports the transverse and longitudinal arches and actively stabilizes the first ray during push–off in the late stance phase. The brevis stabilizes the mid tarsal joint, allowing the longus to work efficiently over the "cuboid pulley" (Fig 9–14). The cuboid pulley is

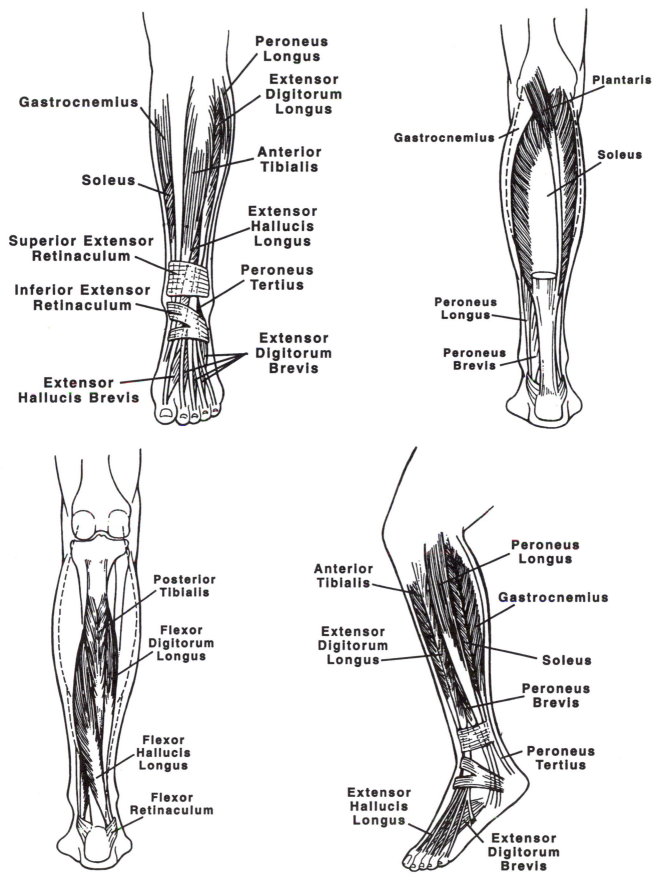

Figure 9–13A. The muscles of the foot and ankle.

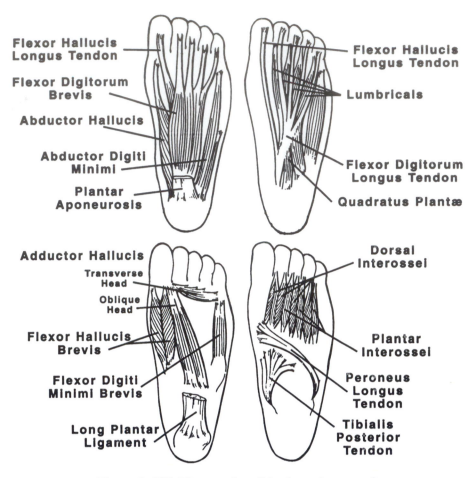

Figure 9–13B. The muscles of the foot, plantar surface.

formed by the tendon of the longus passing through the bony groove on the plantar surface of the cuboid.

Anterior Muscles

The anterior muscles are the anterior tibialis, extensor digitorum longus (EDL), and extensor hallucis longus (EHL). In the open kinematic chain, the EHL and EDL extend the toes and dorsiflex the ankle. In the closed kinematic chain, these muscles contract eccentrically to decelerate plantar flexion and pronation of the subtalar joint after heel strike in gait.

The EHL helps stabilize the first MTP and the EDL helps stabilize the IP joints during push–off. The anterior tibialis acts eccentrically to decelerate the posterior shear of the tibia on the talus at heel strike. During the swing phase of gait, the anterior tibialis contracts concentrically to dorsiflex the ankle to aid ground clearance. It also slightly supinates the foot during late swing phase before heel strike.

Intrinsic Muscles

There are six intrinsic muscles in the foot (Fig 9–13B). The flexor digitorum brevis, flexor hallucis brevis, abductor hallucis, adductor hallucis, and the lumbricals are on the plantar surface, and the extensor hallucis brevis is on the dorsal surface. The intrinsic muscles stabilize the mid tarsal joint and forefoot, and keep the toes flat during the final stages of the stance phase of gait.

Table 9–2 lists the muscles of the lower leg, ankle, and foot; their actions; and their peripheral and segmental innervations.

Neural Structures

There are several nerves passing through the lower leg into the foot and ankle. The nerves discussed here are the peroneal nerves, the tibial nerve and the sural nerve.

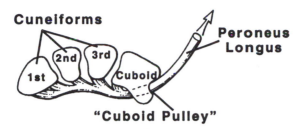

Figure 9–14. The peroneus longus passes through a bony groove on the cuboid, called the "cuboid pulley."

Table 9–2. Muscles of the Foot and Ankle, Their Actions, Peripheral Nerve Supplies, and Nerve Roots

Muscles	Actions	Peripheral Nerve Supply	Spinal Segment
Abductor digiti minimi	Toe abduction	Tibial (lateral plantar branch)	S2-S3
Abductor hallucis	Toe abduction, toe adduction	Tibial (medial plantar branch)	S2-S3
Dorsal interossei	Toe abduction	Tibial (lateral plantar branch)	S2-S3
Extensor digitorum brevis	Toe extension	Deep peroneal (lateral terminal branch)	S1-S2
Extensor digitorum longus	Dorsiflexion, eversion, toe extension	Deep peroneal	L5, S1
Extensor hallucis longus	Dorsiflexion, inversion, toe extension	Deep peroneal	L5, S1
Flexor accessorius	Toe flexion	Tibial (medial plantar branch)	S2-S3
Flexor digiti minimi brevis	Toe flexion	Tibial (medial plantar branch)	S2-S3
Flexor digitorum brevis	Toe flexion	Tibial (medial plantar branch)	S2-S3
Flexor digitorum longus	Plantar flexion, inversion, toe flexion	Tibial	S2-S3
Flexor hallucis brevis	Toe flexion	Tibial (medial plantar branch)	S2-S3
Flexor hallucis longus	Plantar flexion, inversion, toe flexion	Tibial	S2-S3
Gastrocnemius	Plantar flexion	Tibial	S1-S2
Interossei	Toe flexion	Tibial (medial plantar branch)	S2-S3
Lumbricals (interphalangeal joints)	Toe extension	Tibial (1st medial plantar branch; 2nd–4th by lateral plantar branch)	S2-S3
Lumbricals (metatarsophalangeal joints)	Toe flexion	Tibial (1st medial plantar branch; 2nd–4th by lateral plantar branch)	S2-S3
Peroneus brevis	Plantar flexion, eversion	Superficial peroneal	L5, S1-S2
Peroneus longus	Plantar flexion, eversion	Superficial peroneal	L5, S1-S2
Peroneus tertius	Dorsiflexion, eversion	Deep peroneal	L5, S1
Plantar interossei	Toe adduction	Tibial (lateral plantar branch)	S2-S3
Plantaris	Plantar flexion	Tibial	S1-S2
Soleus	Plantar flexion	Tibial	S1-S2
Tibialis anterior	Dorsiflexion, inversion	Deep peroneal	L4-L5
Tibialis posterior	Plantar flexion, inversion	Tibial	L4-L5

Peroneal Nerves

The common peroneal nerve divides at the proximal head of the fibula to form the deep and superficial branches. The deep peroneal nerve courses medially to the fibula and exits beneath the extensor hallucis muscle belly several centimeters proximal to the ankle. It continues distally, passing beneath first the superior and then the inferior extensor retinaculum. This area between the retinacula, sometimes referred to as the anterior tarsal tunnel,[5,26,55] is a site of potential neural entrapment. [48] The nerve continues distally, giving off the medial sensory branch. This branch passes between the first and second cuneiforms and the extensor hallucis brevis tendon, another potential site for nerve entrapment.[51] Tight shoes may contribute to compression of this branch of the deep peroneal nerve.[5,26] The medial sensory branch continues distally, supplying the web space between the first and second toes.

The superficial peroneal nerve courses distally from the fibular head, passing under the peroneus brevis muscle. It pierces the deep fascia of the lower leg ≈10–12 cm proximal to the lateral malleolus. From there, it travels over the superior extensor retinaculum and branches into the intermediate and medial dorsal cutaneous nerves. These nerves supply cutaneous sensation to most of the dorsum of the foot; the web space between the first and second toes is supplied by the deep peroneal nerve. Compression injury is possible with tight fitting shoes; this nerve may be overstretched in chronic inversion sprains. [32]

The peroneal nerve may be subject to injury via compression, entrapment, or stretch at the following sites (Fig 9–15): deep peroneal nerve—either the anterior tarsal tunnel or between the extensor hallucis brevis tendon and the first and second cuneiforms; superficial peroneal nerve—over the superior extensor retinaculum distally to the dorsum of the foot.

Tibial Nerve

Posterior Tibial Nerve

The posterior tibial nerve courses distally down the midline of the calf under the soleus muscle. It then passes under the flexor retinaculum, which bridges the space between the calcaneus and medial malleolus. This area is called the tarsal tunnel and is analogous to the carpal tunnel at the wrist. The posterior tibial nerve passes through the tunnel with the posterior tibial artery and the flexor tendons of the foot. The tarsal tunnel is a site of potential nerve entrapment.

The nerve branches into the medial and lateral plantar nerves and the medial calcaneal branch. The medial calcaneal branch supplies the cutaneous sensation on the medial heel and the plantar surface of the heel. Here it may be subject to overstretch with excessive heel valgus during weightbearing. It may also be compressed within the medial fat pad of the heel.

The medial plantar nerve passes between the abductor hallucis and flexor digitorum brevis muscles. "Jogger's foot" is compression of the nerve at this site.[67] The nerve then branches into many cutaneous nerves that pierce the plantar aponeurosis. These nerves supply the cutaneous sensation to the medial sole of the foot.

The lateral plantar nerve passes laterally from the tarsal tunnel, piercing the plantar aponeurosis and supplying the cutaneous sensation to the lateral sole of the foot. The medial and lateral nerves join near the plantar surface of the fourth MTP joint, between the third and fourth metatarsals. These nerves are subject to compression here, a condition called Morton's Neuroma, or metatarsalgia.

The posterior tibial nerve and its branches are subject to injury at the following sites (Fig 9–16): 1) tarsal tunnel; 2) medial heel; 3) between the abductor hallucis and flexor digitorum brevis; and 4) between the third and fourth metatarsals.

Sural Nerve

The sural nerve is a cutaneous branch of the tibial nerve. It passes between the two heads of the gastrocnemius and pierces the deep fascia approximately halfway down the calf. Just below the muscle bellies of the gastrocnemius, the sural nerve is joined by the lateral sural nerve, a branch of the common peroneal nerve. The nerve then courses laterally to the Achilles tendon, posterior to the lateral malleolus. It continues distally to the lateral foot, coursing along the fifth metatarsal. The sites of

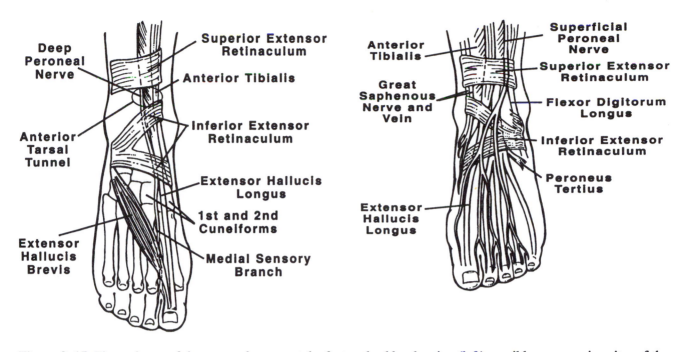

Figure 9–15. The pathway of the peroneal nerves at the foot and ankle, showing (left) possible compression sites of the deep peroneal nerve at the anterior tarsal tunnel and in the region between the flexor hallucis brevis and the first and second cuneiforms; and (right) possible compression sites of the superficial peroneal nerve over the superior extensor retinaculum distally into the foot.

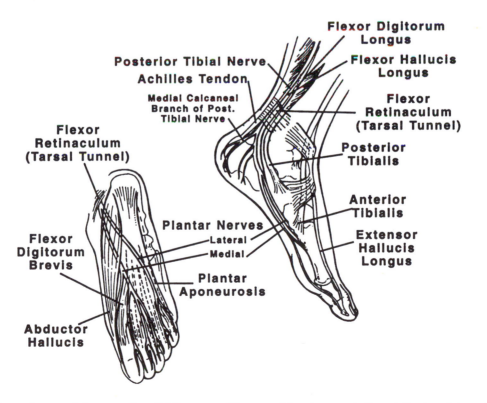

Figure 9–16. The pathway of the posterior tibial nerve, with potential entrapment sites at the tarsal tunnel, medial heel, between the abductor hallucis and the flexor digitorum brevis; and between the third and fourth metatarsal heads.

potential compression, entrapment, or stretch of the sural nerve are 1) where the nerve emerges from the deep fascia; 2) beside the Achilles tendon; and 3) along the lateral foot and ankle (Fig 9–17).

Increased pressure in any muscular compartment of the lower leg may interfere with nerve function due to compression, and cause symptoms in the foot and ankle.[32] Increases in compartment pressure can be caused by repetitive muscular stress.

EVALUATION

Subjective Examination

The subjective evaluation should proceed as outlined in Chapter 2, Principles of Extremity Evaluation. The patient's main complaints give the clinician valuable clues about the patient's current problems and help plan the objective examination. The mechanism of an acute injury can help identify the structures involved. For example, the clinician should suspect a lateral ligamentous sprain if the patient reports twisting the ankle into inversion.

Repetitive trauma can affect many structures at the foot and ankle, including the tendons, bones, and

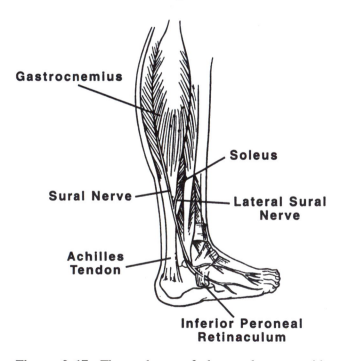

Figure 9–17. The pathway of the sural nerve with potential entrapment sites where the nerve emerges from the deep fascia (between the bellies of the gastrocnemius), beside the achilles tendon, and along the lateral foot.

joints. Even the skin in this region is subject to repetitive stresses, resulting in corns, calluses, and blisters. Abnormal foot and ankle biomechanics can be detrimental to the entire proximal kinematic chain. The specific demands of daily activities will help identify potential sources of repetitive trauma.

Many problems at the foot and ankle cause specific patterns of shoe wear; therefore, the clinician should ask about the type of footwear the patient uses and the types of surfaces the patient usually walks on. If there is a history of surgical procedures at the foot and ankle, it is important to note the specific procedure performed and the mechanical consequences it may have on function of the foot and ankle.

Planning the Objective Examination

The objective examination of the foot and ankle should be based on the subjective examination clues. Symptoms felt at the foot can be referred from the lumbar spine, hip, knee, and lower leg. These areas should be considered if they are suspected contributors to the patient's problems. If there is significant pain after acute trauma to the foot and ankle, the clinician should suspect a fracture, which should be confirmed or ruled out with diagnostic examination.

Information regarding the severity, irritability, and nature (SIN) of the problem is important when planning the objective examination. If pain prevents the patient from attaining and maintaining normal foot and ankle positions, the problem is severe. The movements and positions causing pain should be avoided during the objective examination, if possible. If the problems are easily provoked by weightbearing, the problem is irritable. This may limit the movements and positions included in the examination. The nature of the problem—for example, progressive weakness in the foot and ankle, which may be caused by central nervous system problems—may make a neurological examination essential.

Objective Examination

The objective examination should be carried out as outlined in Chapter 2, Principles of Extremity Evaluation. The proximal areas that may contribute to the symptoms felt at the ankle and foot should be screened first to rule out the need for a more extensive examination. The lower quarter screening examination and clearing tests (see Chapter 2, Principles of Extremity Evaluation) can initially define problem areas. More extensive evaluation of these areas may be needed if they contribute to complaints.

Structural Observation

Since the shape and alignment of the foot and ankle change with the weightbearing status, the foot and ankle should be observed in both the open and closed kinematic chain. The patient's gait pattern upon entering the examination room will give the clinician initial clues about the patient's problem. Gait deviations may reflect compensation due to pain, joint stiffness, or joint instability. Any structural deviations from the normal bony or soft tissue contours should be noted. This includes examination of the skin, where calluses, corns, blisters, or sores may develop. Evidence of vascular changes should be noted; discoloration may represent vascular insufficiency or early changes from reflex sympathetic dystrophy (RSD). Bilateral comparison of any abnormalities in alignment should be made in weightbearing and non–weightbearing.

Weightbearing

The weightbearing examination should include anterior, posterior, medial, and lateral views. The examination of gait is discussed in Chapter 10, Gait Evaluation.

Anterior View

The patient is asked to stand with the feet ≈6 in apart with toes pointing straight ahead. The clinician should observe the relation of the entire lower extremity to the foot. This establishes a baseline alignment and helps the clinician sort out the relations between the functional segments. The tibial alignment should be checked for internal or external torsion and tibial valgum or varum. Likewise, the alignment of the femur, pelvis, and sacrum should be examined.

Normal alignment of the foot to the ankle equally distributes the weight on all metatarsal heads. The metatarsal heads should all lie in the same transverse plane. The alignment of the first ray should be noted; metatarsus adductus is a common deformity in this area (Fig 9–18). The alignment of the toes, especially the great toe, should be noted; hallux valgus is a common deformity here (Fig 9–19). The forefoot may have different alignments, based on the lengths of the metatarsal bones.[41] Any splaying of the forefoot or loss of transverse arch height should be noted. Bony exostoses are common in the foot and ankle, as are corns and calluses.

Posterior View

As the patient continues to stand with the feet ≈6 in apart and pointed straight ahead, the clinician

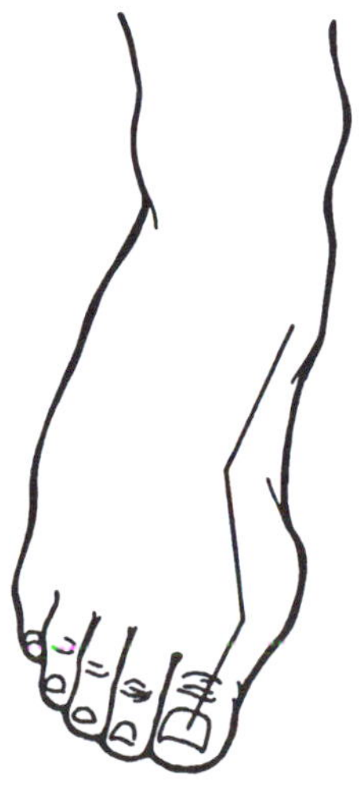

Figure 9–18. Metatarsus adductus.

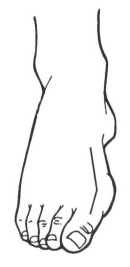

Figure 9–19. Hallux valgus.

observes from behind. In normal alignment, a line bisecting the calcaneus runs parallel to a line bisecting the distal 1/3 of the lower leg.[69] Deviations from this alignment are calcaneal eversion or inversion—referred to as calcaneal valgus and calcaneal varus, respectively (Fig 9–20).

The position of the heel influences the contour of the Achilles tendon. A calcaneal valgus with a low arch is a pronated foot. This heel position causes a relative convexity of the medial foot, the ankle, and the Achilles tendon. The opposite will occur with calcaneal varus and a high arch—a supinated foot (Fig 9–21). If all five toes are visible from the posterior view, the patient has a "too many toes sign." This occurs when there has been a trauma to the posterior tibialis tendon, resulting in a collapse of the subtalar joint and subsequent flatfoot.[16]

There are many other structural changes observable from the posterior view. Thickening of the Achilles tendon is often noted in patients with Achilles tendinitis. Many patients have a bony exostosis and callus build up on the heel, named a "pump bump." This term was coined after those patients who acquired this problem from the wearing high heel shoes, but many running shoes can also cause this deformity.

Medial View

The medial view lets the clinician observe the medial longitudinal arch of the foot. The height of the arch should be noted. An excessively high arch is called a pes cavus deformity, and an excessively low arch is called a pes planus deformity. The relation of the first ray to the midfoot should be noted. A relatively plantarflexed first ray usually coincides with a supinated foot and a forefoot valgus. A relatively dorsiflexed first ray usually coincides with a pronated foot and a forefoot varus position (see "Biomechanical Assessment" section of this chapter). The relative position of the navicular bone should be noted. The navicular bone is often referred to as the keystone of the medial longitudinal arch because of its position between the first MTP and the calcaneus (Fig 9–22).

Lateral View

The lateral view lets the clinician observe the lateral longitudinal arch. The position of the cuboid should be noted. The cuboid is the keystone of the lateral longitudinal arch, analogous to the navicular of the medial arch (Fig 9–23).

Non–weightbearing

The clinician should also observe the foot and ankle in a non–weightbearing position. With the patient supine, the clinician should check for calluses, plantar warts, etc., on the sole of the foot. Any edema should be noted. The shape and contours of the toes should be examined and any deformities noted. The contour of the transverse arches can be assessed in this position and correlated to the position of the arches in weightbearing.

With the patient prone, the clinician should inspect the posterior lower leg, ankle, and foot. Most

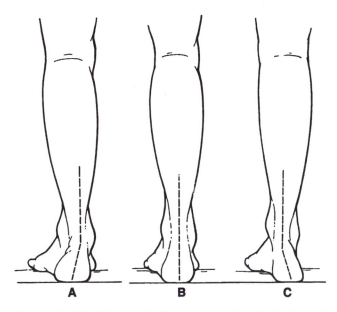

Figure 9–20. Calcaneal alignment, right; A) Calcaneal varus; B) normal alignment; C) Calcaneal valgus.

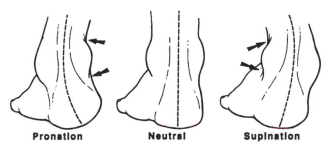

Figure 9–21. Influence of heel position on foot contours and Achilles tendon alignment with the foot in; A) pronation, B) neutral; C) supination

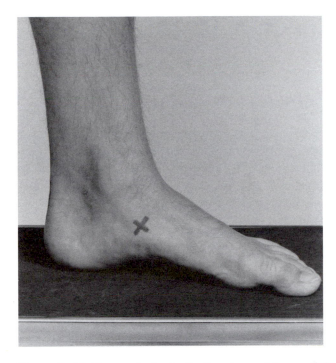

Figure 9–22. The navicular is the keystone of the medial longitudinal arch.

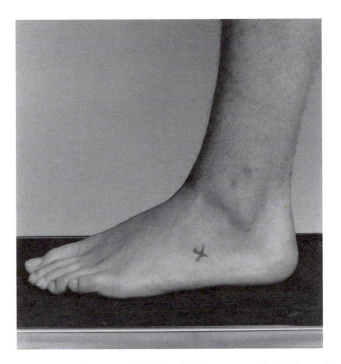

Figure 9–23. The cuboid is the keystone of the lateral longitudinal arch.

of the items to look for have been mentioned in the "Posterior View" section of this chapter. In non–weightbearing, it is important to note the positional relations of the lower leg to the calcaneus and the relation of the forefoot to the rearfoot. Tibial torsion can be observed in sitting, supine, or prone. Measurement of these relations is discussed in the "Special Tests" section of this chapter.

Other deformities of the toes include (Fig 9–24):

- Claw Toe
- Mallet Toe
- Hammer Toe
- Morton's Toe

Footwear

The clinician should critically evaluate the patient's footwear. The wear pattern of shoes often reflects the biomechanical stresses applied to the foot and the responding compensations made by the foot and ankle. Work, dress, recreational, and sport shoes should be checked. Heel heights should be noted. Patients who frequently wear high heel shoes bear increased pressure on the ball of the foot and often have tightness in the gastroc–soleus complex.

Excessive wear and material breakdown should be noted. The shape of the forefoot and rearfoot should be checked. Bulging on the medial side of the footwear suggests excessive pronation or a flatfoot deformity. Bulging on the lateral side of the footwear suggests excessive supination or a rigid foot deformity. The width of the rearfoot should be compared bilaterally. An increased width reflects increased rearfoot motion. Footwear with a bulging dorsum usually correlates with complaints of corns or blisters from a tight toebox. Outersole wear may reflect abnormal mechanics of the foot and ankle.

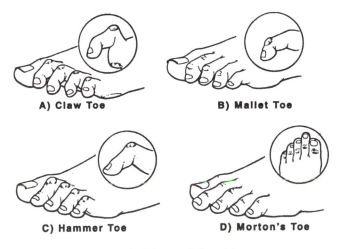

A) Claw Toe   B) Mallet Toe

C) Hammer Toe   D) Morton's Toe

Figure 9–24. Toe deformities.

Scuffed toes suggest a neuropathic weakness of the dorsiflexors. Medial heel wear may mean early pronation.

Because technology has improved the outersole's resistance to wear, the amount of time spent on the shoes; the frequency and duration of their use; and the surfaces they are used on should be considered together. Waiting for shoes to "wear out" before obtaining new ones may not be a wise practice for good foot and ankle health.

Mobility

Physiological Mobility

Physiological mobility refers to the movement of the foot and ankle in standard planes and functional combinations. The clinician should assess active and passive physiological mobility.

Active Mobility

Active mobility assesses the patient's willingness and ability to move the lower leg, ankle, and foot. Overpressure should be applied at the end of the available active range of motion, if tolerated. The important findings that should be noted include: the available active range of motion; the symptom response during the motion; any crepitus felt or heard; and the response to overpressure. Overpressure may increase the range of motion or alter the symptom response.

The order and number of motions tested should be determined by the subjective clues. The motions suspected of causing severe symptoms or irritability should be checked last, and the examination should initially include only those motions that won't exacerbate the symptoms. Bilateral and normal active range comparison should be noted. The motions that should be tested include: plantar flexion, dorsiflexion, inversion, and eversion of the ankle; supination and pronation of the forefoot; and flexion and extension of the toes. Testing can be done with the patient sitting, supine, or prone.

Common findings include limited first MTP extension; limited and painful ankle dorsiflexion in the patient with anterior talar spurring; limited dorsiflexion in the post–operative Achilles tendon rupture patient; and painfully limited plantar flexion/inversion in the lateral ankle sprain patient.

Passive Mobility

Passive mobility testing assesses the integrity of the non–contractile components of the foot and ankle. These should be examined for any active motion that was not within normal limits or where the clinician is unable to test the end–feel. The following should be noted: range of motion, symptom response, end–feel, and the pattern of any motion restriction. Bilateral comparison should be made.

The pattern of motion restriction can be considered capsular or non–capsular. The capsular patterns at the foot and ankle are:

- talocrural joint:
  plantar flexion limited more than dorsiflexion

- subtalar joint:
  supination limited more than pronation

- first MTP:
  extension limited more than flexion.

- second through fifth MTP:
  variable pattern

- IP joints:
  extension limited more than flexion

The symptom response to passive motion can reveal the stage of the problem (see Chapter 2, Principles of Extremity Evaluation). Passive mobility can be tested with the patient sitting or supine as needed (Fig 9–25).

Accessory Mobility

Accessory mobility refers to component motion and joint play. Accessory mobility should be assessed for each movement in which the physiological range of motion was limited or abnormal in some way. Accessory mobility of the foot and ankle is usually examined in the supine position but can be checked in prone or sidelying (see Chapter 11, Mobilization Techniques). The accessory motions that should be tested at the foot and ankle include:

Tibiofibular joint

- anterior and posterior glide

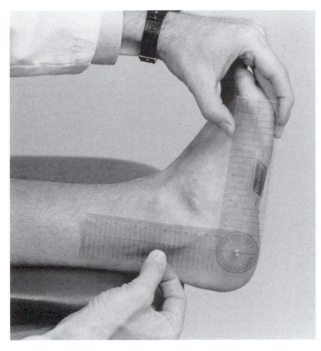

Figure 9–25A. Passive mobility testing: ankle dorsiflexion.

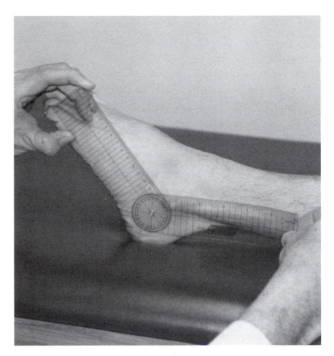

Figure 9–25B. Passive mobility testing: ankle plantar flexion.

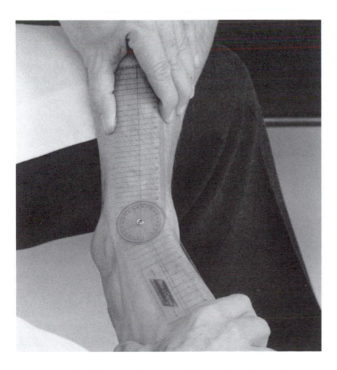

Figure 9–25C. Passive mobility testing: inversion.

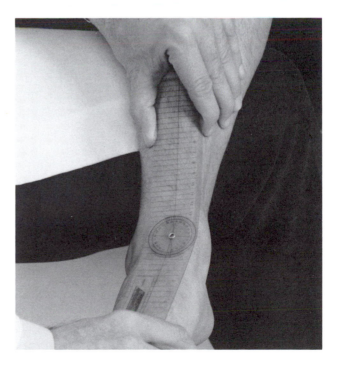

Figure 9–25D. Passive mobility testing: eversion.

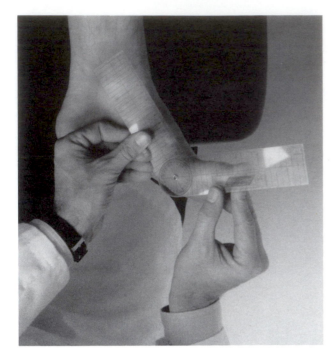

Figure 9–25E. Passive mobility testing: toe extension.

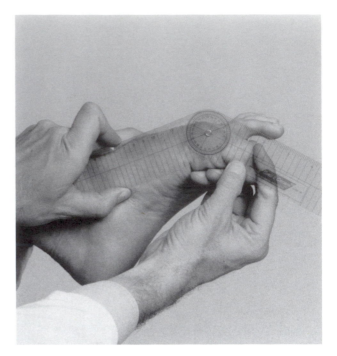

Figure 9–25F. Passive mobility testing: toe flexion.

Talocrural joint

- distal distraction (traction)
- anterior and posterior glide

Subtalar joint

- medial and lateral tilt

Mid tarsal joints

- anterior and posterior glide

TMT and IMT joints

- anterior and posterior glide

MTP and IP joints

- distal distraction (traction)
- anterior and posterior glide
- medial and lateral glide

The clinician should compare findings bilaterally and to normal. These findings include the available range of motion, the end–feel, any crepitus noted, and any symptoms provoked. The results should be consistent with the findings of the physiological mobility examination. For example, decreased anterior glide of the talocrural joint is consistent with limited plantar flexion.

Strength

Manual muscle testing (MMT) assesses the status of the contractile elements of the foot and ankle. These tests are performed in the mid range of motion to avoid stress on the non–contractile structures. The patient is told to gradually increase effort to a voluntary maximum contraction, which the clinician resists isometrically. The muscle strength should be graded and any symptom response noted. Any muscle acting on, acting across, or influencing the foot and ankle should be included in the muscle test. Cyriax's four patterns of response (see Chapter 2, <u>Principles of Extremity Evaluation</u>) can help with assessment and the eventual treatment plan.

It can be useful to assess the functional strength of the foot and ankle muscles. These can be tested by repeated rising up on the toes and by lifting the foot and toes in dorsiflexion while standing. These should be performed with the patient standing on one leg, using one hand to maintain balance. A typical criterion for normal function is ability to perform 10–15 repetitions of each movement.[69] The functional strength of the toe flexors is tested by having the patient put a foot on a towel and scrunch it up or by having patients pick up small objects with their toes.

Neurological

The neurological examination should be carried out as outlined in Chapter 2, Principles of Extremity Evaluation. Indications for the examination include complaints of functional weakness, paresthesias, anesthesias, or other symptoms suspicious of neurological involvement. The neurological examination includes testing motor function, light touch sensation, and deep tendon reflexes (DTR's). Motor function is tested in the lumbosacral myotomes, per the lower quarter screening examination (see Chapter 2, Principles of Extremity Evaluation). Light touch sensation should be checked in the L3–S2 dermatomes and in the cutaneous nerve distributions (Fig 2–12). The relevant DTR's include the knee jerk (L3–L4), the medial hamstring reflex (L5–S1), and the ankle jerk (S1–S2). Unilateral and bilateral comparisons should be made.

Ankle proprioception should be checked in any patient with an ankle or foot injury,[23,46,90] especially those with a history of recurrent ankle sprains.[30] While the patient stands on one foot, the clinician observes any difficulties the patient has maintaining balance. Proprioception tests can be made more difficult by having the patient stand on a pillow or a balance board.

Neural tension tests can also help confirm or rule–out neurological involvement. The important tests for the foot, ankle, and lower leg include the straight leg raise (SLR), prone knee bend (PKB), and the Slump test. These tests are shown in Chapter 2, Principles of Extremity Evaluation.

Palpation

The palpation examination should proceed as discussed in Chapter 2, Principles of Extremity Evaluation. Palpation should begin with surface tissues and progress as tolerated to deeper structures. Bilateral comparisons should be made. The patient can be supine, sitting, or long sitting, as needed. The following structures of the lower leg should be palpated:

Anterior (Fig 9–26)

- anterior tibia
- anterior tibialis tendon
- superficial peroneal nerve
- extensor retinaculum
- extensor hallucis longus tendon
- extensor digitorum longus tendons
- neck of the talus
- cuneiforms
- metatarsals
- toes

Posterior (Fig 9–27)

- gastrocnemius and soleus muscles
- Achilles tendon
- sural nerve
- retrocalcaneal bursæ
- calcaneus
- metatarsal heads
- plantar aponeurosis
- flexor hallucis longus tendon
- sesamoid bones of the first MTP joint

Medial (Fig 9–28)

- posteromedial muscles
- medial malleolus
- tarsal tunnel
- deltoid ligamentous complex
- talus

Lateral (Fig 9–29)

- peroneal muscles
- lateral malleolus of the distal fibula
- anterior and posterior tibiofibular, calcaneofibular, and anterior talofibular ligaments
- sinus tarsus
- peroneus longus and brevis tendons

It is important to correlate the palpation findings with the rest of the objective examination. Proximal structures thought to contribute to the patient's problems should be palpated.

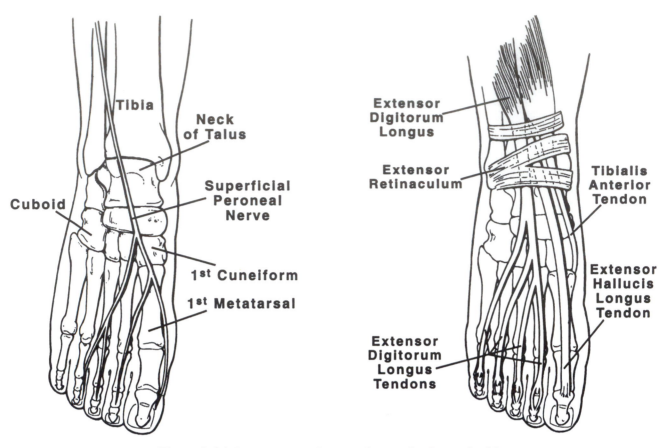

Figure 9–26. Structures to palpate on the anterior foot and ankle.

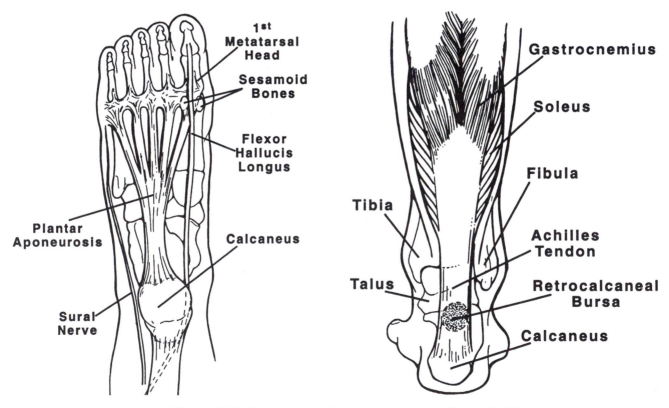

Figure 9–27. Structures to palpate on the posterior foot and ankle.

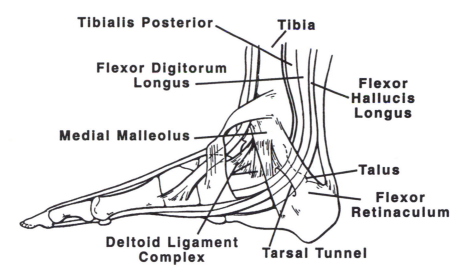

Figure 9–28. Structures to palpate on the medial foot and ankle.

Special Tests

This section describes tests that can help the clinician identify structures contributing to the patient's problem. The special tests for the foot and ankle are summarized in Table 9–3. These tests are discussed in three sections: Musculotendinous, Joint and Ligamentous, and Miscellaneous.

Musculotendinous Tests

Thompson Test

This is the classic test to confirm or rule out a rupture of the gastroc–soleus complex at the Achilles tendon. The patient is prone or kneeling. With the patient's foot and ankle unsupported, the clinician squeezes the muscle bellies of the gastroc–soleus complex (Fig 9–30). The test is negative if there is equal plantar flexion on the injured and uninjured sides. The test is positive if the foot does not passively plantarflex. If the response on the injured side is sluggish or less than the uninjured limb, there is probable musculotendinous injury, perhaps implicating a partial tear of the tendon.

Joint and Ligamentous Tests

Functional ankle stability in the closed kinematic chain depends on several factors. These include the dynamic control of muscle action,[59] the congruity of the articular surfaces, and the orientation of the ligaments.[86] The lateral ligaments are the primary

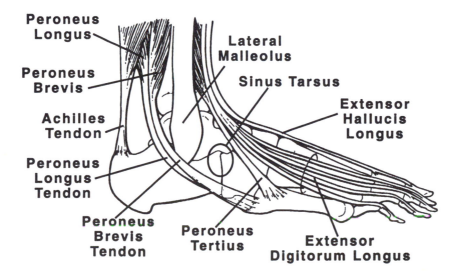

Figure 9–29. Structures to palpate on the lateral foot and ankle (for ligaments, refer to Fig 9–2).

Table 9–3. **Special Tests for the Foot and Ankle**

Test Type	Test Name	Purpose
Musculotendinous	Thomas Test	Achilles tendon tear
Joint/Ligamentous	Anterior drawer	Anterior ankle stability
	Inversion stress	Lateral ankle stability
	Talar tilt	Medial and lateral stability
Miscellaneous	Homan's Sign	Deep vein thrombosis
	Swelling and effusion	Swelling or joint effusion
	Biomechanical assessment	Biomechanical alignment of the lower limb

restraints to varus stress and anterior excursion of the talus. The medial ligaments are the primary restraints to a valgus stress of the talus.

There are two types of instability at the ankle: straight and anterolateral. Straight instability is caused by injury to medial and lateral capsuloligamentous structures. Anterolateral instability is caused by injury to lateral capsuloligamentous structures.

Anterior Drawer Test

The anterior drawer test is the standard stability test for the ankle. The base test is performed in ≈20°

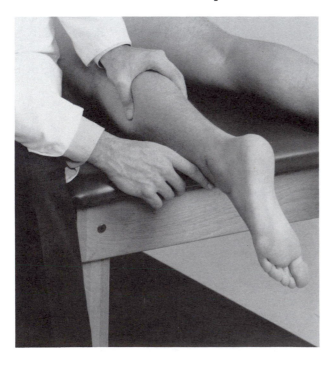

Figure 9–30. Thompson test.

of plantar flexion (Fig 9–31, left). The talus and calcaneus are pulled in an anterior direction. The test is positive if there is increased laxity when compared bilaterally.

To selectively test the integrity of the anterior talofibular ligament, the foot is positioned in inversion and plantar flexion. The talus and calcaneus are pulled anteriorly. The test is positive there is increased laxity and no firm end–feel. To test the medial and lateral structures simultaneously, the foot is dorsiflexed.

An optional method of testing is shown in Figure 9–31 (right). Here, the heel is stabilized on the examination table, fixing the talus and calcaneus. The distal tibia is pushed posteriorly.[31] The test is positive if there is excessive laxity when compared bilaterally.

Inversion Stress Test

The inversion stress test assesses the integrity of the lateral ligament structures. The tibia and fibula are stabilized. The clinician grasps the midfoot and forces the calcaneus into an inversion stress position (Fig 9–32). The test is positive if there is excessive laxity when compared bilaterally. When positive with the foot in neutral, this test implicates injury to the calcaneofibular ligament.

Talar Tilt Test

This test assesses the lateral and medial ligamentous structures individually. The patient is supine, sidelying, or long sitting, and the clinician applies a varus or valgus stress to the calcaneus (Fig 9–33). A varus tilt tests the calcaneal fibular ligament,

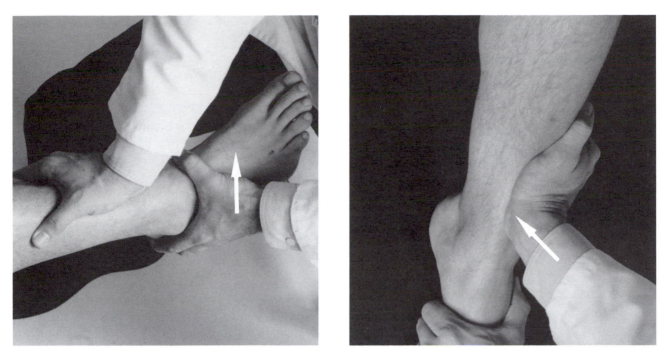

Figure 9-31. Anterior drawer test. Left: standard test. Right: with the heel stabilized.

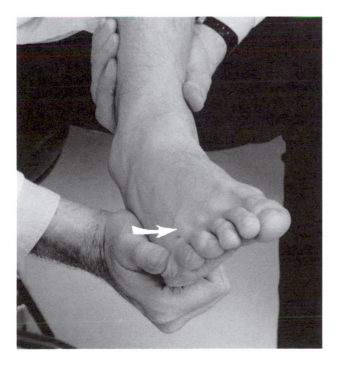

Figure 9-32. Inversion stress test.

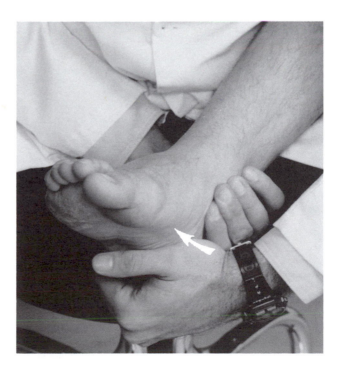

Figure 9-33. Talar tilt test. A valgus stress is shown.

while a valgus stress tests the integrity of the deltoid ligament complex. The test is positive if the ligament is excessively lax when compared bilaterally.

Miscellaneous Tests

Homan's Sign

Patients who have had surgery in the lower extremity should be checked for thrombosis, a common condition in the deep veins of the calf. The clinician tests for thrombosis by squeezing the calf firmly and deeply while passively dorsiflexing the ankle (Fig 9–34). The test is positive if the patient has excessive pain complaints or an asymmetrical response (more pain on one side than the other). Findings should be correlated with dorsal pedal pulse palpation.

Swelling and Effusion Tests

Effusion can be assessed objectively with two common techniques: volumetric displacement and "figure–8" girth measurements (Fig 9–35). The volumetric methods are highly reliable compared to the girth measurements.[65] The technique for volumetric measurement is described in the "Special Tests" section of Chapter 6, The Wrist and Hand. The test is positive if either volumetric displacement or

girth measurements increase when compared bilaterally.

Biomechanical Assessment

The following steps assess the biomechanical alignment of the lower leg, ankle, and foot. Only the static measurements are discussed here. The procedures for dynamic assessment of gait are presented in Chapter 10, Gait Evaluation.

1. Establish subtalar neutral position

Subtalar joint neutral position is the mid–position of joint play at the sub–talar joint. This position can be found in prone, supine, or weightbearing.[60,65,69,72,74,92] Subtalar neutral can be assessed manually with palpation,[60,65,69,74] or by calculation based on range of motion measurements.[72,92] The palpation method has fair intratester reliability but poor intertester reliability;[18] the calculation method has good intratester and intertester reliability.[9,22]

Palpation Technique

The talus is grasped between the finger and thumb on the medial and lateral surfaces. Stabilizing the talus, the foot is moved side to side into supination

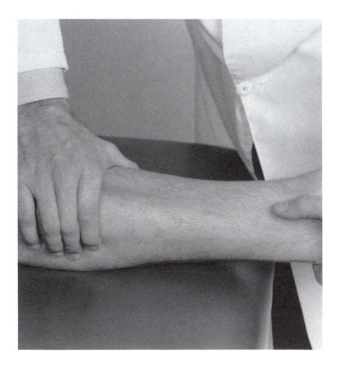

Figure 9–34. Homan's Sign.

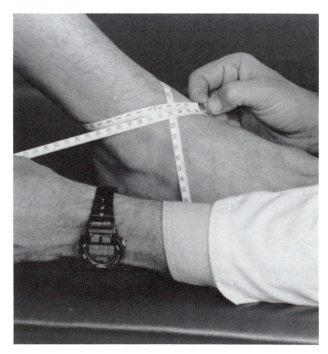

Figure 9–35. Figure-8 girth measurement.

and pronation. When the foot is positioned so the talus does not bulge medially or laterally, the subtalar joint is in the neutral position. (Fig 9–36) [60,65,69,74] This can be done in non–weightbearing or weightbearing.

Calculation Method

This test is performed in a non–weightbearing position. The distal third of the lower leg and the calcaneus are each bisected with vertical lines. These lines are aligned to create a reference point (Fig 9–37). Passive inversion and eversion are measured from this reference point. The subtalar neutral position is calculated by summing the two measurements (inversion + eversion), dividing by 3, and subtracting this number from end–range eversion. [72,92]

The calculation method involves goniometric measurement and is more objective than the palpation method. It provides numerical data for comparisons with the relative rearfoot and forefoot position, for comparisons with the calcaneal and tibial positions in weightbearing, and for reassessment when orthotics are used for biomechanical correction. [92]

2. Establish the relation between the rearfoot and forefoot

Abnormal alignment of the forefoot can affect the weightbearing position of the subtalar joint. [16,17,72] Two forefoot deformities are possible: forefoot varus and forefoot valgus (Fig 9–11). When present, these deformities cause compensations in weightbearing; forefoot varus causes compensatory subtalar joint pronation, and forefoot valgus causes compensatory subtalar joint supination.

Forefoot varus and valgus are measured goniometrically by comparing two lines. The first line runs perpendicular to the line bisecting the lower leg and calcaneus, parallel to the plantar surface of the calcaneus. The second line runs parallel to the metatarsal heads (Fig 9–38). The clinician stabilizes the foot in the subtalar neutral position and holds the foot by the base of the fifth metatarsal, moving the foot into plantar flexion. The angle between the two lines is measured. The axis of the goniometer is held laterally to measure forefoot varus (Fig 9–39); it is held medially to measure forefoot valgus. [92]

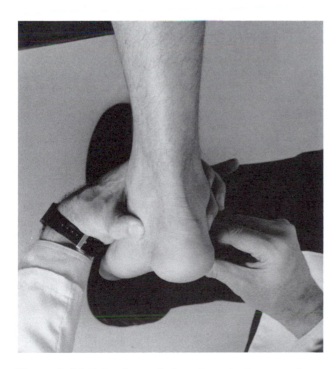

Figure 9–36. Palpation technique for subtalar neutral.

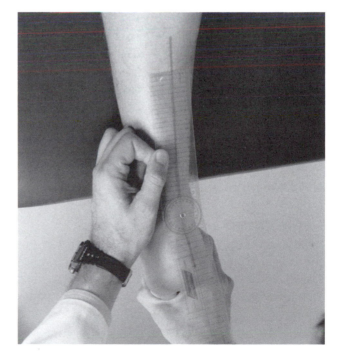

Figure 9–37. Calculation method for determining subtalar neutral. Measurement of passive calcaneal inversion is shown.

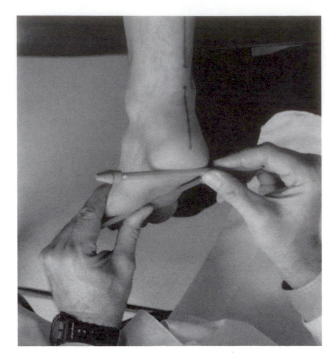

Figure 9–38. Comparing forefoot and rearfoot position.

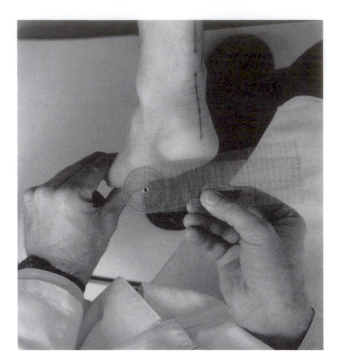

Figure 9–39. Goniometric measurement of forefoot varus.

3. Measure ankle dorsiflexion

The subtalar joint compensates for limited ankle dorsiflexion with excessive pronation in weightbearing.[16,72,88] To measure ankle dorsiflexion, the patient lies prone and the subtalar joint is held in neutral. Ankle dorsiflexion is measured with the knee extended and with the knee flexed to 90° (Fig 9–40). Forefoot hypermobility can cause inaccurate measurement, so dorsiflexion pressure is applied at the midfoot rather than at the forefoot. Normal dorsiflexion with knee extension is ≈10°; normal dorsiflexion with knee flexion is ≈15–20°.

4. Assess tibial alignment

Tibial alignment can affect the position of the subtalar joint in weightbearing. It can contribute to a compensated subtalar, forefoot, and rearfoot position. Tibial varus causes compensatory subtalar joint pronation in weightbearing.[72] With the patient standing, the clinician places one edge of a goniometer on the floor and the other edge along the line bisecting the distal lower leg. A line perpendicular to the floor serves as the reference point for measuring varus (medial) and valgus (lateral) deviations (Fig 9–41).

5. Assess calcaneal alignment

The position of the calcaneus should be measured in weightbearing because the weightbearing position reflects the compensated position of the subtalar joint. Calcaneal alignment is assessed by measuring the angle of the calcaneus relative to the floor. One edge of the goniometer is aligned on the floor and the other edge along the calcaneal line (Fig 9–42). The neutral or reference position is a line perpendicular to the floor. Calcaneal varus (medial) and valgus (lateral) angles deviate from this position.

This measurement assumes the subtalar joint is in a neutral position. If the calculated subtalar neutral was 2° of varus (inversion), and the calcaneus is measured at 6° of valgus (eversion), the subtalar joint is actually in a total of 8° of valgus from subtalar neutral.

The position of the calcaneus relative to the tibia can be assessed in non–weightbearing. The subtalar joint is held in neutral while the clinician measures the calcaneal deviation from the vertical line bisecting the lower leg. The reference point is line perpendicular to the bottom of the heel that runs up the leg. Any varus (inverted) or valgus (everted)

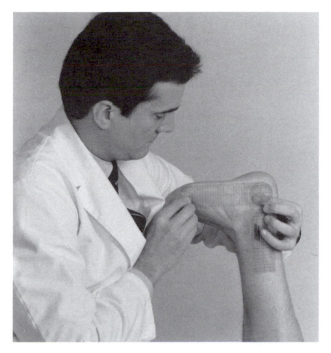

Figure 9–40. Measurement of ankle dorsiflexion with the knee flexed.

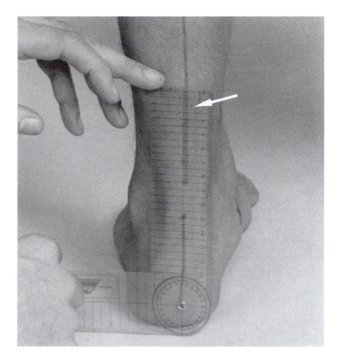

Figure 9–41. Measurement of tibial alignment.

deviations of the calcaneus are measured from this point.

6. Measure the first MTP range of motion

Limited motion at the first MTP can cause abnormal pronation during gait.[72] The first ray helps maintain the longitudinal arch via the windlass effect. Normal MTP extension is 65–70°.[16] The passive range of motion is measured with one edge of the goniometer along the line of the first metatarsal and medial cuneiform (the first ray) and the other edge along the proximal phalanx of the great toe (Fig 9–43).

7. Determine the first ray position.

The relative position of the first ray can influence the mechanics at the forefoot and the position of the subtalar joint in weightbearing. A plantar flexed first ray is usually hypomobile and rigid. This first ray position usually occurs with forefoot valgus, subtalar supination, and an externally rotated tibia—the components of a high arch. A dorsiflexed first ray is usually hypermobile and flexible. A dorsiflexed first ray is consistent with a forefoot varus position, subtalar pronation, and an internally rotated tibia. These are all components of a low arch.

The position of the first ray is assessed with the patient prone and the subtalar joint held in neutral. The clinician stabilizes the other metatarsals while gliding the first ray dorsally and plantarly (Fig 9–44). The direction of greater mobility reflects the relative position of the first ray. If the first ray is dorsiflexed,

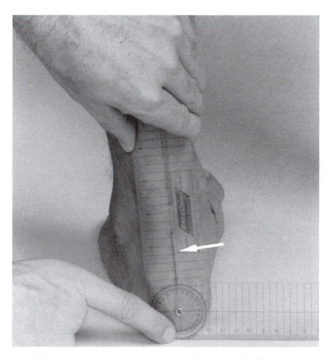

Figure 9–42. Measurement of calcaneal alignment.

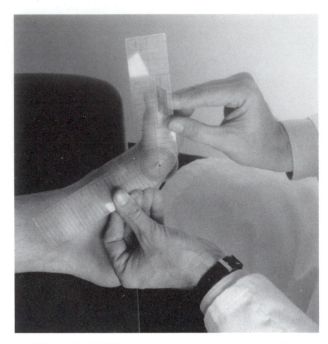

Figure 9–43. Measurement of great toe extension.

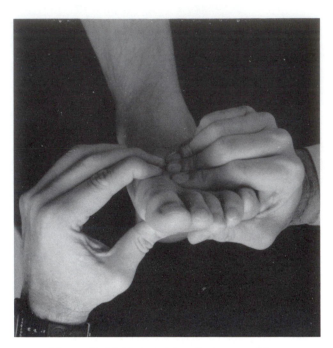

Figure 9–44. Determining first ray position.

it will move more in the dorsal direction than the plantar direction. If the first ray is plantarflexed, it will move more in a plantar direction.

8. Identify any rotational abnormalities of the lower limb

Tibial torsion is a rotation of the tibia along its longitudinal axis. Tibial torsion changes the axial relationship of the foot to the thigh.[72,83] Normal adult external tibial torsion is 20°;[37] >20° is considered excessive external tibial torsion, and <0° is considered excessive internal tibial torsion.[16] When there is excessive external tibial torsion, there will be pronation at the subtalar joint.[72] Internal tibial torsion is consistent with metatarsus adductus and in–toeing posture of the lower extremity.[83]

Tibial torsion can be measured with the patient sitting, supine, or prone. Using a goniometer, the clinician measures the angle between a line through the knee axis and a line through the ankle axis (Fig 9–45).

Other torsions are also important in lower extremity biomechanics. Rotational abnormalities of the hip and thigh were discussed in Chapter 7, The Hip. Rotational deformities of the thigh are 1) version—an altered relationship between the femoral

head and neck and the acetabulum;[58] 2) femoral torsion—rotation of the femur along its longitudinal axis; and 3) a twist in the femur.[16] It can be difficult to differentiate between version and bony torsion. If rotational asymmetry is found in all four possible positions—hip and knee extended, hip and knee

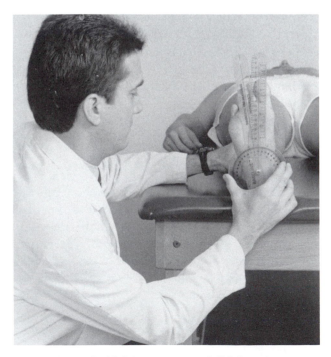

Figure 9–45. Measurement of tibial torsion.

flexed, hip flexed and knee extended, hip extended and knee flexed—then bony torsion is present.[64]

9. Determine limb lengths

A leg length discrepancy (LLD) can influence the alignment of the lower extremity and spine. If there is an LLD, there will be an alignment compensation somewhere along the kinematic chain.[16] The procedures to measure for an LLD were discussed in Chapter 7, The Hip. Comparison of leg lengths in standing is probably most useful clinically, since it considers all parts along the kinematic chain.

Compensations for an LLD do not always follow a consistent pattern. The clinician should be aware that different compensations exist.[6,87] One of the more significant compensation for an LLD occurs at the subtalar joint.[3,6,68] Generally, the subtalar joint on the long–limb side pronates to reduce the vertical height of the limb; however, the subtalar joint on the short–limb side may supinate to effectively lengthen the limb and balance the pelvis.[3] It is important to recheck the compensations of a suspected LLD after treatment intervention.

10. Determine the navicular position

The navicular bone is the key bone in the medial longitudinal arch of the foot. To determine its position, the clinician palpates the navicular tuberosity and places a mark on it. Then the medial plantar aspect of the first MTP and the apex of the medial malleolus are marked, and a line is drawn connecting these two marks (Fig 9–46). This helps the clinician observe the rise and fall of the medial arch during dynamic gait evaluation.[92] A normal arch allows the navicular bone to deviate downward only slightly in standing. During gait, a patient with a rigid supinated foot may begin with the navicular bone above this line, and it may move downward only slightly at midstance. The patient with a flat foot deformity may begin with the navicular bone much lower than the line. During midstance, excessive pronation may cause the navicular bone to deviate markedly lower than normal. Patients with excessive pronation may fail to resupinate (the navicular bone

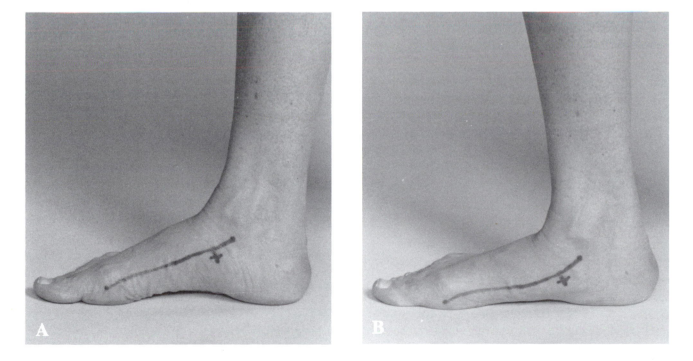

Figure 9–46. The position of the navicular bone A) non-weightbearing; and B) weightbearing. Note the dramatic fall of the medial arch during weightbearing. This patient shows excessive pronation.

stays down too long) or may pronate at push–off when they should resupinate.

Objective Examination Summary

A thorough evaluation of the lower leg, foot, and ankle is essential to effective management of patients with problems in this area. Problems can stem from injury to the bones, ligaments, muscles, or nerves. All these structures should be considered in a comprehensive evaluation. A biomechanical assessment determines whether there are biomechanical problems with the foot itself. Problems at the distal joints can cause adaptive changes throughout the lower kinematic chain.

Other sources of foot and ankle complaints that should be considered include the lumbar spine, hip, and knee. These areas should be screened in the initial evaluation to confirm or rule–out their involvement. Reassessments should include any of these areas, especially if the patient is not benefiting from treatment.

At the conclusion of the evaluation the clinician determines what problems the patient has and develops a problem list. This list is used to set goals and plan treatment.

TREATMENT STRATEGIES

The clinician should consider recommending a gait assistive device for any patient who has problems that are significantly worse with weightbearing. The assistive device should be used until symptoms resolve and gait pattern is symmetrical. Ankle splints or braces can limit range of motion and protect the joint. Protective taping, shoe inserts, or orthotics for cushioned support or biomechanical correction may be needed to control symptoms.

The patient's daily routines and activities should be reviewed. Special attention should be paid to the weightbearing stresses that may contribute to the patient's problems. Patients should be told to avoid prolonged standing, excessive walking, running, pivoting, and jumping. Footwear should be examined, and suggestions for modification should be made based upon the structure of the patient's foot, the current symptoms, and the physical demands of daily activities. Shoe inserts may be needed to relieve the stresses causing symptoms and tissue breakdown.

General treatment strategies are discussed in Chapter 3, Pathology and Treatment Principles. Refer to Chapter 11, Mobilization Techniques and to Chapter 12, Exercise, for mobilization techniques, stretching, strengthening, and proprioceptive training exercises for the foot and ankle.

COMMON CLINICAL CONDITIONS

Ankle Sprain

Traumatic injury to the ankle ligaments is probably the most common injury to the foot and ankle.[11,21,65] Most frequently, the injury involves the lateral ligaments of the ankle. The usual mechanism of injury is trauma in a position of plantar flexion and inversion. Eighty to ninety percent of ankle sprains result from this type of trauma.[24,65] The anterior talofibular ligament is the primary restraint to plantar flexion–inversion stress, so it is the first ligament to be injured. The calcaneal fibular ligament is a secondary restraint; it is also frequently involved in ankle sprains. The posterior talofibular ligament may also be injured, especially if the injury involves lower extremity rotation.[65] Injury to the anterior and posterior tibiofibular ligaments can also result from rotational stresses. Damage to these ligaments may lead to widening of the ankle mortise; this is called a "high ankle sprain."[84] Fractures should be ruled out by x–rays before evaluation and treatment begins.

Injury to the medial ankle ligaments is less common. Such injuries usually involve an eversion stress. Both the medial and lateral ligaments can suffer moderate to severe sprains. In moderate and severe sprains, the peroneal nerves can be injured.[66] Neural tension tests such as the SLR may provoke symptoms in patients with a history of chronic inversion sprains.[57]

Even with adequate non–operative treatment, chronic functional instability of the ankle occurs in 10–20% of patients with acute lateral ankle ligament ruptures.[45] Long term ankle instability can lead to osteoarthritis of the talus and tibial plafond.[33,78] Proprioceptive training is critical to the success of rehabilitation. These exercises are needed to compensate for the damage to the joint and ligament mechanoreceptors.[1,20,23,25,30,45,46,78,90]

History

The onset is usually a traumatic twisting injury of the ankle. The patient can usually identify the specific mechanism of injury, such as the plantar flexion–inversion stress. The patient with an acute injury may report hearing a pop or snap, with immediate pain on weightbearing and a rapid onset of effusion. The patient with chronic ankle instability complains of episodic sprains. These episodes are associated with the ankle intermittently giving way followed by effusion and pain on weightbearing.

Signs/Symptoms

The patient usually presents with an antalgic gait pattern and may already be using an assistive device. There may be significant swelling, which may be resolving, depending on time since injury. Gait and active movements may be guarded and apprehensive, and the patient may complain of an unstable feeling at times. Pain complaints will correlate with the site of ligament injury.

Objective examination will reveal measurable swelling over the site of ligament injury. Palpation may also reveal tenderness and warmth over the injured area. Range of motion will be limited and painful. Ligament testing may reveal mild, moderate, or severe laxity. The peroneal tendons should be palpated to ensure they are intact. Often these may sublux when the retinacular tissues are injured near the lateral malleolus in a lateral ankle sprain.

The clinician should always look for signs of fracture during examination of patients with acute sprains. These signs include inordinate focal pain, pain distant from the site of percussion along the same bone, and distal pain on compression of the proximal tibial–fibular joint.[74] Fracture signs should not be present, since fractures should be ruled out with diagnostic tests before objective examination.

Diagnostics

Routine x–rays should be sufficient to rule out fractures at the foot and ankle; however, stress views may be needed to define the severity of the injury

more specifically; arthrography can be used in difficult cases.[76] Widening of the mortise is commonly seen when the tibiofibular ligaments are involved (Fig 9–47). MRI can be used for more specific soft tissue assessment, and tomograms help investigate specific bony injury.

Problem List

Patients with ankle sprains may present with the following problems:

1. Post–traumatic edema

2. Pain with weightbearing

3. Instability or "giving way" of joint

4. Tenderness on palpation of injured ligaments

Treatment

Initially, the symptoms and weightbearing forces need to be controlled. Crutches should be used with weightbearing as tolerated. Ankle supports can limit the range of motion and provide early protected weightbearing. Physical agents should be used to decrease pain, prevent or reduce effusion, and promote healing. Vasopneumatic devices and compressive sleeves can prevent and reduce effusion.

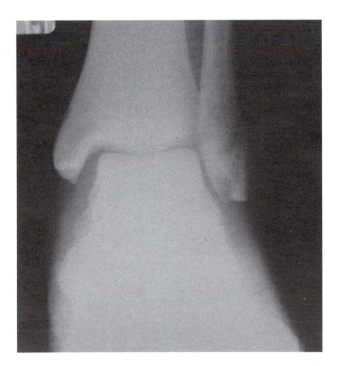

Figure 9–47. Radiograph showing widening of the ankle mortise due to an acute ankle sprain.

Felt horseshoe pads can also help keep the edema under control around the malleoli and sinus tarsi region (Fig 9–48).

Cold treatments alternated with exercises can help patients tolerate early mobility exercises. Proprioceptive exercises can begin while sitting and eventually progress to full weightbearing.[25] Open kinematic chain strengthening exercises using elastic band or tubing can help rehabilitation. Closed kinematic chain exercises should be progressed as the symptoms and healing constraints allow. Gastroc–soleus stretching should be a part of the rehabilitation process since tightness in these structures may predispose the patient to recurrent sprains. Pool exercises can progress weightbearing. Prophylactic braces can help return the patient to usual daily activities. These braces may help prevent chronic ankle instability.[19,44]

Severe sprains are often treated surgically with good results. Surgery may include primary anatomical repair for acute injuries and ligamentous reconstruction for chronic instability.[37,42,66] Rehabilitation after these procedures should be consistent with the healing constraints and established post–operative guidelines.

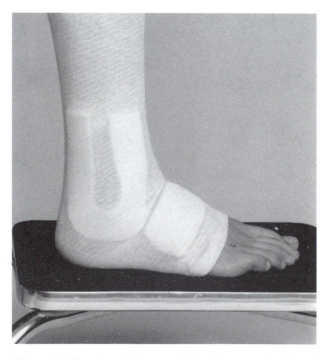

Figure 9–48. Felt padding can be used to control edema in the ankle.

Achilles Tendinitis

Achilles tendinitis is a common problem in athletes but can occur in any patient who subjects the tissues to overuse.[12,13,49,80] The Achilles tendon is the tendon common to the gastrocnemius and soleus muscles. The tendon is surrounded by a structure called the paratenon, which functions like an elastic sleeve and increases freedom of movement against surrounding tissues. The paratenon also provides the major blood supply to the Achilles tendon. There is a zone of hypovascularity 2–6 cm proximal to the insertion at the calcaneus, and it is thought this predisposes the tendon to injury at this area.[80] Either the tendon or paratenon (or both) can become inflamed and symptomatic, resulting in tendinitis or peritendinitis.[13] Patients with symptoms in this region may also have retrocalcaneal bursitis. This condition causes symptoms and tissue thickening in the area of the Achilles tendon.

The sural nerve lies close to the gastroc–soleus complex, ≈16 cm proximal to the lateral malleolus. It can be palpated near the Achilles tendon laterally.[8] This nerve may be involved in problems with the gastroc–soleus/Achilles tendon complex.[8,81] Abnormal alignment or mechanics at the lower leg, ankle, or foot may predispose the Achilles tendon to injury.[13,65]

History

The patient usually complains of a gradual onset of symptoms. The etiology is sometimes identified as an unaccustomed activity, but it may be insidious. Initially mild symptoms may have come on after activity. These symptoms can progress to moderate pain during activity and can eventually progress to severe complaints that prevent activity. This problem can become chronic if left untreated.

Signs/Symptoms

The patient often complains of a dull aching pain in the area of the Achilles tendon, usually proximal to its insertion into the calcaneus. Pain may be present at rest but most often occurs with activity. There may be observable, palpable edema and thickening of the Achilles tendon. Crepitus may be felt on repeated plantar flexion and dorsiflexion.[65] There is usually pain with passive dorsiflexion and on active and resisted plantar flexion. Pain with palpation is also common, usually 2–6 in proximal from the calcaneal insertion. This should be differentiated from retrocalcaneal bursa tenderness, which is anterior to the tendon but posterior to the talus.

If there is an acute strain, the clinician should palpate for a partial tear or rupture. The Thompson Test will be positive if there is a complete tear of the tendon. Palpation of the sural nerve lateral to the Achilles tendon may provoke symptoms similar to the patient's complaints. This should be considered when performing a follow–up neural tension test.

Diagnostics

There are no routine diagnostic tests for Achilles tendinitis; however, lateral radiographs may show changes or a loss of a distinct outline of the tendon, possibly due to local edema or tendon thickening. MRI examination will show soft tissue changes in the patient with Achilles tendinitis or with a tear.

Problem List

Patients with Achilles tendinitis may present with some of the following problems:

1. Achilles tendon pain with weightbearing

2. Crepitus on palpation

3. Swelling around the tendon

4. Pain on palpation

Treatment

Treatment is initially geared toward controlling the symptoms, edema, and inflammation using PRICE. The physician may prescribe drugs to decrease inflammation and pain. Physical agents can control symptoms and promote healing. Transverse friction massage may promote healing. Soft tissue mobilization of the muscle–tendon junction and of the tendon may reduce tension on the sural nerve.

A heel lift can decrease stresses on the tendon by effectively shortening it during weightbearing. Foot orthotics may be needed if abnormal mechanics at the foot and ankle contribute to the onset or recurrence.

Daily activities should be modified according to the severity of the tendinitis. The program should eventually include active stretching to improve tendon extensibility and strength. Gastroc–soleus strengthening exercises should include eccentric exercises to improve the tendon's tension resistance.[14] Balance boards can introduce activities on uneven surfaces and add stresses to mimic function in weightbearing. Pool exercise can be an appropriate adjunct to promote progression in weightbearing activities.

The patient should ice the tendon area after activities until he or she has returned to normal activities. Prevention can be facilitated with appropriate footwear; maintenance of strength and flexibility; monitoring activities; and balancing any mechanical abnormalities at the foot and ankle. Counterforce straps may decrease symptoms and tension to the Achilles tendon. Their use should be based on clinical experience; we are not aware of any research supporting their use.

Plantar Fasciitis

The plantar fascia (aponeurosis) acts as a tension band that supports the medial longitudinal arch. It helps generate power for push–off in running and jumping.[89] This structure is responsible for resisting as much as 60% of the stress applied to the foot during midstance.[35] Dorsiflexion of the first MTP joint at toe–off tightens the plantar fascia and helps resupinate the foot via the windlass effect,[29,35,56,81] sustaining 1.7–3.0 times body weight.[35]

Some authors believe plantar fasciitis is the most common cause of heel pain in runners.[7] Limited range of motion at the first MTP has been associated with the onset of plantar fasciitis in runners.[81]

The suspected etiology of plantar fasciitis is repetitive microtrauma at the insertion of the fascia at the medial tubercle of the calcaneus. This may be related to a high arch foot with an abnormally tight plantar fascia, which is unable to tolerate the stresses applied to it. Alternatively, it may be caused by prolonged eversion at midstance of gait, which can overstretch the plantar fascia.[50]

Symptoms felt near the proximal attachment of the plantar fascia may be caused by tibial nerve entrapment at the tarsal tunnel[15,51] where the posterior tibial nerve bifurcates to form the medial and lateral branches of the plantar nerve. The medial plantar nerve may be entrapped or injured under the abductor hallucis muscle—a condition called "jogger's foot."[67] The mobility of these nerves may be restricted in the fascia.[8] Careful differential examination is essential to successful treatment.

History

Most often the patient has a gradual, insidious onset of complaints. A patient occasionally complains of an acute onset or "strain" of the arch during vigorous activities. The symptoms may progress if unattended and are usually provoked during the first steps in the morning and with excessive weightbearing activities.

Signs/Symptoms

The classic complaint is acute pain after prolonged sitting or with the initial weightbearing in the morning. This is thought to be related to the phenomena called "physiological creep," where the tissues contract when non–weightbearing and then are forcefully stretched with initial weightbearing.[65] The pain may be localized at the proximal attachment of the fascia and may radiate along the length of the fascia distally. The patient may have an antalgic gait pattern, depending on the severity of the symptoms. The symptoms can decrease after the initial steps but may increase after activity.

Objective findings include limited range of motion at the first MTP. Passive stretch of this joint can increase the symptoms along the plantar fascia. Deep palpation may provoke symptoms at the medial tubercle of the calcaneus and at other areas along the plantar fascia. The patient usually has pain on weightbearing. Differential examination includes palpation of the tarsal tunnel for posterior tibial nerve involvement and neural tension testing using the SLR. This test should be performed with dorsiflexion and eversion of the ankle and either pronation to implicate the lateral plantar branch or supination to implicate the medial plantar branch. These findings should be correlated with the rest of the examination findings.

Diagnostics

Routine radiographs may reveal a hypertrophied spur formation at the medial calcaneal tubercle (Fig 9–49). This finding should be correlated with the patient's complaints and the duration of the problem.

Problem List

Patients with plantar fasciitis can present with any of the following problems:

1. Heel pain in weightbearing

2. Increased pain with first steps in the morning when walking barefoot

3. Pain on palpation of the medial tubercle of the calcaneus

4. Limited extension of the first MTP joint.

5. Excessively rigid foot or an excessively mobile foot.

Treatment

The initial treatment should consist of reducing symptoms and decreasing the stresses on the plantar fascia. Physical agents and anti–inflammatory drugs

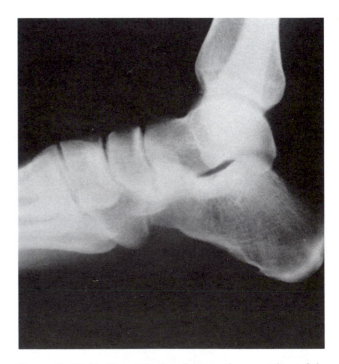

Figure 9–49. Radiograph showing traction spurring of the calcaneus at the proximal attachment of the plantar fascia.

can control symptoms. Temporary taping and foot orthotics can splint the plantar fascia during the healing process. Long term use of orthotics may be required to prevent reinjury. Shock–absorption shoe inserts can be used for the rigid foot. Some patients benefit from an insert with a heel cut–out.

An immobile first MTP should be mobilized. The gastroc–soleus complex should be stretched to prevent undue tension on the plantar fascia at midstance. Stretching exercises should be performed in a pain free range. Treatment of any neural tension signs may be needed to decrease symptoms. Plantar fasciitis is often resistant to standard therapy; a treatment approach that considers all related structures is essential for successful treatment.

Medial Tibial Stress Syndrome

A common problem in active people is irritation of the posteromedial border of the tibia. Medial tibial stress syndrome can be caused by tendinitis or periosteal irritation.[65,74,84] This syndrome is often called "shin splints."

The muscles that may be involved include the posterior tibialis, soleus,[63] flexor hallucis, and flexor digitorum. This condition may be caused by excessive pronation at the subtalar joint.[29,65,91] Excessive pronation stretches the muscles in this area. The muscles must work to control pronation from this stretched position. This can cause irritation and inflammation of the muscles or the tibial periosteum.

Precipitating factors include inappropriate footwear, malalignment of the lower kinematic chain, poor flexibility, muscle imbalances, and repetitive microtrauma. It can be difficult to differentiate this problem from tibial stress reaction or tibial stress fracture.[65,74,79] Differential diagnosis requires a thorough examination[74] and possibly a bone scan (Fig 9–50) and radiograph.

History

This problem usually has a gradual onset. Medial tibial stress syndrome is usually brought on by unaccustomed activities or by overuse. The patient notices a gradual progression of symptoms that interfere with weightbearing activities.

Signs/Symptoms

The patient usually reports dull, aching pain at the posteromedial tibia. This pain can become sharp in vigorous weightbearing activities. The pain may be focal or diffuse. The objective findings include palpation tenderness at the posterior medial tibia, along the soft tissues, or along the tibia itself. Crepitus may be palpable with repeated movements of the foot and ankle, and there may be mild effusion. Percussion of the bone and vibration over the bone should be negative.[40,74] Positive results with percussion and vibration may indicate a tibial stress fracture. Resisted testing of the posterior tibialis, soleus, flexor hallucis, and flexor digitorum muscles may be painful. Dynamic gait evaluation may show excessive pronation on the involved limb.

Diagnostics

Diagnostic testing rules out a tibial stress reaction or stress fracture. Standard radiographs will be negative initially. Radiographs taken several weeks to several months after the onset of injury may show healing. Bone scan testing will usually pick up a diffuse pattern of uptake (stress reaction) or focal uptake (stress fracture). A fracture line is not commonly seen.

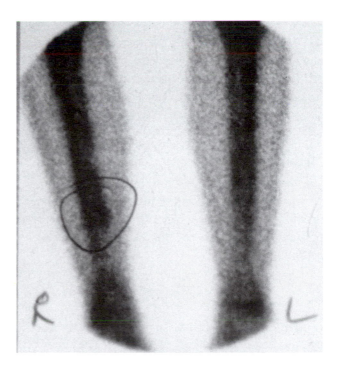

Figure 9–50. Bone scan evidence of a stress fracture at the posteromedial tibia.

Problem List

1. Posteromedial shin pain with weightbearing activities, especially running

2. Tenderness to palpation on the posteromedial distal third of the tibia

3. Excessive pronation at the subtalar joint

4. Tight soleus

5. Pain with resisted muscle testing

Treatment

Symptoms can be controlled by using ice, decreasing weightbearing, and modifying activities; if there is swelling, compression can help. Physical agents can decrease pain and inflammation. The physician usually prescribes anti–inflammatory drugs. Activity modifications may include cross–training to decrease stresses. In severe cases, gait assistive devices may be needed for a short time. Flexibility and strengthening exercises should be added as needed. Orthotic devices may help decrease excessive pronation and absorb shock. The clinician should closely monitor gradual return to stressful activities.

Interdigital Neuroma

The terms "Morton's Neuroma," metatarsalgia, and interdigital neuroma are synonymous. The bifurcation of the neurovascular bundle between the metatarsal heads makes it susceptible to excessive compression and shearing forces with weightbearing. This can result in the formation of benign fibrous tissue called a neuroma. These stresses result from excessive pronation during the stance phase of gait.[65,74] The most common site for the neuroma is between the third and fourth metatarsals. Initially, the problem is caused by a lack of neural mobility. If the problem is left untreated, the nerve may enlarge and form a neuroma.

History

Patients may complain of a gradual onset of symptoms under the ball of the foot. They may state they feel as if there is a stone in their shoe. The symptoms may progress and limit weightbearing.

Signs/Symptoms

The patient's main complaints are of pain in the metatarsal heads on the plantar surface of the foot. The pain is often described as a dull, burning sensation that can radiate into the toes like an electric shock. These symptoms are aggravated by weightbearing, especially if the patient is wearing worn–out shoes, is barefoot, or is on a hard surface. Palpation near the involved metatarsal interspace produces pain. Percussion of this area may provoke symptoms that radiate into the toes. Crepitus and clicking may be provoked with gliding of the IMT joints and with toe flexion. The two involved metatarsals may be immobile or hypermobile. Toe extension may aggravate the symptoms. A Slump test will confirm any neural tension component.

Diagnostics

There are no standard diagnostic tests for this condition.

Problem List

1. Pain between the third and fourth metatarsal heads, aggravated by weightbearing

2. Excessive pronation at the subtalar joint

3. Pain on palpation between third and fourth metatarsal heads

4. Hypomobility or hypermobility of the metatarsals

5. Radiating pain on percussion of involved area (positive Tinel's Sign)

Treatment

Physical agents should be used as needed to control symptoms. Anti–inflammatory drugs may be prescribed. Joint mobilization may be needed to improve IMT joint glide. Neural mobilization may be attempted if there are neural tension signs. The patient's footwear should be checked, and orthotics should be used to control any forefoot hypermobility or any excessive pronation. It may be necessary to surgically remove the neuroma in severe or chronic cases. Early post–operative mobility exercises are necessary to prevent scar tissue formation and problem recurrence.

SUMMARY

The foot and ankle comprise an intricate arrangement of joints that undergo many complex interactions. They are subjected to repetitive stresses due to their position at the terminal end of the lower extremity kinematic chain. The mechanics of the foot and ankle significantly influence the proximal structures. Injury and disruption of normal mechanics can cause local tissue breakdown and compensations at the proximal structures. These adaptations have potentially disabling consequences on the function of the lower limb.

Symptoms at the foot and ankle can be referred from the lumbopelvic area, hip, knee, and lower leg. Effective management of problems at the lower leg, ankle, and foot includes treatment of all involved neuromusculoskeletal structures.

REFERENCES

1. Baldwini FC, Vegso JJ, Torg JS, Torg E: Management and Rehabilitation of Ligamentous Injuries to the Ankle. Sports Med: 364-380, 1987.

2. Basmajian JV and Stecko G: The Role of Muscles in Arch Support of the Foot. JBJS 45A:1184, 1963.

3. Blustein SM, D'Amico JC: Leg Length Discrepancy: Identification, Clinical Signs, and Management. J Am Podiatr Assoc 75:200, 1985.

4. Bordelon RL: Surgical and Conservative Foot Care. Slack, Thorofare NJ 1988.

5. Borges LF, Hallett M, et al: The Anterior Tarsal Tunnel Syndrome. Journal of Neurosurgery 54: 89-92, 1981.

6. Botte RR: An Interpretation of the Pronation Syndrome and Foot Types of Patients with LBP. J Am Podiatr Assoc 72:595, 1982.

7. Bujsen-Muller F, Flagsted KE: Plantar Aponeurosis and Integral Architecture of the Ball of the Foot. Anat 121:599, 1976.

8. Butler DL, Noyes FR, Grood ES, et al: Ligamentous Restraints in the Human Knee: Anterior-Posterior Stability. Orthop Trans 2:161, 1978.

9. Cantu R, Catlin PA, Wooden MJ: A Comparison of Two Measurement Tools and Two Techniques for Measuring the Forefoot-Rearfoot Relationship. Emory University Physical Therapy Department, 1987. Unpublished material.

10. Cavanagh PR: Pressure Distribution under Symptom-free Feet during Barefoot Standing. Foot Ankle 7:262, 1987.

11. Cedell CA: Ankle Lesions. Acta Orthop Scand 46:4250445, 1976.

12. Clancy WE, et al: Achilles Tendinitis in Runners: A Report of Five Cases. Am J Sports Med 4:46-57, 1976.

13. Clement DB, et al: Achilles Tendinitis and Peritendinitis: Etiology and Treatment. Am J Sports Med 12:179-184, 1984.

14. Curwin S, Standish WD: Tendinitis: Its Etiology and Treatment. Collamire Pren, Lexington MA 1984.?

15. Dellon AL, MacKinnon SE: Tibial Nerve Branching in the Tarsal Tunnel. Archives of Neurology 41:645-646, 1984.

16. Donatelli R: The Biomechanics of the Foot and Ankle. FA Davis, Philadelphia PA 1990.

17. Duckworth T: The Hindfoot and its Relation to Rotational Deformities of the Forefoot. Clin Orthop 177:39, 1983.

18. Elveru RA, Rothstein JM, Lamb RL: Goniometric Reliability in a Clinical Setting: Subtalar and Ankle Joint Measurements. Phys Ther 68(5):672, 1988.

19. Feurbach J, Grabiner M: Effect of the Aircast on Unilateral Postural Control: Amplitude and Frequency Variables. JOSPT 7(3):149-154, 1993.

20. Freeman MAR, et al: The etiology and Prevention of Functional Instability of the Foot. JBJS Br 47B:678-685, 1965.

21. Fulp MJ: Ankle Joint Injuries. J Am Podiatr Med Assoc 65:8890911, 1975.

22. Garbalosa J, et al: The Forefoot/Rearfoot Relationship in the Normal Population. Emory University Physical Therapy Department, 1988. Unpublished material.

23. Garbalosa JC: Physical Therapy. In The Biomechanics of the Foot and Ankle. R Donatelli, ed. FA Davis, Philadelphia PA 1990.

24. Garrick JG: The Frequency of Injury, Mechanism of Injury, and Epidemiology of Ankle Sprains. Am J Sports Med 5:241-242, 1977.

25. Gauffin H, Tropp H, Odenrick P: Effect of Ankle Disk Training on Postural Control in Patients with Functional Instability of the Ankle Joint. Int J Sports Med 9:141-144, 1988.

26. Gessini L, Jandolo B, Pietrangeli A: The Anterior Tarsal Tunnel Syndrome. JBJS 66A: 786-787, what year?

27. Gray G: When the Foot Hits the Ground, Everything Changes. Practical Programs for Applied Biomechanics. Toledo, OH 1984. Seminar manual.

28. Gray's Anatomy. PL Williams PL and R Warwick, ed. 36th ed. WB Saunders Co, Philadelphia PA

1980.

29. Greenfield B: Evaluation of Overuse Syndromes. In The Biomechanics of the Foot and Ankle. R Donatelli, ed. FA Davis, Philadelphia PA 1990.

30. Gross MT: Effects of Recurrent Lateral Ankle Sprains on Active and Passive Judgements of Joint Position. Phys Ther 67(10):1505, 1987.

31. Gungor T: A Test for Ankle Instability: Brief Report. JBJS 70B:487, 1988.

32. Hargens AR: Measurement of Tissue Fluid Pressure as related to Nerve Compression Syndromes. Nerve Compression Syndromes, RM Szabo, ed. Slack Thorofare, 1989.

33. Harrington KD: Degenerative Arthritis of the Ankle Secondary to Longstanding Lateral Ligament Instability. JBJS 61A:3540361, 1979.

34. Hicks JH: The Mechanics of the Foot, I. The Joints. J Anat 87:345, 1953.

35. Hicks JH: The Mechanics of the Foot, II. The Plantar Aponeurosis. J Anat 88:55, 1954.

36. Hicks JH: The Mechanics of the Foot, IV. The Action of Muscles on the Foot in Standing. Acta Anat 27:180, 1956.

37. Hutter CG, Scott W: Tibial Torsion. JBJS 31A:511, 1949.

38. Hutton WC, Dhaneddran M: The Mechanics of Normal and Hallux Valgus Feet: A Quantitative Study. Clin Orthop 157:7, 1981.

39. Inman VT: The Joints of the Ankle. William and Wilkins 1976.

40. Jackson DW: Shin Splints: Common, Painful, and Confusing. Consultant 16:75-79, 1976.

41. Jahss MH: Disorders of the Foot. WB Saunders 1991.

42. Kannus P, Renstrom P: Current Concepts Review: Treatment of Acute Tears of Lateral Ligaments of the Ankle. JBJS 73A:305-311, 1991.

43. Kapandji I: The Physiology of the Joints, 5th ed. Churchill-Livingstone, New York NY 1982.

44. Karlsson J, Andreasson GO: The Effect of External Ankle Support in Chronic Ankle Instability. Am J Sports Med 10:257-261, 1992.

45. Karlsson J, Lansinger O: Lateral Instability of the Ankle Joint. Clin Orthop and Rel Res 276:253-260, 1992.

46. Kay DB: The Sprained Ankle: Current Therapy. Foot Ankle 6(1):22, 1985.

47. Kisner C, Colby LA: Therapeutic Exercise: Foundations and Techniques, 2nd ed. FA Davis, 1990.

48. Kopell HP, Thompson WAL: Peripheral Entrapment Neuropathies. Williams and Wilkins, Baltimore MD 1963.

49. Leach RE, et al: Achilles Tendinitis. Am J Sports Med 9:93-98, 1981.

50. Lutter LD: Running Athletes in Office Practice. Foot Ankle 3:153, 1982.

51. MacKinnon SE, Dellon AL: Surgery of the Peripheral Nerve. Thieme, New York NY 1988.

52. Magee D: Orthopedic Physical Assessment, 2nd ed. WB Saunders, Philadelphia PA 1992.

53. Mann RA, Hagy JL: The Function of the Toes in Walking, Jogging, and Running. Clin Orthop 142:24, 1979.

54. Mann RA, Inman VT: Phasic Activity of Intrinsic Muscles of the Foot. JBJS 46A:469, 1964.

55. Marinacci AA: Neurological Syndromes of the Tarsal Tunnels. Bulletin of the Los Angeles Neurological Society 33: 90-100, 1968.

56. Marshall RN: Foot Mechanics and Jogger Injuries. NZ Med J 88:288, 1978.

57. Mauhart D: The Effect of Chronic Inversion Ankle Sprains on the Plantar Flexion/inversion SLR (Straight Leg Raise) Test. South Australian Institute of Technology, Adelaide Australia 1989. Unpublished thesis.

58. McCrea JD: Pediatric Orthopaedics of the Lower Extremity. Futura Publishing, New York NY 1985.

59. McCullough CL, Burge PD: Rotatory Instability of the Loadbearing Ankle. JBJS 62B:410, 1980.

60. McPhoil TG, Brocato RS: The Foot and Ankle: Biomechanical Evaluation and Treatment. In Orthopædic and Sports Physical Therapy. JA Gould and GJ Davies, ed. CV Mosby, St. Louis MO 1990.

61. Mennell J: Joint Pain. Little-Brown, Boston MA 1964.

62. Mereday C, et al: Evaluation of the University of CA Biomechanics Lab Shoe Insert in Flexible Pes Planus. Clin Orthop 82:45, 1972.

63. Michael RH, Holder LE: The Soleus Syndrome: A Cause of Medial Tibial *Illegible* (Shin Splints). Am J Sports Med 13:87, 1985.

64. Mittleman G: Transverse Plane Abnormalities of the Lower Extremities: Intoe and Outtoe Gait. J Am Podiatr Med Assoc 61:1, 1971.

65. Mulligan E: Lower Leg, Ankle, and Foot Rehabilitation. In Physical Rehabilitation of the Injured Athlete. JR Andrews and GL Harrelson, ed. WB Saunders 1991.

66. Nitz AJ, Dobner JJ, Kersey D: Nerve Injury and Grade II and III Ankle Sprains. Amer Jour Sports Med 13:177-182, 1985.

67. Oh SJ, Lee KW: Medial Plantar Neuropathy. Neurology 37:1408-1410, 1987.

68. Okun SJ, et al: Limb Length Discrepancy: A New Method of Measurement and its Clinical Significance. J Am Podiatr Assoc 72:595, 1982.

69. Palmer M, Epler M: Clinical Assessment Procedures in Physical Therapy. JB Lippincott, Philadelphia PA 1990.

70. Perry J: Anatomy and Biomechanics of the Hind-

foot. Clin Orthop 177:9, 1983.

71. Phillips RD, Phillips RL: Quantitative Analysis of the Locking Position of the Midtarsal Joint. J Amer Podiat Med Assoc 73:518, 1983.

72. Root ML, Orien WP, and Weed JH: Normal and Abnormal Function of the Foot. Clinical Biomechanics Corporation, Los Angeles CA 1977.

73. Rovere GD, Clarke TJ, Yates CS, et al: Retrospective Comparison of Taping and Ankle Stabilizers in Preventing Ankle Injuries. Am J Sports Med 16(3):228-233, 1988.

74. Roy S, Irving R: Sports Medicine: Prevention, Evaluation, Management, and Rehabilitation. Prentice Hall, Englewood Cliffs NJ 1983.

75. Sarrafian SK: Anatomy of the Foot and Ankle: Descriptive Topographic, Functional. JB Lippincott, Philadelphia PA 1983.

76. Sauser DD, et al: Acute Injury of the Latera Ligaments of the Ankle: Comparison of *Illegible* Radiographs and Arthrography. Radiology 148:653-657, 1983.

77. Seibel MO: Foot Function. Williams and Wilkins 1988.

78. Seidl RK: Chronic Lateral Ankle Instability. Seminar handout: Minneapolis Sports Medicine Center, Minneapolis MN 1993.

79. Slocum DB: The Shin Splint Syndrome. Medical Aspects and Differential Diagnosis. Am J Surg 114:875, 1967.

80. Smart GW, et al: Achilles Tendinitis and Peritendinitis. Med Sci Sports Ex 17:731-743, 1980.

81. Smith BE, Litchy WJ: Sural Mononeuropathy: A Clinical and Electrodiagnostic Study. Neurology 39(Suppl 1):296, 1989.

82. Soderberg G: Kinesiology - Application to Pathological Motion. William and Wilkins, Baltimore MD 1986.

83. Staehli LT: Rotational Problems of the Lower Extremities. Orthop Clin North Am 18:503, 1987.

84. Standard Nomenclature of Athletic Injuries. American Medical Association, Monroe WI 1976.

85. Stokes IAF, et al: Forces Acting on the Metatarsals during Normal Walking. J Anat 129:579, 1979.

86. Stormont DM, et al: Stability of the Loaded Ankle. Am J Sports Med 13:295, 1985.

87. Subotnick S: Case History of Unilateral Short Leg with Athletic Overuse Injury. J Am Podiatr Assoc 70:255, 1980.

88. Subotnick S: Podiatric Sports Medicine. Futura Publishing, Los Angeles CA 1975.

89. Tanner S, Harvey J: How We Manage Plantar Fasciitis. Physician Sports Medicine 16:39-48, 1988.

90. Tropp H, Askling C, Gillquist J: Prevention of Ankle Sprains. Am J Sports Medicine 13(4):259, 1985.

91. Viitasale JT, Kvist M: Some Biomechanical Aspects of the Foot and Ankle in Athletes With and Without Shin Splints. Am J Sports Med 11:125, 1983.

92. Wooden MJ: Biomechanical Evaluation for Foot Orthotics. In The Biomechanics of the Foot and Ankle. R Donatelli, ed. FA Davis, Philadelphia PA 1990.

CHAPTER 10

GAIT EVALUATION

INTRODUCTION

Human gait is the result of many coordinated muscle and joint interactions. Normal gait is highly efficient, the result of motor responses programmed at the spinal cord level.[27] During normal walking and running, muscle activation does not require higher order cognitive function.[29]

Many neuromusculoskeletal disorders can disrupt the sequence of actions during gait. Abnormal function at any joint in the lower kinematic chain can also disrupt the normal pattern of gait.[29] Theoretically, these forces can affect the entire neuromusculoskeletal system, causing fatigue, repetitive trauma, and other harmful effects; thus, a basic understanding of gait and the ability to analyze and treat gait dysfunction are important for the clinician treating neuromusculoskeletal disorders.

Detailed gait analysis is beyond the scope of this textbook. Excellent resources are available for a more comprehensive discussion of gait mechanics, analysis, and treatment.[13,26,29] The purpose of this chapter is to impart a basic knowledge of normal gait mechanics so the clinician can recognize significant gait deviations and to present simple concepts important to the management of gait abnormalities.

DEFINITIONS

Step Width

The distance between the two feet is called *step width*. The normal step width is 5–10 cm (Fig 10–1).

Step and Stride Length

The distance between successive contact points on opposite feet is called *step length* (Fig 10–1). Step length is usually symmetrical and is normally 35–41 cm. The *stride length* is the distance between successive contacts of the same foot. Stride length is normally 70–82 cm.

Cadence

The number of steps per unit time is called *cadence*. Normal walking cadence is 90–120 steps per minute.

"Toe Out" Angle

Toe out angle is the angle between the line of progression and the second metatarsal (Fig 10-1). This angle is ≈5–18° in normal gait, and decreases as cadence increases.

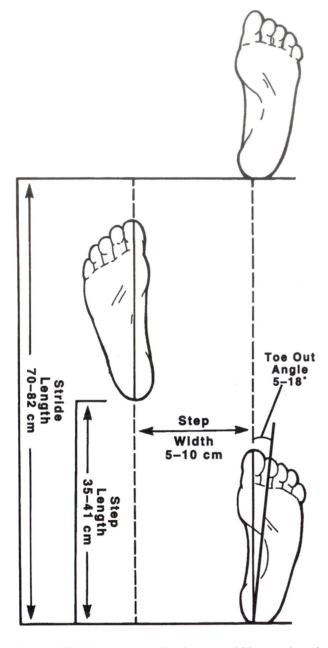

Figure 10–1. Parameters of gait: step width, step length, stride length, and toe out angle.

Ground Reaction Forces (GRF's)

When gravity and muscle forces pull the body toward the ground, the ground exerts a force back, equal and opposite to the force exerted by the body (Newton's Third Law). These are called *ground reaction forces* (GRF's). These forces are potentially deleterious to the joints. The intermittent loading that occurs during gait is a major contributor to fatigue failure of joint tissues.[30]

Gait Cycle

The basic unit of human locomotion is termed the gait cycle.[29] This cycle is repeated during walking and running. The normal cycle is the sequence of motions and the time interval between the heel strike of one foot to the heel strike of the same foot again.

The gait cycle has two phases. *Stance phase* is the time when the foot is in contact with the ground. *Swing phase* is the time when the foot is not in contact with the ground. The stance phase accounts for 60% of the gait cycle and the swing phase accounts for 40%.[20,16] At two points in the gait cycle, there is a period of double limb support—a time when both feet are on the ground. This accounts for ≈30% of the gait cycle.[13] During the remainder of the gait cycle, there is single limb support—one foot is on the ground while the opposite leg swings forward.

Joint Position vs. Joint Motion

The clinician must be familiar with the difference between joint motion and joint position when evaluating a patient's gait pattern. *Joint motion* refers to the movement of the bony segments of a joint toward the end range of motion. The descriptive terms usually include the suffixes *–ion* and *–ing* to indicate motion. For example, prona*tion* describes the action of the subtalar joint prona*ting* during gait. *Joint position* refers to the alignment of the bony segments relative to a reference point. The descriptive terms usually include the suffix *–ed*. For example, the reference point of the subtalar joint is called the neutral position. When the joints are aligned on one side of this reference point, the subtalar joint is prona*ted*; if aligned on the other side the joint is supina*ted*.

The differences between joint motion and joint position are important when analyzing gait. The subtalar joint can be supinating from a pronated position, or the joint can be pronating from a supinated position.

Open Kinematic Chain Motion

Joint motion is traditionally described in the context of an open kinematic chain. Open kinematic chain motion takes place when the proximal bony segment of a joint is fixed and the distal bony segment is free to move. Many upper extremity functional movements are performed in an open kinematic chain. Most lower extremity functional movements are performed in a closed kinematic chain.

Closed Kinematic Chain Motion

Most functional movements in the lower extremity take place when the foot is on the ground. When the distal segment is fixed and proximal segments move, the motion is called closed kinematic chain motion. Muscle contractions in closed kinematic chain motion are different from those in open kinematic chain motion at the same joint.

The clinician must understand the importance of closed kinematic chain gait mechanics. Joint motion in the lower extremity is caused by many controlled muscle contractions that are the opposite of those in the open kinematic chain. For example, in the open kinematic chain, knee flexion is caused by concentric contraction of the hamstring muscles, which moves the tibia towards the femur. During closed kinematic chain motion, knee flexion is caused by controlled eccentric contraction of the quadriceps muscles which moves the femur towards the tibia.

GAIT CYCLE TERMINOLOGY

There are two well known schools of thought that describe the events of the gait cycle: the "traditional" terminology and the Ranchos Los Amigos terminology (Table 10–1). While both nomenclatures are useful, we find it practical to describe the gait cycle more simply by using the terms "stance phase"

and "swing phase" (Fig 10–2). Both phases can be divided into early, mid, and late subphases. We will use these terms throughout the rest of this chapter.

Stance Phase

The stance phase of gait occurs when the foot is in contact with the ground during weightbearing. [24,25,29] This phase has three basic subdivisions which are defined as early, mid-, and late stance phases.

In the *early stance phase*, the foot makes contact with the ground. This phase lasts from the time of heel contact until the foot is flat on the ground. The *mid-stance phase* is a response to the load of the weightbearing limb. It lasts from the time the foot is flat on the ground until the heel rises from the ground. The *late stance phase* is a preparation to propel the limb forward. It lasts from the time the heel rises until toe–off.

Swing Phase

The swing phase of gait occurs when the foot is not in contact with the ground. Swing phase of one limb and midstance of the opposite limb occurs simultaneously. This phase has three basic subdivisions which are defined as early, mid, and late swing phase.

In the *early swing phase*, the hip and knee rapidly flex to accelerate the lower limb forward and the foot is lifted off the ground. In *mid–swing phase*, the forward momentum of the swing limb continues and the swing limb becomes parallel to the opposite limb,

Table 10–1. Comparison of Gait Terminology

Traditional	Ranchos Los Amigos	Our Terminology
Heel strike	Initial contact	Early stance
Heel strike to foot flat	Loading response	
Foot flat to midstance	Midstance	Mid stance
Midstance to heel off	Terminal stance	Late stance
Toe off	Preswing	
Toe off to acceleration	Initial swing	Early swing
Acceleration to midswing	Midswing	Mid swing
Midswing to deceleration	Terminal swing	Late swing

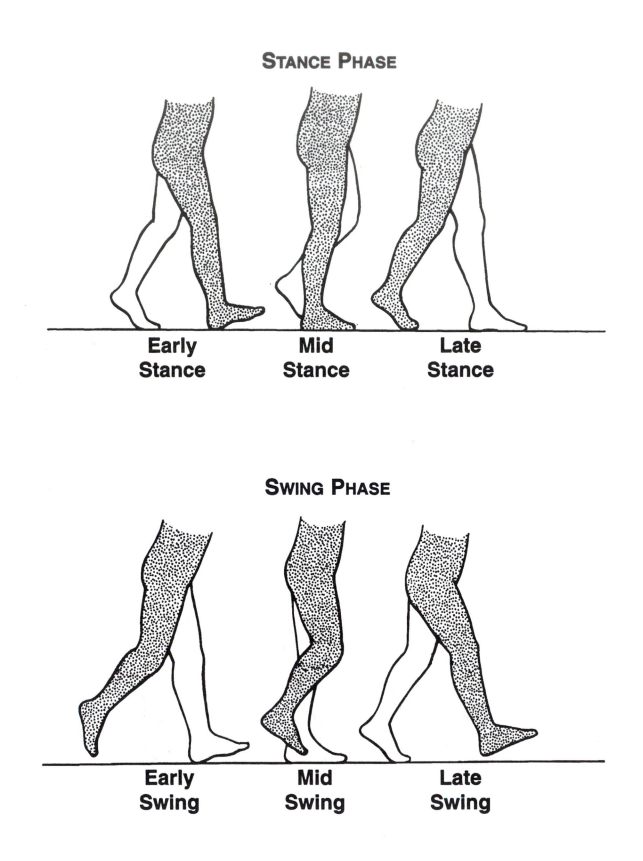

Figure 10–2. The phases of gait.

which is simultaneously in midstance phase. In *late swing phase*, the swing limb begins to decelerate for initial contact with the ground.

DETERMINANTS OF GAIT

The body makes several adjustments to keep its center of gravity (COG) from moving. These adjustments, called the *determinants of gait*, minimize the vertical and horizontal movements of the COG.[29,13,16,19,26]

The COG in humans is ≈5cm anterior to the second sacral vertebra in the standing position. The vertical displacement of the COG is ≤5cm total motion. The horizontal displacement of the COG is 2.5–5.0cm total motion.

Pelvic Rotation

The pelvis rotates ≈8° in the transverse plane (4° forward on the swing limb and 4° backward on the stance limb) during the gait cycle. This rotation has four purposes:

1. It effectively lengthens the femur as it lessens the angle between the femur and the ground.

2. It decreases the COG "dip" or inferior displacement of the pelvis (see pelvic tilt).

3. It helps maintain balance.

4. It regulates the speed of walking. Balance and the speed of walking are functions of the rotations of the pelvis and trunk, which occur in opposite directions (Fig 10–3).

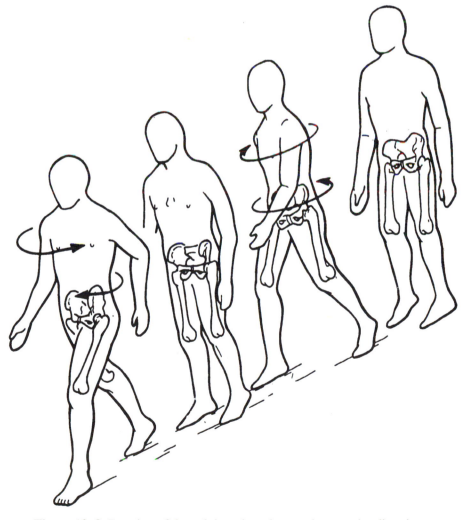

Figure 10–3. Rotation of the pelvis and trunk occur in opposite directions.

Pelvic Tilt

The pelvis tilts up and down in the frontal plane during the gait cycle, minimizing the rise and fall at the COG. The high point of this vertical tilt occurs during midstance and the low point during early stance.

Pelvic List

The pelvis lists (shifts) side-to-side during the gait cycle. Pelvic listing centers the upper body and trunk over the stance leg to maintain balance and controls the lateral movement of the body's COG.

Knee Flexion

Knee flexion during midstance helps reduce the energy requirements during gait by smoothing abrupt changes in the path of the body's COG, keeping the COG from rising excessively. Knee flexion during early stance phase also helps shock absorption.

Knee, Foot, and Ankle Mechanisms

The knee, foot and ankle interact to control the rise of the body's COG. If the leg was rigid there would be a large rise of COG during midstance as the COG shifts toward the stance limb. Knee flexion, ankle dorsiflexion, and subtalar joint pronation at mid-stance control the rise in COG by shortening the stance limb.

The closed kinematic chain motion of the subtalar joint is important because of its effect on the proximal bony segments of the lower quarter.[29] Motion of the subtalar joint influences the height of the longitudinal arch; the rotation of the lower extremity; and the motion of the pelvis. During closed chain pronation, the head of the talus plantarflexes and adducts, causing the arch height to decrease. During closed chain supination, the head of the talus abducts and dorsiflexes, causing a relative increase in arch height.[24,25]

The lower extremity rotates during the gait cycle due to pronation and supination of the subtalar joint and due to movements of the proximal hip and pelvis. During closed chain pronation (early and mid-stance phases), the body of the talus internally rotates, causing the ankle and lower leg to internally rotate. During closed chain supination (mid-stance and late stance phases), the body of the talus externally rotates, causing the ankle and lower leg to externally rotate.[13,14,24,31] Both the change in arch height and the accommodating rotation of the lower extremity help decrease the vertical displacement of the COG.

NORMAL GAIT PATTERN

Walking

To evaluate a patient with gait problems, the clinician must understand how individual joints and muscles normally function during the various phases of gait. Basic kinematic (joint) and kinetic (muscle) functions during gait are summarized in Tables 10–2 and 10–3.[1,6,8,9,11,12,13,17,20,22,29,31]

Running

There are several similarities and differences between walking and running that should be considered when evaluating a patient with gait dysfunction or symptoms. In running, the time for one gait cycle decreases, but running is not simply fast walking. The stance time decreases both in absolute terms and as a percentage of the gait cycle.[29] Joint range of motion is greater during running, and the speed of joint motion increases.[17] The demands on the muscles are greater during running because they must control more motion in a shorter period.[29] There is no period of double support during running. GRF's increase as running speed increases.[3,5,10,29]

The difference between the mechanics of walking and running varies with running style. Based on the way the foot contacts the ground, there are three styles of running:[4] heel–to–toe; simultaneous heel–toe; and toe–to–heel. Heel–to–toe running most closely parallels normal gait patterns. Running with simultaneous heel–toe or toe–to–heel patterns distributes forces differently from normal gait.

The primary function of the lower limb remains the same during walking and running: the limb must accept body weight, the foot must adapt to the ground, the GRF's must be dispersed, and the body must be propelled forward.[29]

Table 10–2. Joint Motions and Muscle Contractions of the Lower Extremity during the Stance Phase of Gait

JOINT	EARLY STANCE		MID STANCE		LATE STANCE	
	Motion	Contractions Concentric/Eccentric	Motion	Contractions Concentric/Eccentric	Motion	Contractions Concentric/Eccentric
Rearfoot Midfoot	Pronate from a supinated position	Posterior Tibialis Gastroc-Soleus	Begin to supinate from pronated position	Posterior Tibialis Gastroc-Soleus Peroneus Longus Peroneus Brevis	Continue to supinate	Posterior Tibialis Gastroc-Soleus
Forefoot	From pronated position, begins to supinate; 1st ray dorsiflexes	Posterior Tibialis Gastroc-Soleus	Anterior metatarsal arch decreases	Posterior Tibialis Gastroc-Soleus Peroneus Longus Peroneus Brevis	Undergoes pronation twist; first ray plantarflexes	Posterior Tibialis Gastroc-Soleus
Ankle	From dorsiflexed position, begins to plantarflex	Anterior Tibialis	Begins to dorsiflex	Flexor digitorum longus Flexor hallucis longus Posterior tibialis Soleus	From dorsiflexed position, begins to plantarflex	Gastroc-Soleus
Knee	From near full extension, begins to flex	Quadriceps Soleus Posterior Tibialis	Continues to flex to about 20 degrees, then begins to extend	Quadriceps Soleus	Continues to full extension, then begins to flex	Gastrocnemius Hamstrings Quadriceps
Hip	From slight abducted, flexed and externally rotated position, begins to adduct, extend and internally rotate	Gracilis Gluteus maximus Hamstrings Gluteus medius External rotators	Continues to extend, begins to abduct and externally rotate	Gluteus maximus External rotators Gluteus medius Adductors Iliopsoas	Begins to flex, continues abduction and external rotation	Gracilis
Pelvis	From neutral position	Adductors Gluteus medius (Less active)	From full forward rotation, begins backward rotation; Full lateral displacement achieved	Gluteus medius	Continues backward rotation; Lateral displacement begins toward opposite limb	Gluteus medius (Less active)
Trunk	Rotates in opposite direction of pelvis	Erector spinae Abdominals Multifidi	Rotates in opposite direction of pelvis	Erector spinae Abdominals Multifidi (All muscles less active)	Rotates in opposite direction of pelvis	Erector spinae Abdominals Multifidi

Table 10–3. Joint Motions and Muscle Contractions of the Lower Extremity during the Swing Phase of Gait

JOINT	EARLY SWING		MID SWING		LATE SWING	
	Motion	Contractions Concentric/Eccentric	Motion	Contractions Concentric/Eccentric	Motion	Contractions Concentric/Eccentric
Rearfoot Midfoot	Continues in a supinated position	Anterior tibialis	Rearfoot begins to pronate from supinated position; midfoot changes little	Anterior tibialis	Little change in position	Anterior tibialis
Forefoot	Continues in pronation twist, first ray is plantarflexed	Anterior tibialis	Little change in position	Anterior tibialis	Little change in position	Anterior tibialis
Ankle	From plantarflexed position, begins to dorsiflex	Anterior tibialis	Continues to dorsiflex	Anterior tibialis	Continues to dorsiflex	Anterior tibialis
Knee	From slight flexion, continues to flex ≈ 60°	Hamstrings *Quadriceps*	From ≈60° flexion, begins to extend	(Hamstrings and quadriceps inactive)	Continues to extend to near full extension	Quadriceps *Hamstrings*
Hip	From neutral position, begins to flex and internally rotate	Iliopsoas	Continues to flex and internally rotate. Begins to adduct	Iliopsoas *Hamstrings*	Continues to flex, internally rotate and adduct	Gracilis *Hamstrings*
Pelvis	From neutral position, backwardly rotates; Lateral displacement away from swing limb begins	*Opposite limb Gluteus Medius (Less active)*	From full backward rotation, begins forward rotation; Full lateral displacement achieved	*Opposite limb Gluteus Medius*	Continues forward rotation; Lateral displacement begins toward swing limb	*Opposite limb Gluteus Medius (Less active)*
Trunk	Rotates in opposite direction of pelvis	Erector spinae Abdominals *Multifidi*	Rotates in opposite direction of pelvis	Erector spinae Abdominals *Multifidi* (All muscles less active)	Rotates in opposite direction of pelvis	Erector spinae Abdominals *Multifidi*

GAIT ANALYSIS

Gait analysis identifies any deviations from the normal gait pattern and provides the clinician with valuable information that can help determine the cause of a patient's problems.

There are many ways to analyze gait. These range from simple observation to complex computerized analysis using videotapes, EMG, and forceplates. Most clinicians use the visual gait analysis method described here. Clinicians use this method when analyzing videotapes of patient's gait. Slow motion and frame–to–frame video displays help show subtle variations in gait.

Visual Gait Analysis

Static Evaluation

Procedures to assess the biomechanical alignment of the lower leg, ankle, and foot were described in Chapter 9, The Foot and Ankle. Static biomechanical analysis is an important part of clinical assessment of gait.

Dynamic Evaluation

Dynamic gait evaluation helps identify the functional problems a patient may encounter in daily activities. Observing the patient walking or running on the ground mimics function, but treadmill–walking greatly increases the convenience of visual gait analysis. The results of a study showed the treadmill may allow more variation in rearfoot motion than walking on the ground, but it does not appear to cause any significant differences when considering four variables of rearfoot motion during gait (maximum pronation, stance phase duration, time to maximum pronation, and time to heel–rise).[15] The slow motion capabilities of videotape further enhance the clinician's ability to identify any gait deviations.

Observations

The clinician should first observe stride length, gait cadence, and duration of each phase of the patient's gait cycle. This general overview of gait also lets the clinician detect any gross deviations in the gait cycle.

Next, the clinician should view the individual joints during successive phases of gait. Marking anatomical landmarks helps in the observation of joint motion (Table 10-4). The actions of the joints and muscles should be compared to normal (Tables 10–2 and 10–3). The clinician should determine:

- the amount of motion present—is it too little, or too much motion for that joint?

- the quality of the motion present—does it occur symmetrically on each limb, and are there any substitutions?

- the timing of the motions—does the motion occur at the correct time in the gait cycle?

The patient should be viewed from the back, the front, and from both sides. The clinician should observe the joints individually, beginning with the foot and ankle and moving up to the knee, hip, and trunk.

During gait analysis the patient should walk in a normal pattern. If using a treadmill, it may take several minutes for patients to familiarize themselves with the equipment. The patient should be observed walking in bare feet, in normal footwear, and with and without any orthotic devices. It may be necessary to change the treadmill's speed to find the patient's most comfortable cadence. Treadmill speed can also be adjusted to provoke gait deviations or symptoms.

Posterior View

The step width can be easily observed. This view also provides the clinician the best view of the motion of the rearfoot and its relation to the tibia. The pelvis list can also be observed. It can be helpful to view

Table 10–4.   Landmarks for Gait Analysis

Joint	Landmarks
Pelvis	Iliac crests, ASIS, PSIS
Hips	Lateral trochanters
Knees	Patellae, tibial tubercles
Ankles	Medial malleoli, vertical midline lower leg
Rearfoot	Vertical midline calcaneous
Midfoot	Medial navicular
Forefoot	Medial first MTP joint

several heel contacts on each limb to see if there is a consistent pattern of joint motion at the rearfoot. The muscle tone and contractions of the posterior muscles can also be observed in this view. The arms should swing symmetrically at the sides. Scoliotic spinal curves or antalgic gait patterns may alter this symmetry.

Anterior View

The step width and the toe out angle can be observed easily. The general joint alignment should be noted: are the joints in varus or valgus? Are the joints rotated abnormally? The reactive movements of the kinematic chain can be observed: is there adequate limb rotation? Does the limb adduct and abduct normally? Muscle tone and action of the anterior muscles of the lower extremity should also be observed. The patellar position during the gait cycle helps the clinician determine the motions occurring at the knee and the effect of the subtalar joint on the patellar position. Pelvic rotation can be observed, and the counterrotation of the trunk on the pelvis should be noted. Lateral pelvic list can be also observed from the anterior view.

Side View

The side view lets the clinician observe joint motion during all phases of gait. The clinician should observe the four events of the stance phase (heel contact, foot flat, heel–rise, toe off). The amount of ankle dorsiflexion at heel strike, the amount of tibial glide over the ankle and foot during midstance, and the dorsiflexion of the first MTP should be observed. The rise and fall of the navicular in the medial longitudinal arch can be correlated with the subtalar joint motion seen from a posterior view. The position of the knee and hip throughout the gait cycle should be noted. Pelvic tilt, lumbar posture, and the general rise and fall of the center of gravity can also be observed from the side. The step and stride length and the symmetry of arm swing should be noted.

Footprint Analysis

Another type of gait analysis focuses on measuring gait parameters, such as step width, step length, stride length, and toe angle. For this method, a strip of paper ≈10x2 feet is laid on the floor (butcher paper is ideal). The patient removes shoes and socks, and the soles of the feet are covered with a marker substance like washable paint or colored chalk. The patient walks the length of the paper in a normal gait pattern. The marker substance leaves footprints that can be used to measure step width, step length, stride length, and toe–angle. If cadence is of interest, a stopwatch can be used to time the period from heelstrike to heelstrike of the same foot.

This method of gait analysis provides limited information about a patient's gait pattern; however, it provides a permanent record of a patient's gait pattern for comparison to changes after treatment.

TREATMENT CONSIDERATIONS

Treating gait dysfunction can be difficult. Many patients with structural malalignments and gait deviations do not have symptoms. Some patients with severe complaints may show no significant findings on static or dynamic gait evaluation. The clinician must take a very common sense approach to gait deviations and correlate gait examination findings with the rest of the objective examination. The question becomes: what are appropriate treatment interventions and the clinical reasons to try them? Gait dysfunction treatment should be consistent with the treatment guidelines in Chapter 3, Pathology and Treatment Principles.

Some gait deviations are caused by *muscle weakness or imbalances*. The weak muscles should be identified and strengthened functionally in a closed kinematic chain.

Limited mobility in muscles or joints can cause gait deviations. The restricted tissues should be identified and treated appropriately (e. g., muscle stretching, joint mobilization treatments).

Joint instability may cause compensatory deviations in gait. The specific joints involved should be identified and treated with proprioceptive exercises, strengthening exercises, and external supports, as needed.

Decreased neuromuscular control due to central nervous system dysfunction can cause gait deviations. Assistive devices and splints or braces (such as ankle–foot orthoses) can be used to decrease these deviations.

The Role of Footwear and Orthotics

Sometimes a patient may need to change footwear or use orthoses to normalize gait and reduce symptoms. The components of a typical athletic shoe are labeled in Figure 10–4. The description and purpose of each shoe component is discussed here:

Outsole

Bottom layer of rubber that contacts the ground. Tread design can enhance stability or traction.

Midsole

Layer between the outsole and upper portion of shoe. Most important part of the shoe. Responsible for cushion and stability.

Last

The infrastructure of the shoe; on top of the midsole. A slip/anatomic last is softer and more accommodating. A board last is firmer and less accommodating.

Upper

Main part of the shoe. Usually made of lightweight, breathable material. Attached to the last.

Toe Box

Important to consider for proper fit. Must be roomy enough to accommodate spreading foot.

Heel Counter

Provides rearfoot support. May be reinforced above midsole.

Achilles Tendon Notch

Provides pressure relief for Achilles Tendon.

Collar

Padded for comfortable fit on rearfoot.

Removable Insole

Provides comfort and cushioning.

Lacing System

Variable widths for comfort, tongue loop to prevent shifting of tongue, lace locks to prevent loosening. Hook and loop–type closure can also be used.

Foot orthotics can increase comfort, absorb shock, control symptoms, or control abnormal foot mechanics. Foot orthotics can be classified as flexible, semi–rigid, and rigid. Flexible orthotics include cushioned inserts for shock absorption, for comfort, and to protect skin from breakdown. Semi–rigid orthotics include corrective inserts made of thermoplastics, leather, and cork. Wedges or posting material can be added to try to control abnormal foot mechanics. Rigid orthotics are used to control abnormal foot mechanics. An excellent text provides

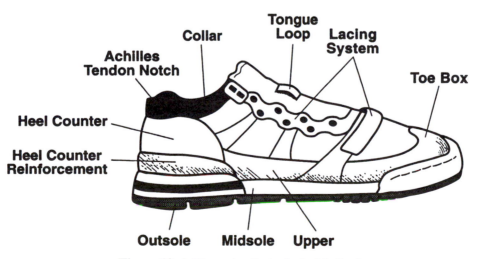

Figure 10–4. The parts of a typical athletic shoe.

more detailed information regarding the treatment of gait using corrective orthotics.[8]

Foot orthotics are becoming more common, but the multitude of orthotic systems available for patients will not be discussed here. When choosing the course of treatment for patients with biomechanical deviations at the foot and ankle, the clinician must determine whether orthotics are clinically necessary. For example, does the patient who presents with an acute iliotibial band (ITB) syndrome need foot orthotics to correct over-pronation when the pronation problem is long-standing? While over–pronation may contribute to ITB syndrome, it may not necessarily be the cause of the syndrome in this patient.

Considering the significant profit that can be made from fabricating or ordering foot orthotics for a patient, these treatment decisions can present ethical questions. To aid the decision making process, we have outlined factors to consider when choosing treatment options for gait deviations (especially those caused by abnormal foot and ankle mechanics).

1. Correlate any gait deviations to the objective examination findings and to the patient's complaints.

2. Check the patient's footwear for excessive wear and proper fit.

3. Match the patient's footwear to their mechanical needs before recommending foot orthoses. For example, a patient with excessive pronation needs a stable shoe; a patient with a rigid foot needs a cushioned shoe to increase shock absorption capabilities (Table 10–5).

4. Consider using temporary foot orthotics before any more permanent orthotics to prove their clinical benefit. These include cushioned inserts, arch supports, wedges, or other devices to control motion or control symptoms by decreasing stress to the involved tissues.

5. Consider other treatment options such as stretching, strengthening, proprioceptive exercises, and symptom relief.

Research on the effects of foot orthotics is evolving. While the results have been inconclusive so far,[2,7,18,21,23,28] many clinicians find these devices help decrease symptoms in patients with abnormal foot mechanics.

SUMMARY

Human gait is a complex set of intricate and coordinated muscle actions and joint motions. The clinician treating patients with neuromusculoskeletal dysfunction should have a basic understanding of gait mechanics and analysis. Identifying gait deviations and determining their causes can be a challenge to the clinician, especially if the cause of a problem is several joints away from the symptom area. The clinician must correlate gait examination findings with findings from the rest of the musculoskeletal examination.

Basic gait terminology and a discussion of the normal gait cycle were presented. The procedure to follow for observational gait analysis was described. Guidelines for determining appropriate treatment options for patients with gait deviations were discussed.

Table 10–5. Recommended Shoe Components for Two Basic Foot Types

Foot Type	Objective	Recommended Components
Supinated/high arch	Accomodate fit, cushion	Curved to semi-curved shape Slip/anatomic last Cushioned midsole (air, gel, foam) Cushioned insole
Overpronated/low arch	Stability, motion control	Semi-curved to straight shape Combination or board last Overpronation device (wedge, bar, etc.) Heel counter reinforcement

REFERENCES

1. Basmajian JV, DeLuca CJ: <u>Muscles Alive: Their Functions Revealed by Electromyograph</u>, 5th ed. Williams & Wilkins, Baltimore MD 1985.

2. Bates BT, Osternig LR, Mason B, James LS: Foot Orthotic Devices to Modify Selected Aspects of Lower Extremity Mechanics. Am J Sports Med 7:338-342, 1979

3. Bates BT: Biomechanics of Running Medithon – A Multidisciplinary Seminar on Running Injuries, 1985. Seminar manual.

4. Brody DM: Running Injuries. Clin Symp 32(4):1, 1980.

5. Cavanaugh PR, La Fortune MA: Ground Reaction Forces in Distance Running. J Biomech 13:397, 1980.

6. Cornwall MW, McPoil TG: The Influence of Tibialis Anterior Muscle Activity on the Pattern of Rearfoot Motion During Walking. Physical Therapy 73(6):S110, 1993.

7. Donatelli R, Hurlbert C, Conaway D, St Pierre R: Biomechanical Foot Orthotics: A Retrospective Study. JOSPT 10:205-212, 1988.

8. Donatelli R: <u>The Biomechanics of the Foot and Ankle</u>. FA Davis Co, Philadelphia PA 1990.

9. Ericson MO, Nisell R, and Ekholm J: Quantified Electromyograph of Lower Limb Muscles During Level Walking. Scand J Rehabil Med 18:159, 1986.

10. Frederick EC, Hagy JL: Factors Influencing Ground Reaction Forces in Distance Running. J Biomech 13:397, 1980.

11. Gray G: Chain Reaction: Successful Strategies for Closed Chain Testing and Rehabilitation. Wynn Marketing, Adrian MI 1990. Seminar manual (revised edition).

12. Gray G: When the Foot Hits the Ground, Everything Changes. Practical Programs for Applied Biomechanics. Toledo, OH 1984. Seminar manual.

13. Inman VT, Ralston HJ, and Todd F: <u>Human Walking</u>. Williams & Wilkins, Baltimore MD 1981.

14. Inman VT: <u>The Joints of the Ankle</u>. Williams & Wilkins, Baltimore MD 1981.

15. Lemke KA, McPoil TG, et al: A Comparison of RF Motion Patterns During Overground Versus Treadmill Walking. Physical Therapy 73:6, 1993.

16. Magee DJ: <u>Orthopaedic Physical Assessment</u>. WB Saunders, Philadelphia PA 1992.

17. Mann RA: Surgical Implications of Biomechanics of the Foot and Ankle. Clin Orthop 146:111, 1980.

18. McCulloch MU, Brunt D, Vanderlinden D: The Effect of Foot Orthotics and Gait Velocity on Lower Limb Kinematics and Temporal Events of Stance. JOSPT 17(1):2-10, 1993.

19. McPoil: The foot, pelvic and lower extremity movement patterns during walking. Presented at Advanced Orthopaedics Competencies Review Meeting. Orthopaedic Section APTA, St. Louis, MO Nove 3-7, 1993.

20. Murray MP: Gait as a Total Pattern of Movement. Am J Phys Med 46:290, 1967.

21. Novick A, Kelley DL: Position and Movement Changes of the Foot with Orthotic Intervention during the Loading Response of Gait. JOSPT 11:301-312, 1990.

22. Prince F, Winter D, Stergiou P: Back EMG: Timing and Amplitude Patterns during Walking. 8th Annual East Coast Clinical Gait Lab Conference, Rochester MN 1993. Seminar manual.

23. Rodgers MM, LeVeau BF: Effectiveness of Foot Orthotic Devices Used to Modify Pronation in Runners. JOSPT 4:86-90, 1982.

24. Root ML, Orien WP, and Weed JH: <u>Normal and Abnormal Function of the Foot</u>. Clinical Biomechanics Corporation, Los Angeles CA 1977.

25. Sarrafian SK: <u>Anatomy of the Foot and Ankle: Descriptive Topographic, Functional</u>. JB Lippincott, Philadelphia PA 1983.

26. Saunders JBM, Inman VT, Eberhart HO: The Major Determinants in Normal and Pathological Gait. JBJS 35A: 543, 1953.

27. Schmidt RA: <u>Motor Control and Learning: A Behavioral Emphasis</u>. Human Kinetics, Champaign, IL 1982.

28. Smith LS, Clarke TE, Hamill CL, Santopeitro F: The Effects of Soft and Semi-rigid Orthoses upon Rearfoot Movement in Running. J Am Podiatr Med Assoc 76:227-233, 1986.

29. Tiberio D, Gray G: Kinematics and Kinetics During Gait. <u>Orthopaedic Physical Therapy</u>. R Donatelli, MJ Wood, ed. Churchill-Livingstone, New York NY 1989.

30. Voldshin AS: Shock Absorption During Running and Walking. J Am Podiatr Med Assoc 78(6):295, 1988.

31. Wright DG, Desai SM, Hengerson WH: Action of the Subtalar and Ankle Complex During the Stance Phase of Walking. JBJS 46(A):361, 1964.

SECTION 4
Specific Treatment and Prevention Techniques

CHAPTER 11

MOBILIZATION TECHNIQUES

Katherine L. Beissner, PhD PT

INTRODUCTION

Joint mobilization has probably been used since prehistoric times. Many medical practitioners, from Hippocrates to Andrew Taylor Still (founder of osteopathy) and Daniel David Palmer (founder of chiropractic) contributed to the early knowledge base in this area. Much of the current practice of joint mobilization relies on the works of James and John Mennell, James Cyriax, Freddie Kaltenborn, and Geoffery Maitland.

Soft tissue mobilization has a much shorter history, with many techniques developing since the 1980's. Osteopaths and rolfers have contributed to our knowledge of soft tissue treatment. Neural mobilization concepts provide us with another way to treat the soft tissues.

We will discuss two forms of mobilization: joint and soft tissue. Soft tissue mobilization techniques discussed here include massage, deep transverse friction massage, myofascial stretching, and neural mobilization.

JOINT MOBILIZATION

Types of Joint Motion

There are two main types of joint motion: physiological and accessory. Physiological motions are gross movements such as flexion, abduction, and rotation that occur between bones in standard planes.

Accessory motions are small movements that accompany physiological motions. Accessory motions are necessary for normal movement, but cannot be performed voluntarily. Limitations of physiological motion can be caused by decreased accessory mobility. Since accessory motions cannot be performed voluntarily, limitations in accessory motion must be treated through passive means.

There are two types of accessory motions: component motions and joint play. *Component motions* are extra–articular motions that occur with active physiological motion, but cannot be performed voluntarily in isolation. For example, the shoulder rotation that accompanies shoulder elevation is a component motion. *Joint play* movements occur within the joint capsule. These motions occur between joint surfaces during physiological motions. Joint play motions are allowed by capsular laxity rather than muscle contraction. Arthrokinematics is the term used to describe the way joint surfaces move in relation to each other. In mobilization and manipulation, joint play movements are reproduced by a clinician passively moving a joint.

There are five types of joint play motion: compression, distraction, slide, roll, and spin (Fig 11–1).

Compression occurs when two joint surfaces approximate each other.

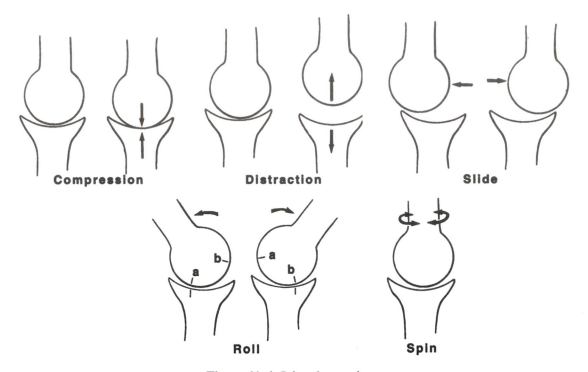

Figure 11-1. Joint play motions.

Distraction occurs when two joint surfaces are separated.

Slide occurs when one joint surface moves across another joint surface so that the same point on one surface continually contacts new points on the second surface.

Roll occurs when joint surfaces are incongruent and new points on one surface meet new points on another surface. Rolling is usually combined with sliding or spinning.

Spin occurs when one bone segment rotates around another bone serving as a stationary axis.

Joint Mobilization Techniques for Testing

Accessory testing is an important part of the objective examination, especially when the patient has limitations in physiological range of motion. The techniques presented in this chapter can be used to evaluate and to treat accessory mobility limitations.

To test joint play the clinician takes the joint through its full accessory range several times. It is important to note the amount of range available, the quality of the movement, the end-feel, and any symptom response. To determine normal accessory mobility for a given patient, the uninvolved extremity is tested first. This demonstrates to the patient what will be done on the involved extremity. Most of the testing techniques require only mild or moderate force to assess joint mobility. The testing techniques often must be done quickly to see or feel joint play.

Joint Mobilization Techniques for Treatment

When joint mobilization is used to restore motion, the normal biomechanics of the joint must be considered. Compression is rarely used in mobilization, because joint surfaces' compression limits motion rather than increasing it. Spinning and rolling do occur with normal movement, but these motions are not easily reproduced during mobilization because they are difficult to control passively. Instead, limitations in accessory mobility are treated with joint glide, which restores normal slide, and with traction, which provides a general stretch of the joint capsule and restores normal distraction.

Principles of Joint Mobilization

Rules of Convex and Concave

Joint surface shape affects joint play motions. For joint mobilization, we will consider two basic shapes: ovoid and sellar. *Ovoid* joints have one convex surface and one concave surface. *Sellar* joints are saddle shaped. One bone is concave in one direction and convex in the other direction; the second bone has convex and concave surfaces in the opposite directions so that the bones fit together congruently.

The direction of slide that normally occurs with physiological movements can be determined with the Rules of Convex and Concave.[3] To use these rules, consider one bone of the joint to be stable, the second bone mobile. The rule used is selected by the shape of the mobile bone.

Concave Rule: Bones with concave surfaces have sliding movement in the same direction as the bone.

Convex Rule: Bones with convex surfaces have sliding movement in the opposite direction as the bone.

For example, consider the motion of glenohumeral abduction. The glenoid fossa is concave, and the proximal humerus is convex. If the scapula is stable and the humerus is mobile, the convex rule applies. As the humerus moves *superiorly* during abduction, The joint surface of the humerus moves in the opposite direction (*inferiorly*) (Fig 11–2).

If the femur is stable during knee flexion, the concave tibia is the moving bone, so the concave rule applies. During knee flexion the tibia moves from an anterior position to a more posterior position. By the

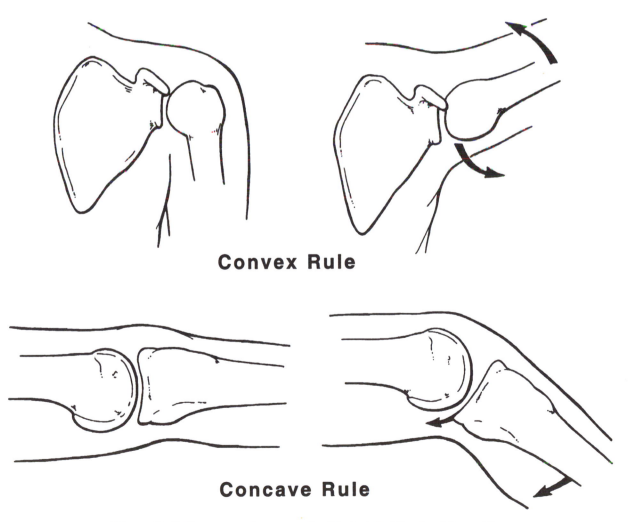

Convex Rule

Concave Rule

Figure 11–2. Concave and convex rules illustrated at the shoulder and knee.

concave rule, the joint surface of the tibia also moves posteriorly (Fig 11–2).

When working with sellar joints, consider the shape of the joint in the plane of motion. At the CMC joint of the thumb, in the plane of palmar abduction, the trapezium is concave and the metacarpal bone is convex. If the trapezium is stabilized, the convex rule applies. In the plane of radial abduction, the trapezium is convex and the metacarpal is concave. If the trapezium is stabilized, the concave rule applies.

Indications for Joint Mobilization

Mobilization is indicated for joints that are painful or hypomobile. These techniques can also be used to reposition subluxed joints.

Contraindications/Precautions for Joint Mobilization

The clinician must be careful when using mobilization techniques on patients with any of the following conditions:

- joint hypermobility
- inflammation or joint effusion
- malignancy
- recent, or unhealed fracture
- degenerative joint disease or rheumatoid arthritis
- osteoporosis
- pregnancy
- total joint replacement
- excessive pain

Grades and Types of Mobilization

There are three types of joint mobilization techniques: oscillations, sustained, and manipulative.

Oscillations are graded, oscillatory movements used to restore joint play and decrease pain. There are four grades of oscillatory mobilizations (Fig 11–3):

Grade 1: Small amplitude oscillations performed at the beginning of available range.

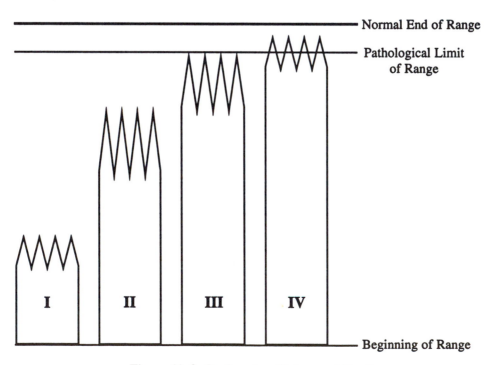

Figure 11–3. Grades of oscillatory mobilizations.

Grade 2: Larger amplitude oscillations performed into available mid–range of a joint.

Grade 3: Large amplitude oscillations performed through the available range of the joint and into the resistance.

Grade 4: Small amplitude oscillations performed into the resistance.

Grades 1 and 2 oscillations maintain joint mobility and relieve pain through neurophysiological pathways. Grade 3 oscillations maintain joint mobility. Grade 4 oscillations increase joint mobility. Grades 1 and 2 are often indicated in the subacute stage of a joint inflammation or sprain to prevent joint motion restriction and to relieve pain. Grade 3 and 4 oscillations are indicated in more advanced stages of hypomobility or in situations involving joint impingement or motion restrictions.

Sustained mobilizations are movements into the accessory range that are held for 20–30 seconds. This type of mobilization is used to restore joint play and increase range of motion. There are three grades of sustained mobilizations (Fig 11–4).

Grade I sustained mobilizations are very small movements into the accessory range.

Grade II sustained mobilizations are movements through the available accessory range without stretching the ligaments and joint capsule. This is sometimes referred to as "taking up the slack."

Grade III sustained mobilizations are movements through the available accessory range stretching into the limitation.

Grade I sustained mobilizations are usually used to separate joint surfaces while other mobilizations are performed. Grade II sustained mobilizations are used to maintain joint mobility when physiological movements are not possible, such as in the case of recent fractures. Grade III sustained mobilizations are used to restore joint play.

Manipulations are advanced techniques that can increase joint motion. They are high amplitude,

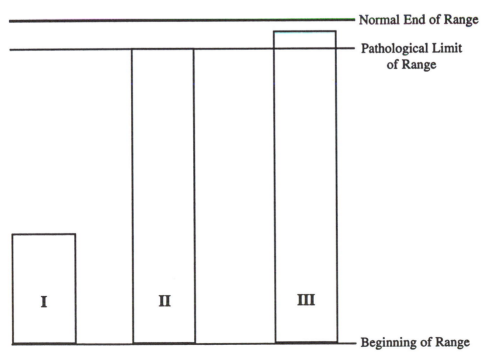

Figure 11–4. Grades of sustained mobilizations.

thrusting movements into the restricted accessory range.

Effects of Joint Mobilization

Neurophysiological Effects

Passive joint mobilization affects joint mechanoreceptors, resulting in decreased pain and decreased muscle tone. Joint mobilization can activate four types of mechanoreceptors.[2] The mechanoreceptor stimulated depends on the grade and type of mobilization applied. Stimulation of types I and II mechanoreceptors reduces pain. These receptors are activated by Grade I and II oscillations. These grades of mobilization are used to control pain. Stimulation of type IV mechanoreceptors causes pain. Grade IV oscillations and Grade III sustained mobilizations can activate type IV mechanoreceptors and cause pain. While this is not desirable, clinicians should recognize that mobilization into the restricted range of motion may cause pain.

Mechanical Effects

Joint mobilization is normally used to increase joint range of motion. As soft tissue injuries and inflammations heal, stiffness is inherent. Left alone, the joints may become hypomobile. The untreated hypomobile joint will eventually begin to show joint degeneration. To avoid this chain of pathological events, mobilization techniques and exercise must be used. The earlier they are started in the treatment regime, the more benefit obtained.

The joint capsule is a richly innervated structure made of two layers: the synovial lining on the inside and a layer of dense, irregular collagen connective tissue on the outside. This outer layer of collagen fiber is thickened and immobile in joints that have a capsular pattern of hypomobility. This thickening can be caused by increased collagen fiber laid down in response to injury or inflammation, or it can be caused by individual collagen fibers binding together. These collagen fibers cannot be stretched like the elastic fibers; rather, they must be mobilized in a more subtle manner and allowed to rearrange and loosen over time.

Mobilization techniques can have mechanical effects because they can cause plastic deformation of the soft tissue when they are used in the range of restriction. If a tissue is stretched in its elastic range, the collagen fibers return to their original length. It is only when the tissue is stretched into the plastic range or beyond that permanent structural changes occur. If stretched beyond the plastic range to the fatigue point, structures may rupture.

Mobilization and passive stretching help rearrange and loosen the collagen fibers.[3] Judiciously applied, mobilization or manipulation techniques can stretch tissues and break adhesions effectively. Indiscriminately applied, they can overstretch tissue and cause joint sprains.

Soft tissue massage, contract–relax techniques, passive stretching, and active and passive range of motion exercises all generally increase the mobility of soft tissue; however, except for certain contract–relax techniques, they only stretch contractile tissues effectively. Joint mobilization techniques usually restore mobility more effectively because they act specifically on the inert structures (capsule, ligament, cartilage and intervertebral disc).

Application of Mobilization

The position of the joint must be considered when performing mobilization.[4] The *close–packed position* is at the extreme of movement at which the concave surface is most congruent with the convex surface. The capsule and ligaments are maximally taut, and the joint surfaces cannot be easily separated by traction. The clinician should not try mobilization with the joint in the maximal close–packed position. If joint motion is to be avoided, the maximal close–packed position can be used to lock the joint during treatment. For example, when applying traction at the talocrural joint, the knee can be "locked" into full knee extension to avoid movement at that proximal segment.

Any position not considered close–packed is considered loose–packed. In a *loose–packed position*, the articular surfaces are not completely congruent and some parts of the capsule are lax. The *maximum loose–packed position* is the best position for early mobilization. In this position, the capsule is most relaxed. The bones of the articular unit can be separated by traction. The maximum loose–packed position is often described as the *resting position* of the joint. Accessory mobility is usually assessed in the maximum loose–packed position. The first treatment for restricted joint movement is also assessed in the maximum loose–packed position. Subsequent treatments may be performed in positions nearer the close–packed position, but they are never performed in the maximum close–packed position.

Generally, rotation will cause a close–packed position. Likewise, extremes of all motions will tend to place the joint into more of a close–packed position; the mid–range of a joint movement will be closer to the loose–packed position.

Joint Mobilization Rules

The rules for joint mobilization are as follows:

1. The patient and the body part being mobilized should be well–supported.

2. The patient and the clinician must be relaxed.

3. Stabilize one bone and mobilize the other. Usually the proximal bone is stabilized and the distal bone is mobilized.

4. Compare the involved extremity to the uninvolved extremity whenever possible.

5. Stop the mobilization testing or treatment if it is too painful for the patient.

6. Check one motion, one joint at a time. It may be necessary to check the accessory movement in different parts of the physiological range.

7. The clinician's hands should be as close to the joint surfaces as possible.

8. Initial mobilizations are usually performed in the loose–packed position.

9. Whenever possible, work with the force of gravity rather than against it.

Treatment Planning and Progression

When assessing accessory mobility, the following scale can be used to grade the amount of motion present:

0—Ankylosed joint

1—Considerable limitation

2—Slight limitation

3—Normal mobility

4—Slight hypermobility

5—Considerable hypermobility

6—Pathologically unstable

Joint mobilization is normally used to treat joints with Grade 1 or 2 mobility; however, patients with painful, hypermobile joints can benefit from gentle, pain reducing joint mobilizations (Grade I and II oscillations).

There are five variables to describe mobilization treatments:

- grade of mobilization

- type of mobilization (sustained or oscillatory)

- direction of mobilization

- position of joint (physiological range)

- length of mobilization

When treating joint tightness, mobilizations are usually performed for 20–30 seconds. When treating pain, oscillatory mobilizations are performed for 60–90 seconds.

Treatment Protocols

The mobilization treatment plan varies according to the patient's condition. Generally, the patient's condition can be classified as joint tightness, pain, or tightness and pain.

Tight Joint Protocol

If the patient's problem is joint restriction caused by adhesions or capsular tightness, the following protocol serves as a good basis for treatment:

Initial treatment: Grade II sustained mobilization applied with the joint in the loose–packed position. Mobilization should be in the direction of limitation (e.g., if posterior slide is limited, perform a posterior glide). The mobilization should be held for 20–30 seconds and repeated 3–5 times.

Progression: At the next treatment session, the patient's physiological and accessory mobility should be reassessed. If the range is improved or unchanged, the treatment should be progressed to a Grade III sustained mobilization with the joint in the loose–packed position. The mobilization should be applied in the direction of limitation and held for 20–30 seconds. If the patient continues improving, the treatment should be progressed to Grade III sustained mobilization in the direction of limitation with the joint at the end of the available physiological range, held for 20–30 seconds.

If the initial treatment causes pain, soreness, or decreased range, the second treatment should follow the painful joint protocol.

Painful Joint Protocol

If the patient's primary problem is joint pain or if a previous joint mobilization caused pain, the following protocol should be applied:

Initial treatment: Grade I oscillations with the joint in loose–packed position. The direction of mobilization should be in the direction of pain. For example, if knee flexion causes pain, the accessory motion associated with flexion (posterior glide) should be used. Oscillations should be continued for 60–90 seconds. If the patient does not tolerate this treatment, mobilization should be performed in the opposite direction. Restoring mobility in one direction will usually increase mobility in other directions, too. Likewise, stimulation of any Type I or Type II mechanoreceptors around the joint can decrease joint pain; therefore, if mobilization in one direction is particularly painful, initially mobilizing in less painful directions is often beneficial.

Progression: At the second treatment session, the patient's pain and range of motion should be reassessed. If the pain or range is improved or unchanged, the treatment should be progressed to Grade II oscillations with the joint in the resting position. The mobilization should be applied in the direction of pain for 60–90 seconds. If the patient responds well to treatment, showing increased range or decreased pain, future treatments should be performed further into the physiological range of motion rather than increasing to stronger oscillations. Stronger oscillations (Grade III or Grade IV) can stimulate nociceptive mechanoreceptors and cause pain rather than stimulating the pain mediating mechanoreceptors; thus, the third step in the pain management progression is Grade II oscillations with the joint positioned at the end available physiological range. The mobilization should be applied in the direction of pain for 60–90 seconds.

Tight and Painful Joint Protocol

Patients frequently have both pain and tightness. In this case, the clinician must decide whether the pain or the tightness is the patient's primary problem. When in doubt, the pain should be treated first. The joint tightness can be treated as the pain resolves.

These protocols for treatment are provided as general guidelines only. Pain can keep the clinician from mobilizing the joint in the direction of restriction. In such a case, it is performed in directions opposite to the direction of restriction. Restoring mobility in one direction will usually increase mobility in other directions, too. If mobilization in one direction is particularly painful, initially mobilizing in less painful directions can be beneficial. The first mobilization treatment performed often consists of gentle traction applied to the joint structures to relieve the pain.

As the clinician gains more experience with mobilization, these protocols can be modified to best meet the patient's needs. Inexperienced clinicians commonly stretch the joints too much during the initial treatment. This causes treatment–induced pain and inflammation and can make the patient very reluctant to continue with mobilization treatments; therefore it is important for the initial treatment to be gentle so the clinician can assess how the joint reacts to mobilization.

Joint Mobilization Techniques

Mobilization, like any other evaluation or treatment skill, cannot be learned or developed entirely by reading a textbook. There is no substitute for clinical practice and experience. It is reasonable to assume the beginner will feel insecure and uncertain when trying these techniques the first time. With perseverance, these techniques can be perfected. It is often beneficial to bring a skeletal model into the treatment room to help with patient education and to remind the clinician where his or her hands should be placed. Patients will appreciate the explanation and will not be aware the clinician is using the model as a guide!

We have found the following techniques are the most helpful in evaluation and treatment of joint dysfunctions. The arrows indicate the directions of the mobilizing forces.

The patient's and clinician's positions should be modified as needed to accommodate to the patient's needs. When modifying mobilization techniques, keep in mind the mobilization rules outlined above.

Shoulder

Glenohumeral Joint

The humerus is convex in the concave glenoid fossa. The greatest challenge to the clinician mobilizing this joint is maintaining adequate stabilization of the scapula.

Glenohumeral *traction* is used for general capsular tightness. It is also used to control pain at the shoulder. The patient is supine with the scapula stabilized and the arm in the loose–packed position. The clinician supports the upper extremity, grasps the proximal humerus in the patient's axilla and pulls the humerus laterally (Fig 11–5A). A belt can be placed around the proximal humerus to help apply this lateral force (Fig 11–5B)

Inferior glide is used for restrictions in glenohumeral abduction and restrictions in the mid range of flexion ($\approx$45–120°). The patient is usually supine and the scapula stabilized. The clinician supports the upper extremity and grasps the humerus, pulling distally (Fig 11–5C). The treatment progression is movement into the restricted range of

motion of flexion or abduction (Fig 11–5D and Fig 11–5E)

Anterior glide is used for restrictions in external rotation, horizontal abduction, and end–ranges of flexion (120–180°). The patient lies prone with a towel roll under the clavicle to support and stabilize. The clinician supports the upper extremity and applies an anterior force to the proximal humerus (Fig 11–5F). To increase anterior glide at the end range of flexion, the clinician brings the patient's arm overhead and applies a downward force (Fig 11–5G). If the patient has a history of shoulder subluxations or dislocations, it is important to avoid mobilizing anteriorly when the arm is in 90° abduction and full external rotation. Excessive anterior force in this position can cause joint subluxation.

Posterior glide is used for restrictions in internal rotation, horizontal adduction and early ranges of flexion (0–45°). The patient is prone and the scapula stabilized. While supporting the upper extremity, the clinician contacts the proximal anterior humerus and pushes posteriorly (Fig 11–5H). An alternate position for this mobilization is with the shoulder flexed to 90° and the elbow flexed. The clinician stabilizes behind the scapula and pushes down through the shaft of the humerus (Fig 11–5I).

Acromioclavicular Joint

Acromioclavicular joint mobility is essential for normal shoulder motion, but accessory motions at this joint are not associated with specific shoulder physiological movements. *Anterior glide* is used to maintain or increase mobility at this joint. The patient is supine or sitting and the scapula stabilized at the acromion process. The clinician stands behind the patient and contacts the posterior aspect of the clavicle with the thumb of the mobilizing hand just medial to the joint line. The mobilizing force is applied by pushing forward with the thumb (Fig 11–6A).

Posterior glide can also be used to increase mobility. With the patient seated, the clinician stabilizes the scapula posteriorly and contacts the lateral aspect of the clavicle close to the joint line. The

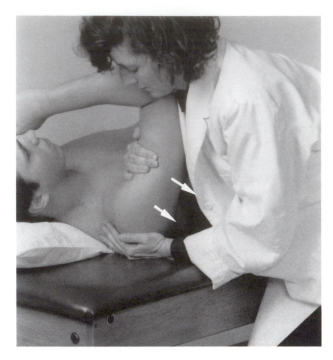

Figure 11–5A. Glenohumeral mobilizations: manual traction.

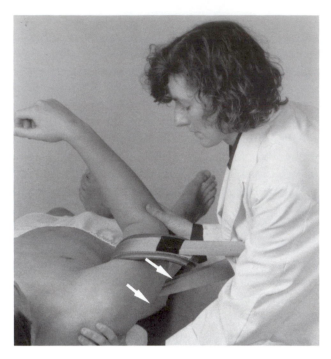

Figure 11–5B. Glenohumeral mobilizations: traction using a belt.

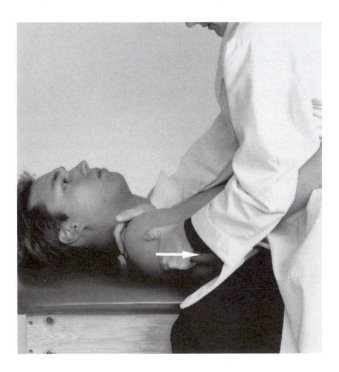

Figure 11–5C. Glenohumeral mobilizations: inferior glide arm at side.

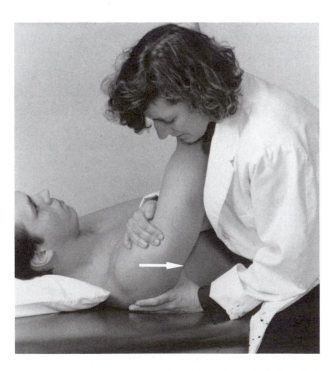

Figure 11–5D. Glenohumeral mobilizations: inferior glide arm in flexion.

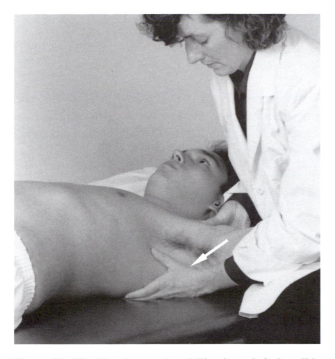

Figure 11–5E. Glenohumeral mobilizations: inferior glide arm in abduction.

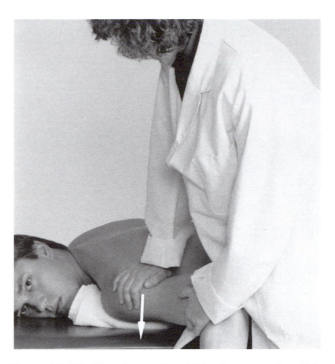

Figure 11–5F. Glenohumeral mobilizations: anterior glide arm at side.

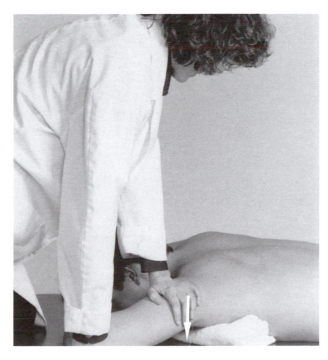

Figure 11–5G. Glenohumeral mobilizations: anterior glide arm overhead.

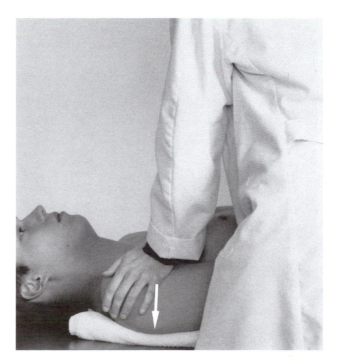

Figure 11–5H. Glenohumeral mobilizations: posterior glide.

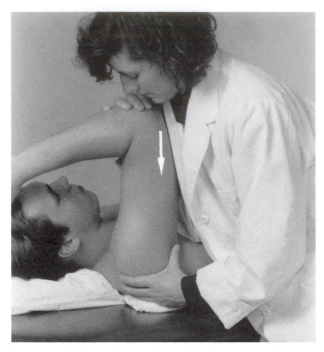

Figure 11–5I. Glenohumeral mobilizations: posterior glide with arm in flexion.

mobilizing force is a posterior pressure through the lateral clavicle (Fig 11–6B)

Sternoclavicular Joint

The clavicle is convex superior–inferior, and concave anterior–posterior. No specific stabilization is needed for mobilization at the sternoclavicular joint because the sternum is inherently stable.

Posterior glide of the clavicle is used to increase scapular retraction. The patient is supine. The clinician contacts the anterior clavicle with the thumb just lateral to the joint line. The mobilizing force is a push posteriorly on the clavicle (Fig 11–7A).

Anterior glide is used to increase scapular protraction. The patient is sitting or supine. The clinician slides the fingertips of the mobilizing hand behind the clavicle lateral to the joint line. The mobilizing force is an anterior pull of the clavicle (Fig 11–7B).

Inferior glide is used to increase scapular elevation. The patient is supine or sitting. The clinician's fingers or thumbs are placed on the superior aspect of the clavicle. The mobilizing force

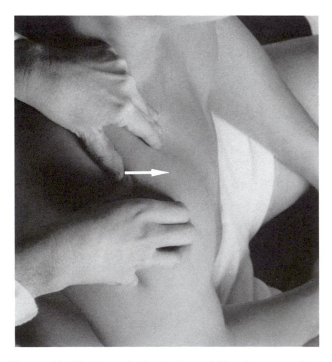

Figure 11–6A. Acromioclavicular mobilizations: anterior glide.

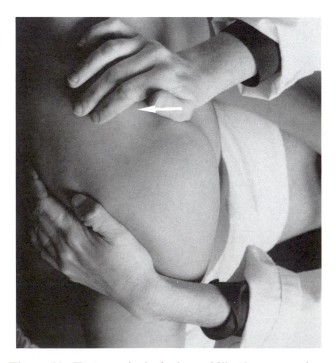

Figure 11–6B. Acromioclavicular mobilizations: posterior glide.

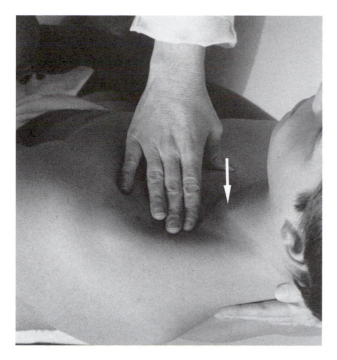

Figure 11–7A. Sternoclavicular mobilizations: posterior glide.

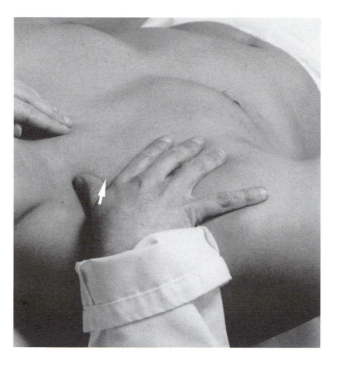

Figure 11–7B. Sternoclavicular mobilizations: anterior glide.

is a downward pressure on the proximal clavicle (Fig 11–7C).

clinician's thumbs contact the inferior aspect of the clavicle just lateral to the joint line. The mobilizing force is an upward pressure on the clavicle (Fig 11–7D). A finger is placed over the superior aspect of the joint to help palpate movement.

Superior glide is used to increase scapular depression. The patient is supine or sitting. The

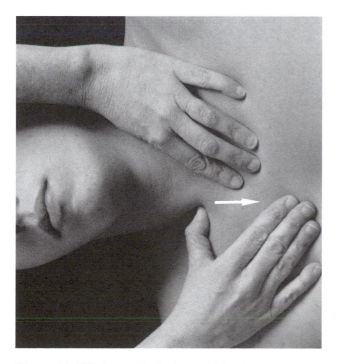

Figure 11–7C. Sternoclavicular mobilizations: inferior glide.

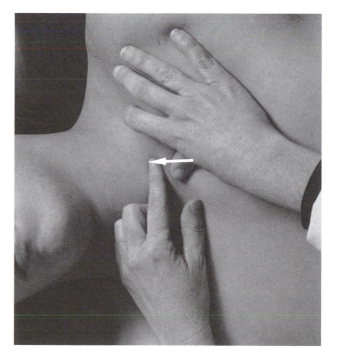

Figure 11–7D. Sternoclavicular mobilizations: superior glide.

Scapulothoracic Joint

The scapulothoracic joint is not a true joint—soft tissue mobility allows gliding movements. Mobilizations at the scapulothoracic joint are used to increase the motions of scapular elevation, depression, upward rotation, downward rotation, protraction, and retraction. The patient is sidelying facing the clinician. The clinician supports the upper extremity by draping it over his or her arm and grasps the inferior angle of the scapula with one hand (Fig 11–8). With the other hand the clinician grasps the superior aspect of the scapula across the acromion process. The scapula is moved in the desired direction.

Elbow

Ulnohumeral Joint

At the ulnohumeral joint the convex humerus articulates with the concave ulna. This joint is congruent, allowing little joint play.

Joint traction is used to increase elbow flexion and extension. The patient is supine with the elbow flexed to about 30°, and the humerus is stabilized with one hand or with a strap. The mobilizing force is a distal pull on the proximal ulna at ≈45° (Fig 11–9A).

Medial and lateral glides are used for general joint mobility and to increase elbow extension. The patient is sitting. For medial glide, the humerus is stabilized on its medial surface as the clinician contacts the ulna from the lateral side and pushes medially (Fig 11–9B). For lateral glide, the humerus is stabilized on the lateral aspect and the clinician grasps the ulna on the medial aspect and pushes laterally (Fig 11–9C).

Radiohumeral Joint

The convex humerus articulates with the concave radius. While elbow motion occurs primarily at the ulnohumeral joint, adhesions that restrict motion between the radius and humerus can decrease elbow mobility.

Joint traction is used for general joint restriction. With the patient supine or sitting, the clinician stabilizes the humerus with one hand and grasps along the length of the radius with the other. The mobilizing force is a distal pull on the radius (Fig 11–10A).

Anterior glide is used to increase elbow flexion. The patient is supine or sitting. The humerus is stabilized with one hand. The fingers of the mobilizing hand are wrapped behind the head of the humerus. The mobilizing force is an anterior pull on the head of the radius (Fig 11–10B).

Posterior glide is used to increase elbow extension. The patient is supine or sitting. The humerus is stabilized with one hand. The palm of the mobilizing hand is positioned on the anterior aspect of the proximal radius. The mobilizing force is a posterior push on the head of the radius (Fig 11–10B).

Proximal Radioulnar Joint

The convex radius articulates with the concave ulna at the superior radioulnar joint.

Posterior glide is used to increase forearm pronation; *anterior glide* is used to increase forearm supination. With the patient supine, the ulna is stabilized with one hand. The clinician grasps the proximal radius with the other hand and applies a posterior or anterior mobilizing force to the head of the radius (Fig 11–11).

Wrist and Hand

Distal Radioulnar Joint

The concave radius articulates with the convex ulna. Although the radius is larger than the ulna at this joint, the ulna is stabilized and the radius is mobilized.

Posterior glide is used to increase forearm supination; *anterior glide* is used to increase forearm pronation. With the patient supine or sitting, the ulna is stabilized with one hand. The radius is grasped with the other hand, and a posterior or anterior force is applied (Fig 11–12).

Radiocarpal Joint

The concave radius articulates with the convex proximal row of carpal bones: the scaphoid, lunate and triquetrum. For all mobilizations of the wrist and hand the patient can be sitting or supine.

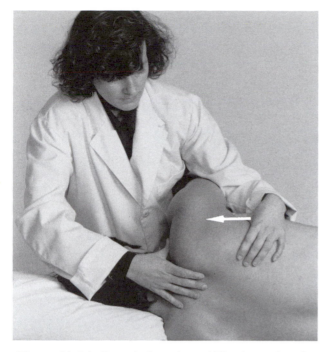

Figure 11–8A. Scapulothoracic mobilizations: elevation.

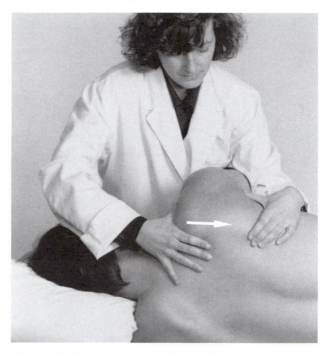

Figure 11–8B. Scapulothoracic mobilizations: depression.

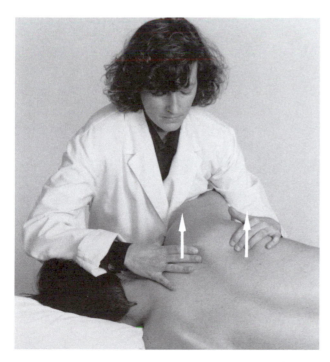

Figure 11–8C. Scapulothoracic mobilizations: protraction.

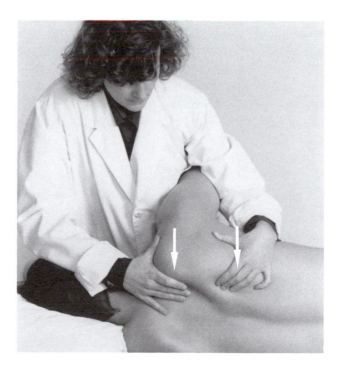

Figure 11–8D. Scapulothoracic mobilizations: retraction.

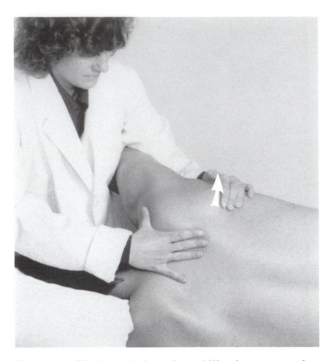

Figure 11–8E. Scapulothoracic mobilizations: upward rotation.

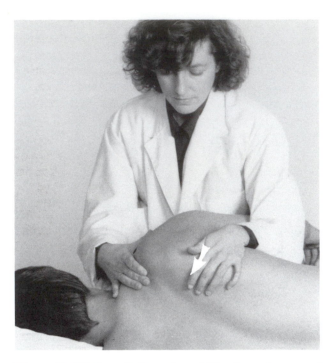

Figure 11–8F. Scapulothoracic mobilizations: downward rotation.

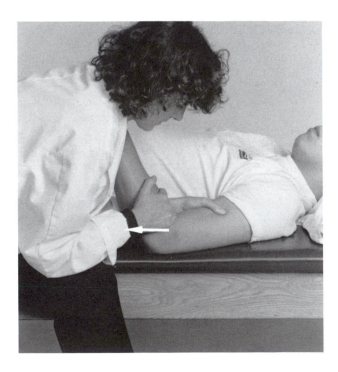

Figure 11–9A. Ulnohumeral mobilizations: traction.

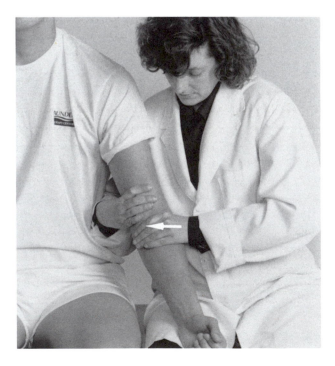

Figure 11–9B. Ulnohumeral mobilizations: medial glide.

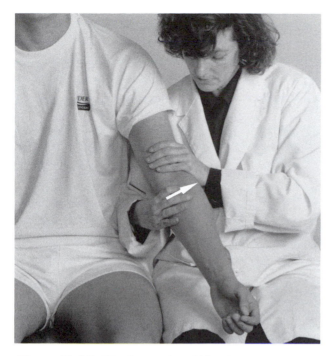

Figure 11-9C. Ulnohumeral mobilizations: lateral glide.

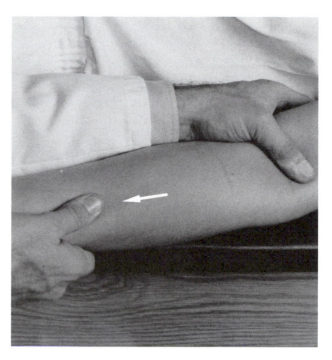

Figure 11-10A. Radiohumeral mobilizations: traction.

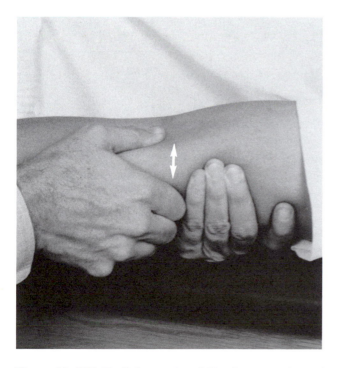

Figure 11-10B. Radiohumeral mobilizations: anterior and posterior glides.

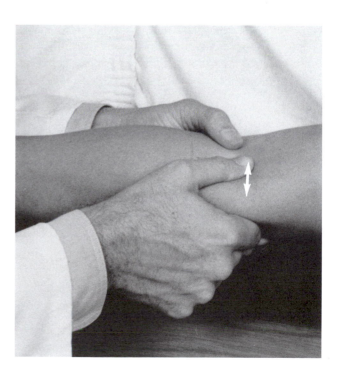

Figure 11-11. Proximal radioulnar mobilizations: anterior and posterior glides.

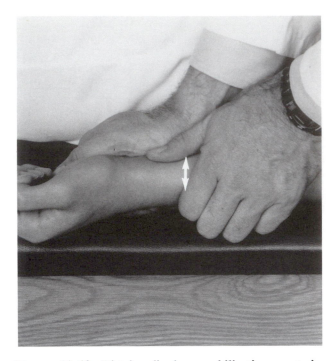

Figure 11–12. Distal radioulnar mobilizations: anterior and posterior glides.

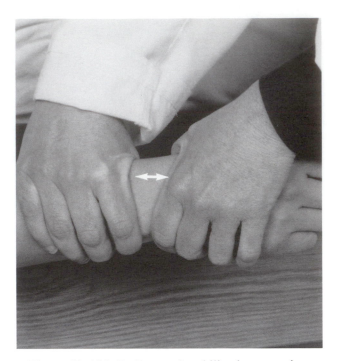

Figure 11–13A. Radiocarpal mobilizations: traction.

Joint traction is used for general joint restrictions. The radius and ulna are stabilized with one hand while the clinician grasps across the first row of carpal bones and pulls distally (Fig 11–13A).

Anterior glide is used to increase wrist extension; *posterior glide* is used to increase wrist flexion. The radius and ulna are stabilized with one hand while the clinician grasps across the first row of carpal bones and pulls anteriorly or pushes posteriorly (Fig 11–13B).

Lateral glide is used to increase wrist ulnar deviation; *medial glide* is used to increase wrist radial deviation. With the radius and ulna stabilized and the forearm in midrange of pronation–supination, the clinician grasps the first row of carpals and applies a medial or lateral force.

Mid Carpal Joint

The concave proximal row of carpals articulates with the convex distal row.

Joint traction is used to increase general mobility. The proximal row of carpals is stabilized with one hand, and the distal row is grasped with the other. The clinician's hands should be very close together to

control this motion. The mobilizing force is a distal pull on the distal row of carpals (Fig 11–14, left).

Anterior and posterior glides are used to increase wrist extension and flexion, respectively. The proximal row of carpals is stabilized, and the distal row is grasped and moved anteriorly or posteriorly (Fig 11–14, right)

Carpometacarpal Joint—Thumb

The trapezium is concave and the proximal metacarpal convex for palmar abduction, and palmar adduction. The trapezium is convex and the proximal metacarpal concave for radial abduction and adduction.

Joint traction is used for general joint restriction. The patient is positioned with the wrist and forearm supported. The clinician stabilizes the trapezium with one hand and grasps the first metacarpal with the other. The mobilizing force is a distal pull of the metacarpal (Fig 11–15A).

Posterior glide is used to palmar abduction; *anterior glide* is used to increase palmar adduction. The triquetrum is stabilized with one hand. With the other hand, the clinician grasps the metacarpal on the

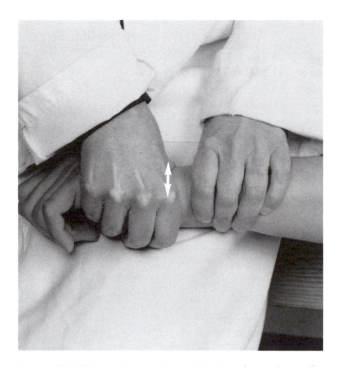

Figure 11–13B. Radiocarpal mobilizations: anterior and posterior glides.

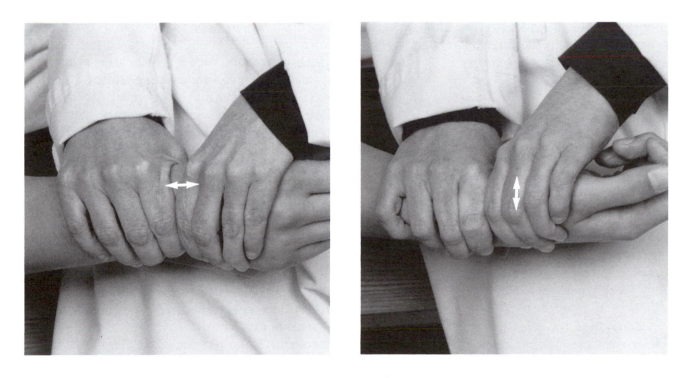

Figure 11–14. Mid carpal mobilizations. Left: traction. Right: anterior and posterior glides.

side opposite the direction of mobilization and applies an anterior or posterior force (Fig 11–15B).

Lateral glide is used to increase radial abduction; *medial glide* is used to increase radial adduction. The triquetrum is stabilized with one hand. With the other hand, the clinician grasps the metacarpal on the side opposite the direction of mobilization and applies a medial or lateral force (Fig 11–15C).

Rotational mobilizations are used to increase opposition and retroposition (Fig 11–15D).

Intermetacarpal Joints of Digits 2–5

These joints are not true joints. Soft tissue mobility allows motion between the metacarpals for cupping and flattening of the hand. The clinician grasps two adjacent metacarpals by lateral pinch grips. Stabilizing one metacarpal, anterior and posterior glides are applied (Fig 11–16, left). General mobilizations across the intermetacarpals can be performed by grasping the patient's hand with one thumb on either side of the posterior aspect of the third metacarpal. The clinician's fingers should be wrapped around the patient's hand, contacting the anterior surface near the first and fifth metacarpals. The mobilizing force is a pressure through the thumbs into an anterior glide while pulling up on the first and fifth metacarpals. Then the first and fifth metacarpals are pushed down as the fingertips contact the third metacarpal on the anterior surface of the hand (Fig 11–16, right).

Metacarpophalangeal Joints

The distal metacarpal is convex, articulating with a concave phalangeal joint.

Joint traction is used for general restricted joint mobility. The metacarpal is stabilized in a lateral pinch grip along the length of the bone. The phalanx is grasped in a lateral pinch grip close to the joint line. Traction is applied by pulling the distal bone away from the proximal bone (Fig 11–17A).

Anterior glides increase finger flexion; *posterior glides* increase finger extension. The clinician stabilizes and grasps the bones as for joint traction. The mobilizing force is in either an anterior or posterior direction (Fig 11–17B).

Medial and lateral glides are used to increase general joint mobility. The metacarpal bone is stabilized and the proximal phalanx is grasped and moved medially or laterally (Fig 11–17C and Fig 11–17D).

Interphalangeal Joints

The proximal joint surface at the IP joints is convex; the distal surface is concave. *Joint traction* is used for general joint restrictions (Fig 11–18, left). *Anterior glides* are used for limitations in flexion; *posterior glides* are used for limitations in extension. The proximal bone is stabilized in a lateral pinch grip. For traction, the distal bone is grasped in a lateral pinch grip and pulled distally. For glides, the distal bone is grasped in a lateral pinch grip and glided anteriorly or posteriorly (Fig 11–18, right).

Hip

Inferior glide is used for general joint restriction and for limitation in abduction. The patient is supine and stabilized against the table with a mobilization belt across the pelvis. In some cases the patient's body weight provides sufficient stabilization. With the patient's knee extended, the clinician grasps around the malleoli. The mobilizing force is applied by shifting weight posteriorly to pull the leg distally. A mobilization belt can be used to bear the weight of the lower extremity during this mobilization (Fig 11–19A). This mobilization is sometimes referred to as a distraction of the weightbearing surface at the hip. Inferior glide can also be performed with the hip in flexion. Here, the clinician grasps around the proximal femur while supporting the weight of the patient's leg, and pulls distally (Fig 11–19B). A mobilization belt can be used to help apply the mobilizing force.

Anterior glide is used for restrictions in hip external rotation and extension. The patient is prone. The clinician supports the weight of the involved extremity or uses a belt to hold the limb. The mobilizing hand contacts the posterior aspect of the femur close to its articulation with the acetabulum. The mobilizing force is a downward pressure to move the femur in an anterior glide (Fig 11–19C). An alternate position for this mobilization is with the patient in single leg stance leaning over the treatment table (Fig 11–19D).

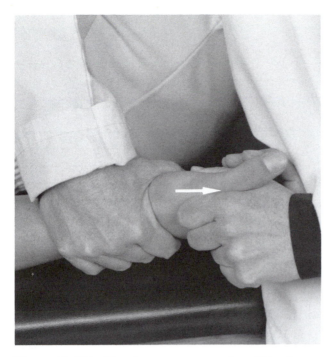

Figure 11–15A. Thumb carpometacarpal mobilizations: traction.

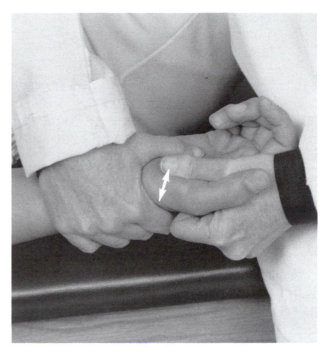

Figure 11–15B. Thumb carpometacarpal mobilizations: anterior and posterior glides.

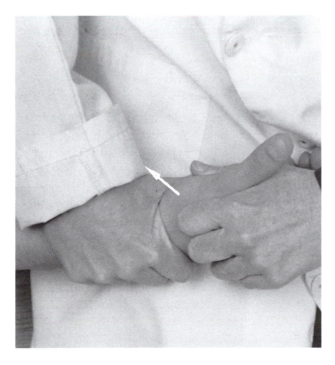

Figure 11–15C. Thumb carpometacarpal mobilizations: lateral glide.

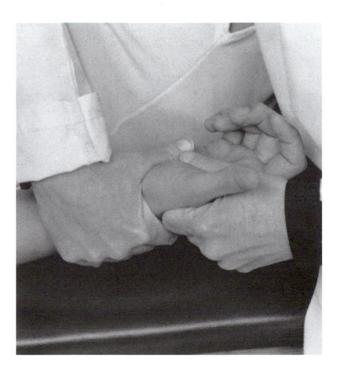

Figure 11–15D. Thumb carpometacarpal mobilizations: rotation.

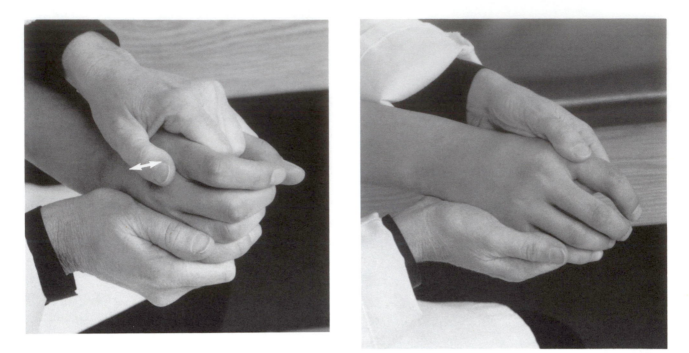

Figure 11–16. Intermetacarpal mobilizations. Left: anterior and posterior glides. Right: general mobilization.

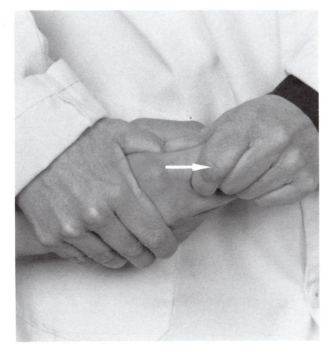

Figure 11–17A. Metacarpophalangeal mobilizations: traction.

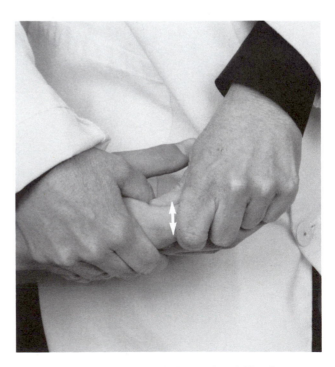

Figure 11–17B. Metacarpophalangeal mobilizations: anterior and posterior glides.

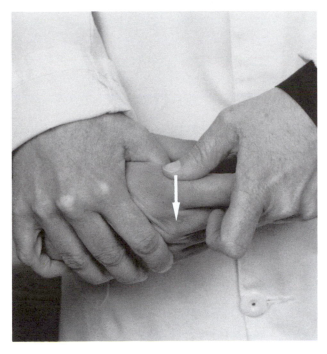

Figure 11–17C. Metacarpophalangeal mobilizations: medial glide.

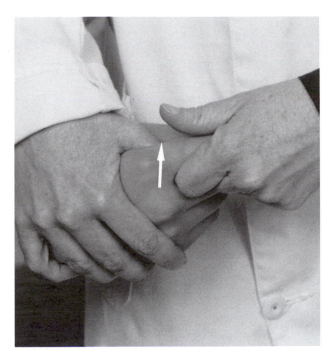

Figure 11–17D. Metacarpophalangeal mobilizations: lateral glide.

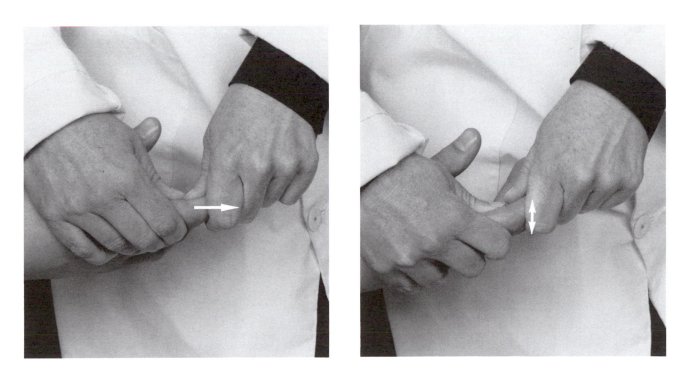

Figure 11–18. Interphalangeal mobilizations. Left: traction. Right: anterior and posterior glides.

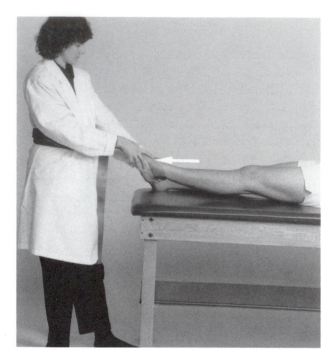

Figure 11–19A. Hip mobilizations: inferior glide using a belt.

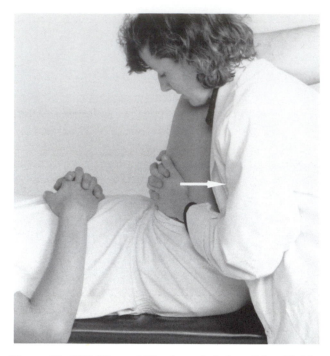

Figure 11–19B. Hip mobilizations: inferior glide with hip in flexion.

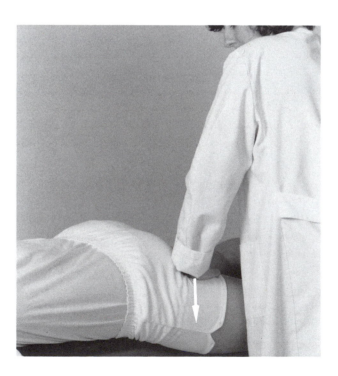

Figure 11–19C. Hip mobilizations: anterior glide.

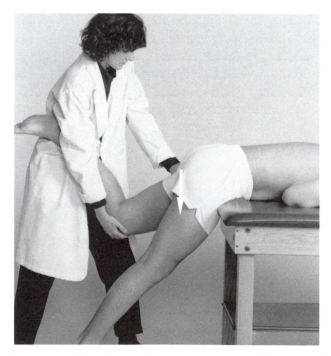

Figure 11–19D. Hip mobilizations: anterior glide with patient in single leg stance.

Posterior glide is used to increase hip internal rotation and flexion. The patient is supine close to the edge of the table. The clinician supports the weight of the limb or uses a belt to support the limb. The mobilizing hand is placed anteriorly over the head of the femur. A downward force causes posterior glide of the femur in the acetabulum. An alternate position for this mobilization is with the hip in 90° of flexion and the knee flexed. A posterior force is applied through the femur (Fig 11–19E). In this position it is important to avoid applying the force through the patella.

Knee

Tibiofemoral Joint

The convex distal femur articulates with the concave tibia. *Joint traction* is used for general joint restrictions. The patient is supine. The femur is stabilized with one hand. The tibia is grasped distally. The mobilizing force is applied by pulling the tibia distally (Fig 11–20A).

Anterior glide is used to increase knee extension. The patient is prone with the femur stabilized and the knee in slight flexion. The clinician places the mobilizing hand along the posterior aspect of the

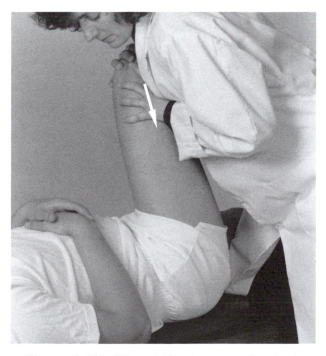

Figure 11–19E. Hip mobilizations: posterior glide.

proximal tibia. The lower leg is supported with the other hand, or with a towel roll under the distal tibia. The mobilizing force is a push anteriorly, parallel to the distal femur (Fig 11–20B).

Posterior glide is used to increase knee flexion. The patient is positioned supine with a towel roll or bolster under the distal femur. The femur is stabilized by the weight of the thigh. The clinician places the palm of the hand along the anterior surface of the patient's proximal tibia. The mobilizing force is a posterior glide performed by straightening the elbow and leaning onto the tibia (Fig 11–20C).

Medial and lateral glides can be used to help increase knee extension. For medial glide, the femur is stabilized on the medial surface, and the tibia is pushed medially (Fig 11–20D). For lateral glide, the femur is stabilized on the lateral surface, and the tibia is pushed laterally (Fig 11–20E)

Patellofemoral Joint

The articulating surface of the patella is irregularly shaped. The shape of the bone does not govern its movements during physiological motion.

Inferior glide is used to increase mobility for knee flexion; *superior glide* is used to increase mobility for knee extension. The patient is supine with the knee extended and the quadriceps relaxed. The clinician cups the superior border of the patella in the web space of one hand and places the other hand at the distal aspect of the patella. The distal glide is performed by pushing the patella inferiorly (Fig 11–21A). A superior glide is performed by pushing up on the patella (Fig 11–21B). With these movements, it is important for the clinician to avoid applying a compressive force through the patella toward the femur.

Medial and lateral patellar glides are used to increase patellar mobility. With the patient supine and the knee extended, the clinician places the thumbs on the medial border of the patella and the index fingers on the lateral border. The mobilization force is applied by pushing laterally with the thumbs or medially with the fingers (Fig 11–21C and Fig 11–21D).

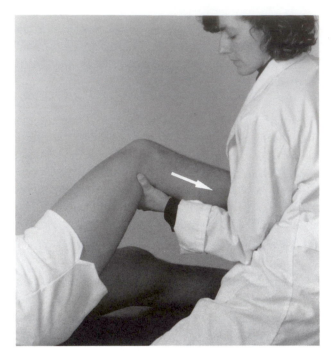

Figure 11–20A. Tibiofemoral mobilizations: traction.

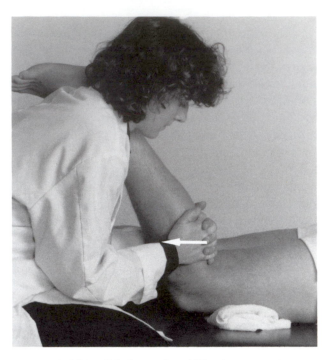

Figure 11–20B. Tibiofemoral mobilizations: anterior glide.

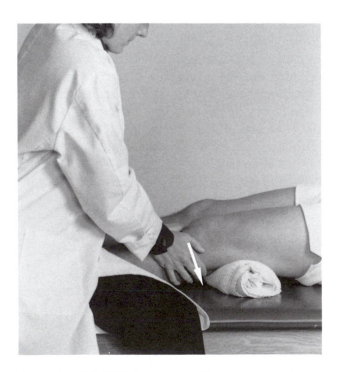

Figure 11–20C. Tibiofemoral mobilizations: posterior glide.

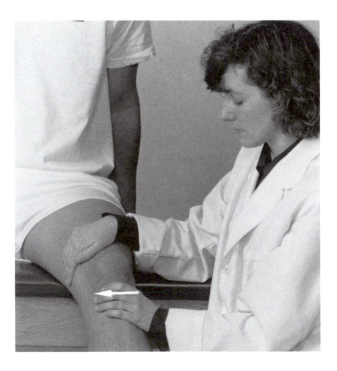

Figure 11–20D. Tibiofemoral mobilizations: medial glide.

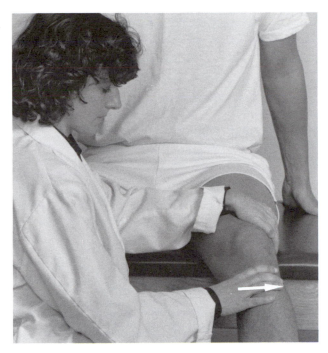

Figure 11–20E. Tibiofemoral mobilizations: lateral glide.

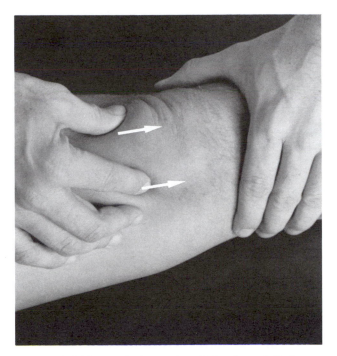

Figure 11–21A. Patellofemoral mobilizations: inferior glide.

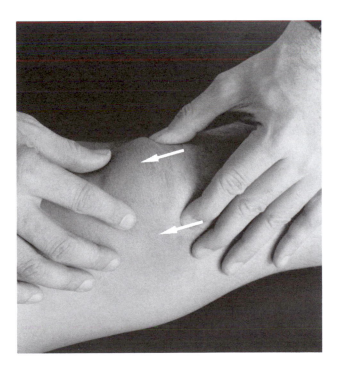

Figure 11–21B. Patellofemoral mobilizations: superior glide.

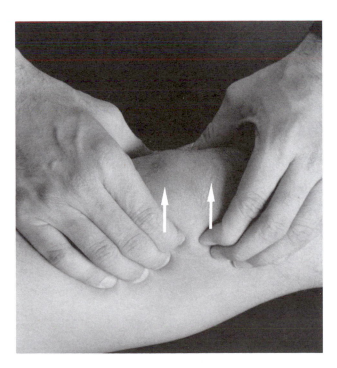

Figure 11–21C. Patellofemoral mobilizations: medial glide, right leg.

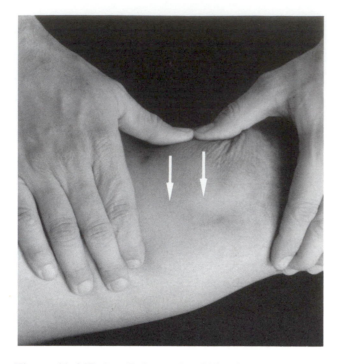

Figure 11–21D. Patellofemoral mobilizations: lateral glide, right leg.

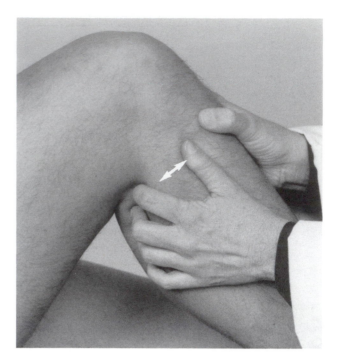

Figure 11–22. Superior tibiofibular mobilizations: anterior and posterior glides.

Superior Tibiofibular Joint

No physiological movements occur at this joint, but some joint play is normal. *Anterior and posterior glides* are used to restore this joint play. The patient is supine or sidelying. The tibia is inherently stable. The clinician grasps the superior fibula and pushes anteriorly or posteriorly (Fig 11–22).

Foot and Ankle

Distal Tibiofibular Joint

This joint must distract slightly to allow full ankle dorsiflexion. It is impossible to replicate the distraction with joint mobilization techniques, so *anterior and posterior glides* are used to restore motion. The patient is supine or sidelying. The tibia is inherently stable. The clinician contacts the anterior or posterior aspect of the lateral malleolus and pushes posteriorly or anteriorly (Fig 11–23).

Talocrural Joint

The convex talus articulates with the concave tibia. *Joint traction* is used for general joint restrictions. The patient is sitting or supine. The clinician stabilizes the tibia with one hand and grasps the talus between the finger and thumb. The

mobilizing force is applied by pulling the talus distally (Fig 11–24A).

Anterior glide is used to restore restricted plantar flexion. The patient is supine with a towel roll under the distal tibia. One hand stabilizes over the distal tibia near the joint line and the clinician grasps the calcaneus with the other hand. The mobilizing force is a pull upward against the calcaneus to glide the talus anteriorly (Fig 11–24B). An alternate technique for this mobilization is stabilization of the calcaneus on a bolster or towel roll as the clinician pushes posteriorly on the distal tibia. This provides a relative anterior glide of the talus.

Posterior glide is used to restore restricted dorsiflexion. The patient is supine with a towel roll under the tibia for stabilization. The clinician contacts the talus with the webspace of one hand, contacting the talus with the index finger and thumb. The other hand can stabilize anteriorly or palpate movement along the joint line. The mobilizing force is a posterior push on the talus (Fig 11–24C).

Subtalar Joint

Movement occurs in the posterior aspect of the joint, where the convex calcaneus articulates with the

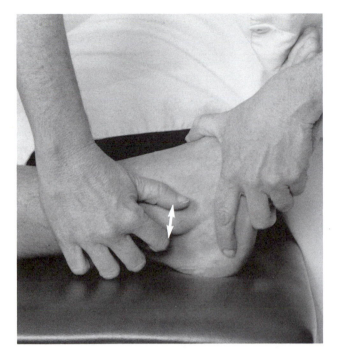

Figure 11–23. Inferior tibiofibular mobilizations: anterior and posterior glides.

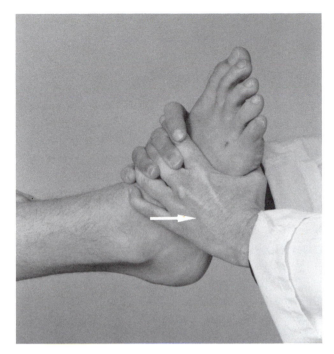

Figure 11–24A. Talocrural mobilizations: traction.

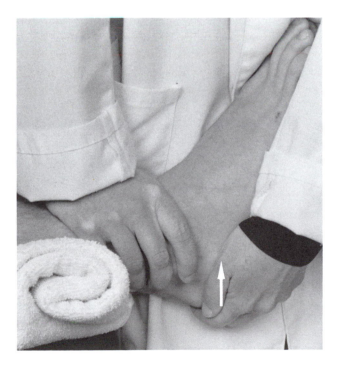

Figure 11–24B. Talocrural mobilizations: anterior glide.

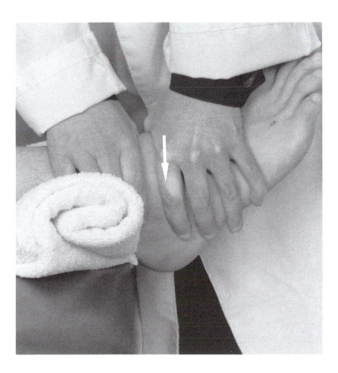

Figure 11–24C. Talocrural mobilizations: posterior glide.

concave talus. *Traction* is used for general joint mobility. The patient is supine with the heel off the edge of the table. The talus is stabilized with one hand. With the other hand the clinician grasps the calcaneus and pulls distally. *Medial and lateral glides* are used to increase eversion and inversion, respectively. The patient is sidelying or prone with the leg supported on a towel roll. The talus is stabilized with one hand. With the other hand, the clinician grasps the calcaneus and pushes medially or laterally (Fig 11–25).

Intertarsal Joints

The tarsal joints are plane joints that allow *anterior and posterior glide* (dorsal and plantar glide). These motions are essential for normal foot function but are not associated with any specific foot motion. The patient is supine or sitting. The proximal bone is stabilized between the index finger and thumb. The distal bone is grasped between the index finger and thumb of the other hand and glided anteriorly and posteriorly. Mobilization of the navicular on the talus is shown in Figure 11–26.

Tarsometatarsal Joints

Accessory movement at the TMT joints is necessary for normal foot motion. *Anterior and posterior glides* are used to restore restricted motions. The tarsal bones are stabilized with one hand, and the shaft of the metatarsal is grasped in the other. The mobilizing force is upward and downward motion (Fig 11–27).

Intermetatarsal Joints

The intermetatarsal joints are not true joints, but soft tissue allows some motion between the bones. This motion is essential for normal foot mobility. Anterior and posterior glides are used to restore normal mobility between these joints. The patient is supine or sitting. One bone is stabilized between the thumb anteriorly and the fingers posteriorly. The adjacent metatarsal is grasped in the same manner and moved anteriorly and posteriorly. Figure 11–28 shows anterior and posterior glide of the fifth metatarsal.

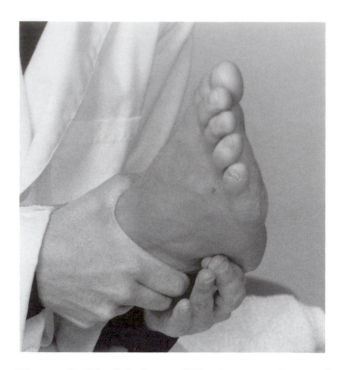

Figure 11–25. Subtalar mobilizations: traction; and medial and lateral glides.

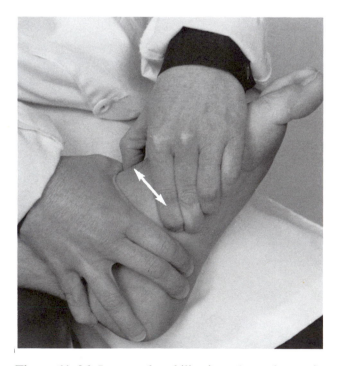

Figure 11–26. Intertarsal mobilization: shown is anterior and posterior glide of navicular on talus.

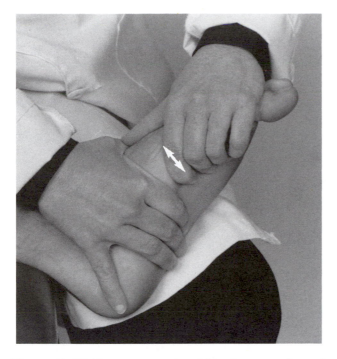

Figure 11–27. Tarsometatarsal mobilizations: anterior and posterior glides.

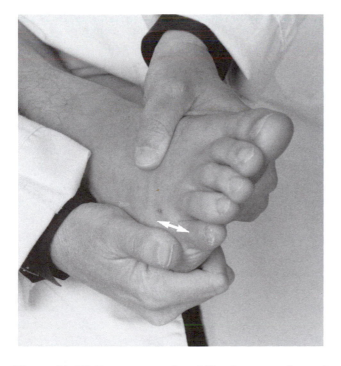

Figure 11–28. Intermetatarsal mobilizations: anterior and posterior glides.

Metatarsophalangeal Joints

The distal surface of the metacarpals is convex, articulating with the concave surface of the proximal phalanx. *Joint traction* is used for general joint tightness. *Anterior glide* is used for restrictions in toe extension; *posterior glide* is used for restrictions in toe flexion. The patient is supine or sitting. The metacarpal bone is stabilized with one hand in a lateral pinch grip. The proximal phalanx is grasped and moved distally (Fig 11–29, left). The same grip is used for anterior and posterior glide, and the phalanx is moved anteriorly or posteriorly (Fig 11–29, right).

Interphalangeal Joints

The proximal joint surface is convex and the distal joint surface is concave. Anterior glide is used to restore extension; posterior glide is used to restore flexion. The proximal bone is stabilized between the finger and thumb of one hand. The distal bone is grasped between the finger and thumb of the other hand, and moved anteriorly or posteriorly.

SOFT TISSUE MOBILIZATION

Massage

The various traditional massage techniques described by such authors as Wood and Becker[6] and Tappan[7] can be quite beneficial when judiciously applied. The theory and practical application of the various techniques will not be repeated here—the reader is referred to those texts.

The temporary physiological effects of massage include increased blood flow, relaxation, decreased muscle spasm, and decreased pain. Because of these temporary effects, massage can help to prepare a patient for other soft tissue or joint mobilization and exercise techniques. Some clinicians believe that massage can result in a permanent elongation of connective tissue, though there is no research evidence to support this belief.

While massage can be an extremely useful tool, the clinician is cautioned to avoid overusing massage, or any other treatment technique, because it "feels good" to the patient, or because temporary relief is obtained. During the objective examination, the clinician applies the skills and principles discussed throughout this text in an attempt to determine the

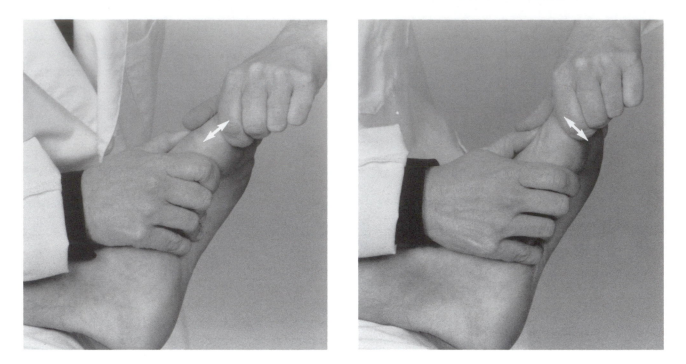

Figure 11–29. Metatarsophalangeal mobilizations. Left: traction. Right: anterior and posterior glides

cause of the patient's complaint. Philosophically, treating the cause of the complaint is always preferred to treating symptoms alone.

Deep Transverse Friction Massage

Deep transverse friction massage is a technique that involves deep massage directly to the site of a lesion, in a direction perpendicular to the normal collagen fiber orientation. It is used to normalize soft tissue modeling in the post–acute phase of injury to tendons and ligaments.

While an acute soft tissue injury is healing, the relative immobility that usually occurs allows new tissue to form. However, the new tissue may not have normal extensibility, or the collagen fibers may not form in a normal orientation. This can occur because of abnormal interfiber bonds (adhesions) that form, decreased mobility between tissue interfaces, or decreased tissue extensibility of individual structures. The decreased tissue extensibility can predispose the soft tissue to further injury. A paradox exists in that the tissue needs to avoid excessive stress while it is healing, but a lack of appropriate stress does not stimulate normal collagen fiber extensibility and orientation.

Deep transverse friction massage appears to work because the perpendicular stress applied to the collagen stimulates interfiber mobility without increasing longitudinal stress that could weaken healing tissue. Appropriate use of friction massage is thought to reflexively relax muscles, restore mobility between tissue interfaces, increase circulation, and increase extensibility of individual structures.[2]

The basic technique involves placing the limb in a position that promotes neutral tension on the tendon or ligament to be massaged. No lubricant is used, as the massage is deep to the skin and subcutaneous layers, and lubricant would cause slippage. The pad of the index or middle finger or thumb is used directly on the site of the lesion. Initially, light transverse (back and forth) pressure is applied with a small amplitude (Fig 11–30). The patient may initially complain of a mild to moderate tenderness, which is acceptable. Massage is continued lightly for 1–2 minutes, then the pressure is increased if tolerated. Often, the patient will report a decrease in symptoms after 1–2 minutes, then an increase again as more pressure is applied. Again, massage is continued for 1–2 minutes, and the pressure is then increased if tolerated. This cycle is repeated for up to 15 minutes, as long as the patient continues to tolerate increased pressure. Treatment times for new patients should usually be much

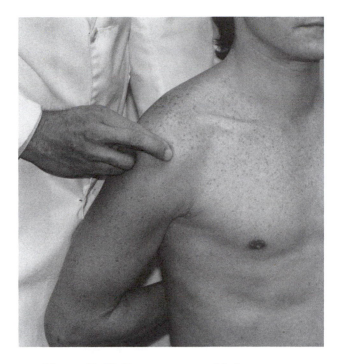

Figure 11–30. Deep transverse friction massage

shorter, perhaps 5 minutes, to avoid latent symptoms. Treatments can take place 2–3 times per week; usually no more than 6–8 treatments are warranted.

Clinicians using deep transverse friction massage in the post–acute phase of tendon or ligament injuries have found it a very useful soft tissue mobilization technique. It is particularly useful with supraspinatus tendinitis, lateral or medial epicondylitis, coronary ligament sprains of the knee and anterior talofibular ligament sprains.[2]

Myofascial Stretching

Myofascial stretching is also referred to as myofascial release, and is often associated with another non–traditional form of treatment— craniosacral therapy. Both myofascial release and craniosacral therapy have been met with some skepticism, mostly from the hypotheses used to explain their usefulness and the emotional, sometimes mystical, component of their use.

We have found myofascial stretching is often a useful tool but prefer to de–mystify its use by thinking of it as simply another type of stretch or soft tissue mobilization technique. The reason it works is no more or less complicated than the reason other soft tissue techniques work. The "release" phenomenon is

perceived by both clinician and patient because the technique is performed slowly and in stages, with great emphasis on the clinician's attentiveness to what he or she is feeling.

There are many different techniques, both for the spine and extremities. A detailed discussion is beyond the scope of this text, but a brief description of five basic techniques that we have found particularly useful will be included. These techniques include the arm pull, leg pull, J–stroking, strumming and stripping.

1) The Arm Pull. The arm pull is used for both generalized upper extremity tightness and specific muscle restrictions. It involves applying a longitudinal traction to the arm with the patient supine in a normal anatomical position. The clinician stands on the same side as the arm being stretched, near the patient's hip. The traction is usually applied through the hand, stretching the lumbricals and finger flexors at the same time by fully extending the fingers, MCP and CMC joints. As the traction is applied, the arm is very gradually moved into abduction, stopping when a soft tissue barrier is perceived by the clinician. External rotation is maintained during abduction. The clinician holds the traction whenever a barrier is felt, waiting for a relaxation or "release" to occur before moving to the next soft tissue barrier. The clinician moves around the table along with the patient's arm to maintain traction at all times. When full abduction (or as much as possible) is obtained, the clinician is standing at the head of the table. Next, the arm is horizontally adducted as the clinician steps to the side of the table opposite the arm being stretched. At the same time, the patient rolls to his or her side facing the clinician. The clinician continues to maintain traction, causing the scapula to protract. Finally, the arm is internally rotated and adducted as the patient rolls back into a supine position, with the final position the same as the starting position except the arm is internally rotated (Fig 11–31).

It is essential to note that the traction is held at all times and the clinician "listens" with both tactile and proprioceptive senses to detect subtle barriers to movement. The patient must be completely relaxed. When a barrier is felt, further motion is stopped until relaxation is felt. If relaxation does not occur, the clinician does not continue beyond the barrier.

Therefore, initial treatments may not be complete as described above.

2) The Leg Pull. This technique is very similar to the arm pull. The basic idea is identical to the arm pull, so the technique will be abbreviated here. The starting position is the supine anatomical position with the foot passively dorsiflexed by the clinician as a longitudinal traction is applied. The leg is moved successively into external rotation, abduction, horizontal adduction (as the patient rolls to his/her side and the clinician steps around to the opposite side of the table), hip protraction, internal rotation, plantar flexion, and back to the supine adducted position.

3) J–Stroking. J–Stroking is so named because of the J–like motion the clinician's fingers draw on the patient's skin. It is a relatively superficial technique and is often used before other deeper techniques. It is applied to a specific area of tissue restriction detected during the palpation examination (e.g., subcutaneous restriction detected during skin rolling). Firm but gentle contact is required. The clinician uses the non–mobilizing hand to stretch the skin and take up slack. The index and middle fingers of the mobilizing hand are flexed slightly and held against each other as firm, short J's are drawn on the patient's skin across the restricted area. Temporary redness will be seen and the patient will complain that the technique is uncomfortable. However, J–stroking should never be performed vigorously enough to cause severe complaints or tissue injury. The technique is repeated several times, with reassessment of tissue mobility performed between each trial.

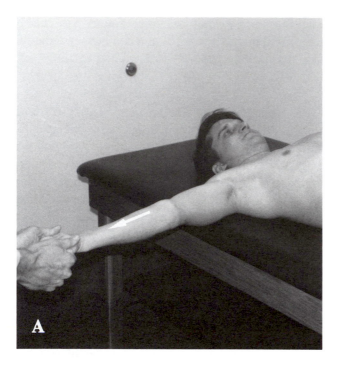

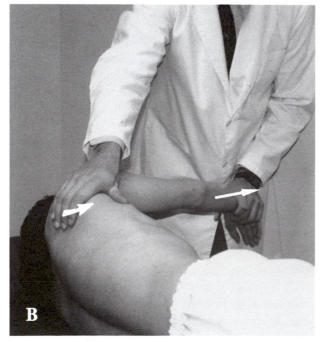

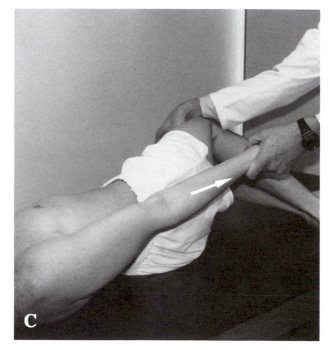

Figure 11–31. Arm pull. A) traction is applied through the hand as the arm is externally rotated and abducted; B) the arm is adducted and the scapula protracted as the patient moves to sidelying; C) the patient is rolled back to supine toward the starting position. The clinician maintains traction at all times.

4) Strumming. Strumming is used to release restrictions deep in the soft tissues and is often uncomfortable for the patient. The clinician positions his or her hand with the fingers flexed at the MCP and extended at the IP joints (Fig 11–32). Pressure is applied to the patient's restricted area through the clinician's fingertips. A back and forth motion running across the muscle or connective tissue fibers is used to break myofascial restrictions.[5] Some clinicians use the elbow or a knuckle to apply the strumming pressure.

5) Stripping. Stripping is another deep release technique that may be uncomfortable for patients. Using an elbow or a knuckle the clinician gradually applies pressure to the involved tissues. The "stripping" force is a slow, deep pressure down the length of the soft tissue.   This   technique   is particularly useful for breaking adhesions associated with chronic hamstring strains.

This section has by no means described all potentially   beneficial   myofascial   stretching techniques. See Manheim and Lavett[5] for a more comprehensive   description   of   these   and   other techniques.

Neural Mobilization

Adverse mechanical neural tension (AMNT) can result in pain and sensory changes in the extremities. Evaluation for potential AMNT was discussed thoroughly in Chapter 2, Principles of Extremity Evaluation.

Painful or dysfunctional neuromusculoskeletal conditions can be irritable or non–irritable. This is true of all neuromusculoskeletal conditions, but is of particular clinical importance in the case of conditions involving AMNT. Since neural tissue is by nature highly irritable, neural mobilization techniques that cause irritability should be approached cautiously.

Neural mobilization techniques are classified according to whether the condition is irritable or non–irritable. The irritable and non–irritable problems discussed here are at opposite ends of a continuum. In reality, the clinician sees varying degrees of irritability; therefore, the treatment guidelines

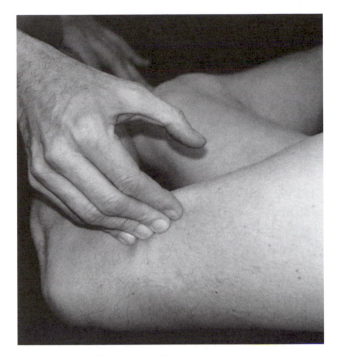

Figure 11–32. Strumming.

presented here are not meant to be definitive "prescriptions." Rather, the clinician is encouraged to continually reassess the patient to determine the appropriateness of the techniques.

Several other considerations will help determine the amount and type of actual mobilization technique. They are:

- What are the sites of altered neural tissue mechanics?

- What are the specific neural tissues involved?

- What structures are juxtaposed with neural tissues along the neural tissue tract that could interfere with their normal mechanics?

Neural Mobilization Techniques

Contraindications to neural mobilization are the same as for AMNT testing outlined in Chapter 2, Principles of Extremity Evaluation. The goals of neural mobilization are decreased symptoms and improved functional mobility of the neural structures. Butler suggests three related ways to treat neural tension   problems   through   movement.[1]   These techniques can be used together to optimize treatment effectiveness.

1. Direct Mobilization

This approach consists of reproducing the neural tension tests described in Chapter 2, <u>Principles of Extremity Evaluation</u>, and gradually stretching into the restrictions. Graded mobilizations can be used in direct mobilizations.

2. Related Tissue Mobilization

This type of treatment involves mobilizing the mechanical interfaces that contribute to neural tension problems. These "related" tissues may include joints, muscles, fascia, and skin interfaces. For example, the sciatic nerve may be entrapped by a tight piriformis. Related tissue treatment involves treating the piriformis muscle tightness. Techniques can involve joint mobilization, physical agents, and exercise, as well as the various other soft tissue mobilization techniques.

3. Indirect Treatment

This approach uses methods such as postural modification and ergonomic assessment to decrease the adverse effects of the patient's work and home activities.

Treating AMNT successfully with mobilization requires considerable skill. The clinician must develop the ability to feel tissue resistance; to assess the patient's symptom response and its relationship to movement; and to decide whether treatment should be strong or gentle. The clinician must continually reassess the patient and compare progress with the goals of decreased symptom response and improved functional mobility.

The grades of joint mobilization presented earlier in this chapter can also be used to describe direct neural mobilization techniques. For example, consider the patient with a positive ULTT (base test), with tightness and symptom onset when the elbow is extended. Grade 3 oscillatory mobilizations would entail using large oscillations through the available range of elbow motion, stopping at the point of resistance. A Grade 2 oscillatory mobilization would stop short of the point where resistance is felt, and a Grade 4 mobilization would involve small amplitude oscillations at the point where resistance is felt.

Neural Mobilization Guidelines for Irritable Problems

Irritable problems usually involve an inflammatory reaction where pathophysiological responses dominate the clinical picture.

1. A direct technique can be used initially, but should be well–removed from the symptom area. For example, the clinician can use a straight leg raise (SLR) or left limb ULTT to treat a patient who has upper extremity symptoms with a neural tension component on the right. This can establish a starting point to which other techniques can be added as tolerated.

2. Initially, the techniques should be non–provoking. Clinically, this means treatment should stop short of symptom response. Most clinicians would agree it is best to "undertreat" or be conservative with any potentially irritable problem. It is important to monitor latent symptom responses.

3. Grade 2 oscillatory mobilizations should be used initially. These mobilizations are performed through the available range with minimal symptom provocation. Eventually, it may be possible to "sneak up" to resistance at a very conservative Grade 4 that gently nudges the resistance, but symptom responses should be monitored.

4. Avoid causing gnawing, deep, constant pain.

5. Proper posture lets the patient be in a position of ease or pain relief. The patient can be taught to replicate the position used in the clinic for self–treatment at home.

6. When the problem becomes less irritable, the clinician can begin applying direct techniques to the symptom area, starting with Grade 2 oscillation mobilizations. If we apply this to the previous example, the patient with right upper extremity symptoms could be mobilized with Grade 2 oscillations into right shoulder depression or elevation with the patient comfortably supine. The cervical spine and distal limbs would be positioned to release neural tension (i.e., right cervical sidebending, right elbow flexion, pillows

under knees, etc.). As the patient improves, tension can be progressively added (i.e., left cervical sidebending, elbow extension, shoulder abduction, etc.).

Neural Mobilization Guidelines for Non–Irritable Problems

Non–irritable problems are usually caused by biomechanical compromise; pathomechanical problems dominate the clinical picture (e.g., stiffness and tissue resistance with abnormal mechanical features).

1. Initially, techniques should be applied into the resistance, but should still stop short of symptom provocation. Grade 3 sustained or Grade 4 oscillatory mobilizations can be used. If symptoms are provoked, they should resolve when the treatment stops. The clinician should monitor any latent symptom provocation.

2. Functional movements that vary from the test positions can be added. Tension on the distal segments can be added. This mimics function better and often provokes symptoms. The limiting factor is the clinician's clinical creativity. The patient should be reassessed in the standard neural tension test positions.

3. Relative irritability should be considered. Treatments should eventually address the symptom source, but the initial treatment may still need to start away from the cause of the problems.

4. Reassessment is critical after neural mobilization techniques have been applied. Take care to note any changes in functional mobility and symptom response.

Neural Mobilization Progression

As clinicians, we understand no two patients' signs and symptoms will be the same. Since each patient will require treatment specific to his or her problem, no precise protocols are available for treatment; however, some suggestions may help the clinician who is just learning to treat AMNT.

1. Gradually increase the length of mobilizations. Oscillatory mobilizations lasting 20–30 seconds may be a good starting point. These may be progressed to sustained mobilizations or longer periods of oscillations.

2. Gradually increase the amount of stretch. This may include adding more resistance until symptoms are reproduced.

3. Symptom response should be continually monitored. Asking the patient if the symptoms are changing or building during treatment is as important as similar questions on follow–up visits. Latency should be monitored.

4. Treatment should progress to adding more tension during treatment while taking into account the irritability of the condition.

5. Muscle energy techniques can help treat related tissues.

6. Soft tissue mobilization techniques can be applied to nerves, where accessible, and to their surrounding myofascial tissues.

7. Frequent reassessment is essential for optimal treatment progression.

Self–Treatment

It usually helps to teach patients to perform self–mobilization stretches. Symptoms should be carefully monitored to avoid an unnecessary flare–up or a latent symptom response. Preventive self–stretches should then be considered for maintaining neural tissue mobility.

SUMMARY

Treatment techniques for mobilizing the joints and soft tissues of the extremities have been presented. These techniques require a great deal of clinical skill, and mastering their application requires practice. Joint and soft tissue mobilization can play a large role in the rehabilitation of patients with extremity problems.

REFERENCES

1. Butler D: Mobilisation of the Nervous System. Churchill-Livingstone, Edinburgh 1991.

2. Hertling D and Kessler RM: Management of Common Musculoskeletal Disorders, 2nd ed. JB Lippincott, Philadelphia PA 1990.

3. Kaltenborn FM: Mobilization of the Extremity Joints. Olaf Norlis Bokhandel, Oslo Norway 1980.

4. MacConaill MA, Basmajian JV: Muscles and Movement: A Basis for Human Kinesiology. Williams & Wilkins, Baltimore MD 1969.

5. Manheim CJ, Lavett D: The Myofascial Release Manual. Slack, Thorofare NJ 1989.

6. Wood EC, Becker PD: Beard's Massage, 3rd edition. WB Saunders, Philadelphia PA, 1981.

7. Tappan FM: Healing Massage Techniques: Holistic, Classic, and Emerging Methods, 2nd edition. Appleton & Lange, Norwalk CT 1988.

CHAPTER 12

EXERCISE

INTRODUCTION

Chapter 12 summarizes some of our favorite exercises—the exercises we use routinely in the clinic. Some of these exercises are the "old standbys" that every clinician will recognize. Others are exercises that some clinicians may not have discovered yet. This chapter is not intended to be a complete source for extremity exercises, or provide a comprehensive discussion of exercise principles for the uninjured person. Instead, this chapter provides the clinician with a basic framework of exercises and exercise principles to use in post–injury rehabilitation.

DESIGNING THE EXERCISE PROGRAM TO FIT INDIVIDUAL NEEDS

Any exercise program the clinician designs should be tailored to fit the patient's specific needs. No two extremity disorders are identical on different patients, so it would be a mistake to prescribe the same exercises for every patient. The evaluation findings are the most important consideration when developing the exercise program.

Each patient responds differently to exercise. In many cases, a patient can progress quite rapidly. Other patients may not progress to more aggressive exercises for several weeks or at all.

The patient's response to exercise may have very little to do with the original diagnosis. For example, some patients with minor sprain or strain injuries progress much slower than expected, while some patients who initially have severe symptoms and pathology progress quite quickly; therefore, the clinician must carefully reassess both subjective and objective findings at each patient visit.

TYPES OF EXERCISE

Three types of exercises will be presented in this chapter: flexibility, strengthening, and proprioceptive.

Flexibility or stretching exercises are performed to increase or maintain soft tissue length and joint range of motion. Most clinicians agree that stretching exercises can help prevent injury recurrence.

Strengthening exercises increase muscle strength and joint stability. Pain and edema can inhibit strength development, so these problems should be addressed before the patient begins a strengthening program, and monitored as rehabilitation progresses.

Proprioception exercises stimulate the nervous system to elicit muscle reflexes that promote neuromuscular control. These exercises are vital after any extremity injury that affects the function of the joint mechanoreceptors.

EXERCISE PROGRAM VARIABLES

There are several basic variables of exercise to be consider when designing a flexibility, strengthening, or proprioceptive exercise program. These variables include intensity, volume, frequency, duration, and mode.

Intensity

Flexibility exercises are usually done gently, avoiding pain, but patients with joint contracture may need to stretch into the pain to achieve lasting results. The hold period of the stretch can vary from short (10–20 seconds) to long (30 seconds to several minutes). Generally, short stretches are more practical for initial patient compliance, especially when the stretches are painful. Longer stretches can be added later as needed.

Intensity is the most important variable of strength training, since the tension developed in the muscle is the mechanical stimulus for strength gains. Loading the tissues safely and progressively restores optimum function. In strengthening programs the intensity is expressed in terms of the amount of the load lifted. Most strengthening programs use light to moderate load intensities, and intensity is increased as the rehabilitation program progresses. Early use of excessively heavy intensity is not indicated in injury rehabilitation. Excessive overloading can damage tissues and prolong pain and edema. Generally, lower repetition, higher intensity exercise is appropriate for basic strengthening needs. Higher repetition, lower intensity exercise is better for endurance training.

The intensity of proprioceptive exercise is varied by the amount of load–bearing on the joint and the complexity of the exercise. Patients with severe or irritable problems may not tolerate much load–bearing initially, but they will gradually improve their ability to control joint motion with increasing loading as the program progresses.

Volume

Volume refers to the total amount of exercise performed and is calculated from the number of repetitions per set, the number of sets, and the intensity of the exercise. When progressing an exercise program, the total volume should be considered. The exercise volume can be increased dramatically by changing only one variable. For example, an increase from six repetitions to eight repetitions causes a volume difference of 120 lb:

6 reps x 3 sets x 20 lb = 360 lb

8 reps x 3 sets x 20 lb = 480 lb

Frequency

The frequency of flexibility exercises depends on the exercise goal. Generally, the patient should stretch before and after any strengthening or aerobic exercise. Patients with specific extremity problems are usually told to stretch several times a day every day. As their condition improves the number of stretches per day may be decreased.

Strengthening exercises are typically performed 1–2 times a day in the early phases of rehabilitation. Later in rehabilitation, it may be useful to train as athletes do, exercising on alternate days, especially if the intensity of exercise is high.

Proprioceptive exercises should be performed with functional strengthening exercises. Usually these exercises are performed once or twice a day initially, and on alternate days as rehabilitation progresses.

Duration

Duration refers to the time that the patient continues to perform the exercises. Some patients may need to exercise for only a few weeks or months to gain and maintain an adequate level of function. Others may need to continue an exercise program for the rest of their lives. With strengthening exercises, neural factors (learning response, increased recruitment of muscle fibers, and increased synchronization) account for increased training responses early in rehabilitation (the first 3–6 weeks) before any change in muscle size. In a rehabilitation program, the minimum time to increase muscle fiber size is usually 8–12 weeks.

If the patient needs a long term exercise program, the clinician will need to find ways to motivate the patient to promote compliance. Keeping the number of different exercises to a minimum can help to foster compliance.

Mode

There are many different ways to exercise. Passive, active, and muscle energy techniques can be used to increase flexibility and range of motion. Ballistic stretching is generally not advisable. For passive stretching, the limb is passively moved to a point in the range of motion to cause a stretch, and it is held there statically. In active stretching, the patient actively moves a limb toward end–range to cause a stretch. Muscle energy techniques using hold/relax PNF principles are commonly used to increase flexibility. The limb is moved to the motion barrier and held there as the patient isometrically contracts the muscle to be stretched for 5–10 seconds. After the isometric contraction, the limb is moved further into the barrier.

The patient can increase strength by using elastic products (tubing, etc.), variable resistance machines, hand-held weights, and isokinetic exercise equipment. Exercises can be performed in isometric, concentric, or eccentric contractions. Muscle functions in daily activities, work, or sport should be analyzed to determine which contraction type to emphasize. Isometric exercises are usually only effective early in a rehabilitation program and are used to re–educate and provide early strengthening responses. Muscles can be strengthened with open or closed kinematic chain exercises. It is best to simulate function as closely as possible. For upper extremities, the choice of open or closed kinematic chain exercises will depend on the function being simulated. For lower extremities, closed kinematic chain exercises are generally preferred unless contraindicated. Table 12–1 summarizes the differences between closed and open kinematic chain exercises.

Proprioceptive exercises should simulate function as closely as possible. The exercises should reflect the functional demands of the involved joint and help restore function in daily activities, work, and sport.

SUMMARY

This chapter has provided basic exercise information. A sampling of our favorite extremity exercises follows. For more comprehensive information consult *Designing Resistance Training Programs*, by Fleck and Kramer,[3] *The Science of Stretching* by Alter,[1] and *Physical Rehabilitation of the Injured Athlete* by Andrews and Harrelson.[2]

REFERENCES

1. Alter MJ: The Science of Stretching. Human Kinetics Books, Champaign, IL 1988.
2. Andrews J, Harrelson G: Physical Rehabilitation of the Injured Athlete. WB Saunders, Philadelphia PA 1991.
3. Fleck SJ, Kraemer WJ: Designing Resistance Training Programs. Human Kinetics Books, Champaign IL 1987.

Table 12–1. Differences between Closed and Open Kinematic Chain Exercises

Factor	Closed Kinematic Chain Exercise	Open Kinematic Chain Exercise
Planes of Motion Used	All three cardinal planes	One plane of motion
Location of Motion	Proximal & distal to joint being exercised	Distal to joint being exercised
Position of End Segment	Fixed	Free
Type of Movement	Usually functional	Often non–functional
Physiological Load	Normal	Artificial
Stabilization	Synergistic muscle action	Artificial
Proprioceptive Feedback	Facilitates functional feedback	Non–functional feedback

SPECIFIC EXERCISE TECHNIQUES

Shoulder Stretching

Shoulder Flexion, Abduction, and Adduction

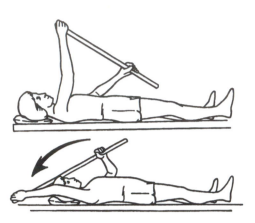

Flexion

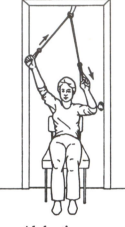

Abduction

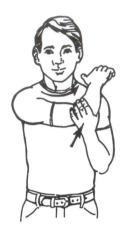

Horizontal adduction

Shoulder Rotation

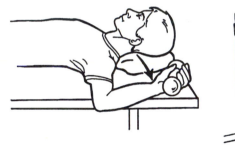

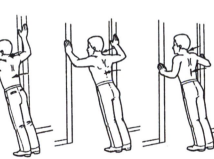

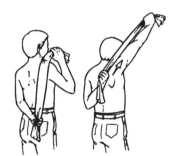

External rotation with abduction

Internal rotation

Shoulder Strengthening

Shoulder Flexion

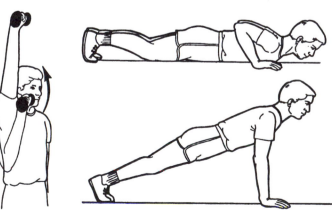

With elbow extension

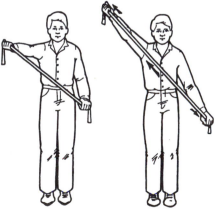

With abduction

Shoulder Strengthening
continued

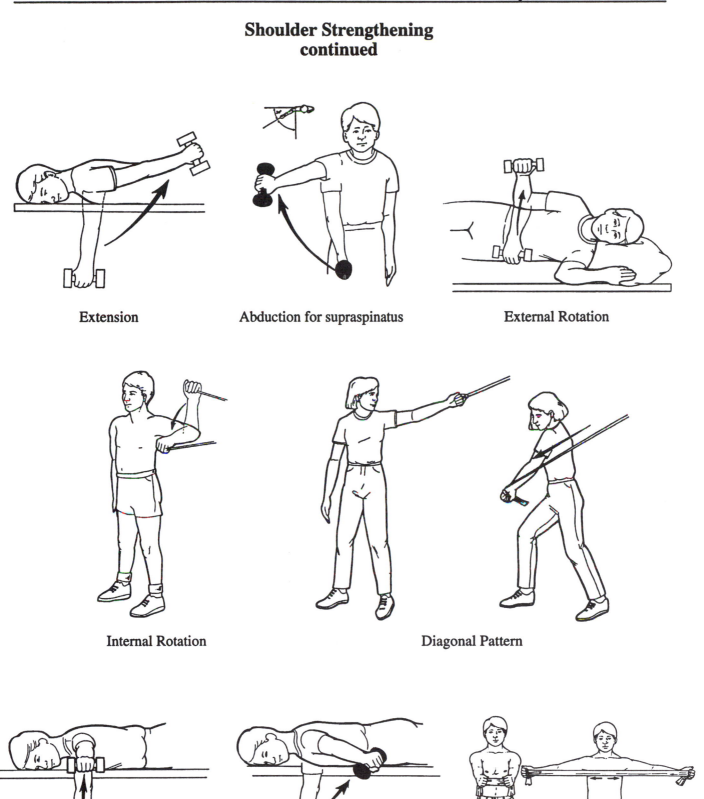

Extension

Abduction for supraspinatus

External Rotation

Internal Rotation

Diagonal Pattern

Horizontal Abduction

Scapular Stability and Shoulder Proprioception Exercises

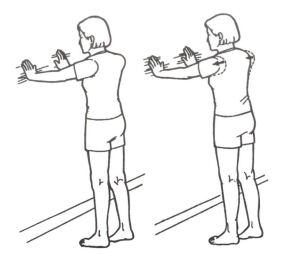
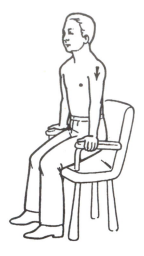
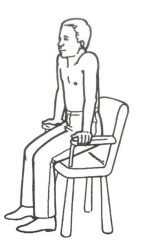
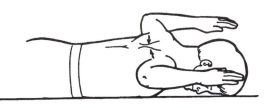
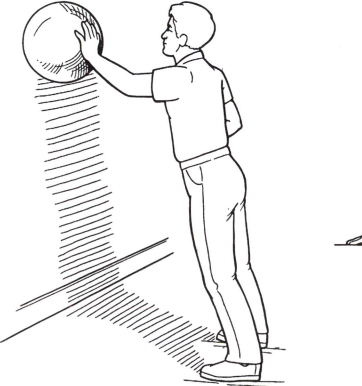
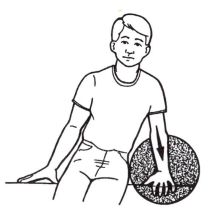
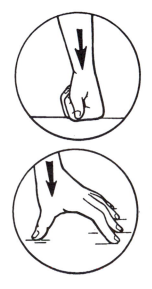

Elbow Stretching

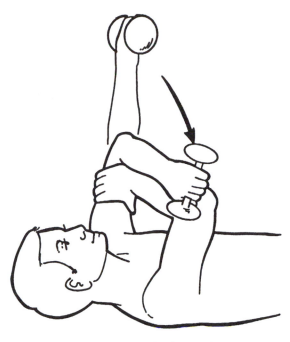

Elbow Flexion

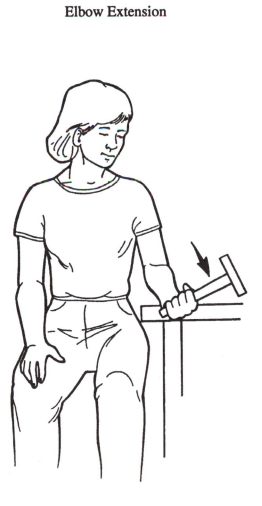

Elbow Extension

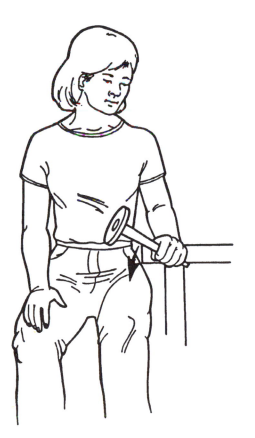

Elbow Pronation

Elbow Supination

Elbow Strengthening

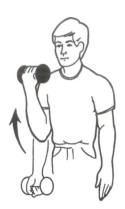
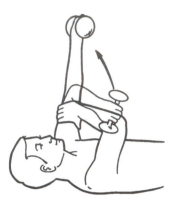
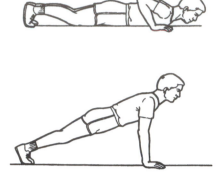

Flexion

Extension

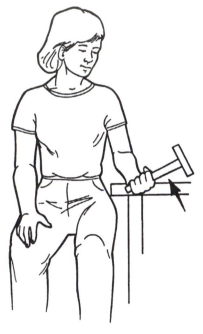
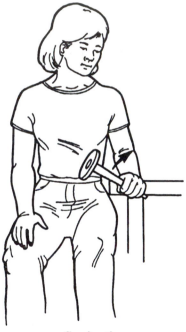

Pronation

Supination

Wrist and Hand Stretching

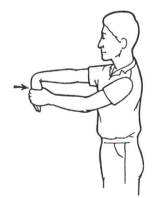
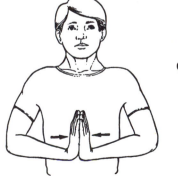
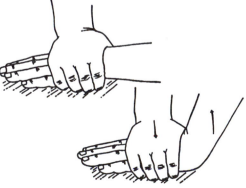

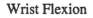
Wrist Flexion

Wrist Extension

Wrist and Hand Stretching
continued

Finger Stretches

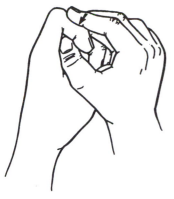

PIP Flexion

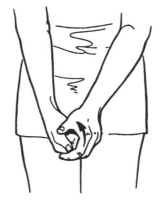

MCP/PIP/DIP Flexion

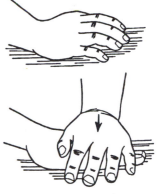

Finger Extension

Thumb Stretches

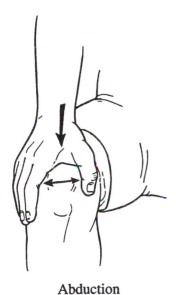

Abduction

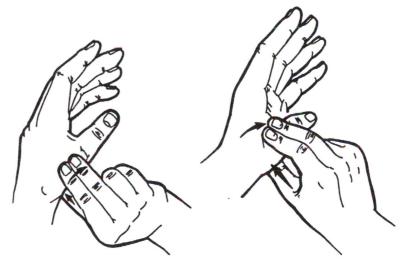

CMC Opposition

Wrist and Hand Strengthening

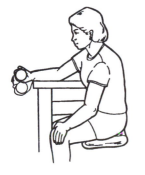

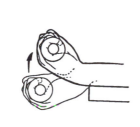

Wrist Flexion

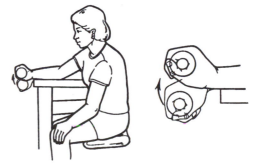

Wrist Extension

Wrist and Hand Strengthening
continued

Ulnar and Radial Deviation

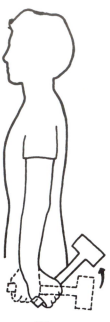

Ulnar

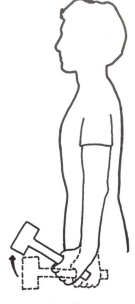

Radial

Finger Exercises

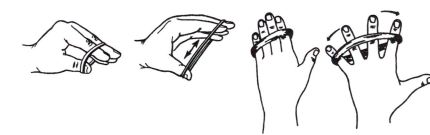

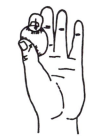

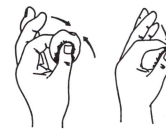

Extension   Abduction   Pinch Grip   Lateral/Key Pinch Grip

Hand Grip Exercises

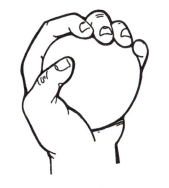

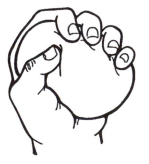

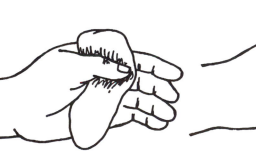

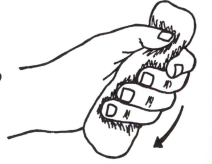

Hip Stretching

Hip Flexion

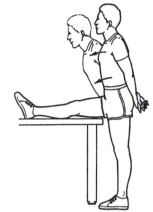

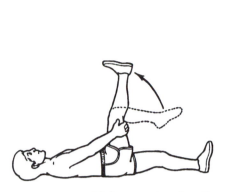

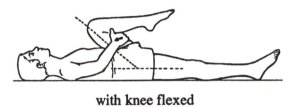

with knee extension (hamstring stretch)   with knee flexed

Hip Extension

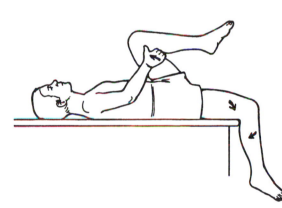

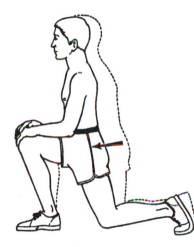

with knee flexion (Quad Stretch)

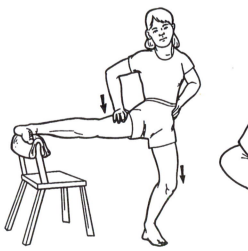

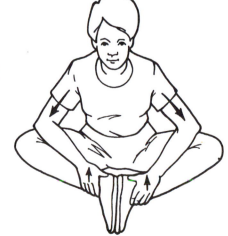

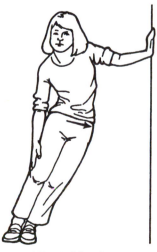

Hip Abduction   Hip Adduction

Hip Stretching
continued

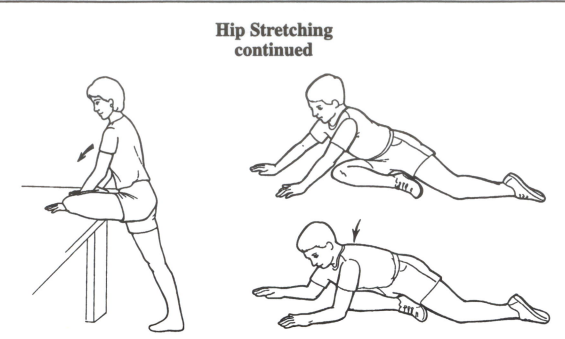

Hip External Rotation with flexion (Piriformis Stretch)

Hip Strengthening

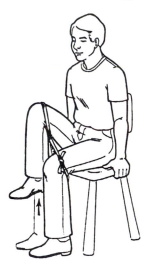

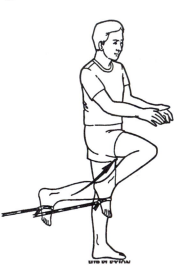

Hip Flexion

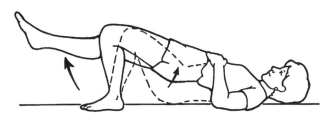

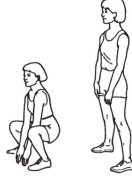

Hip Extension

Hip Strengthening
continued

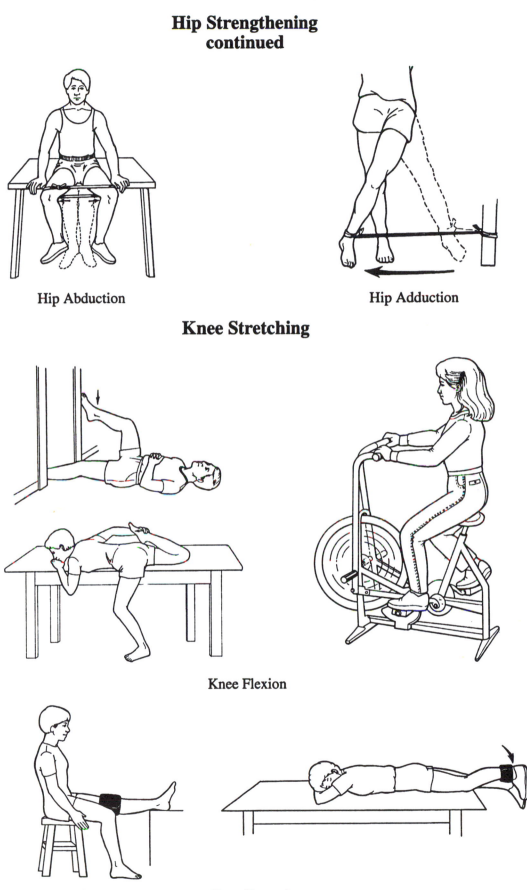

Hip Abduction   Hip Adduction

Knee Stretching

Knee Flexion

Knee Extension

Knee Strengthening

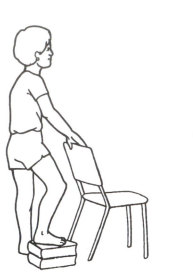
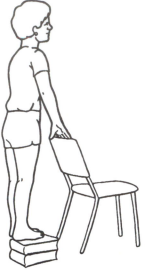
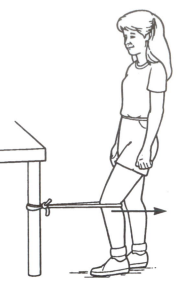

Terminal Knee Extension

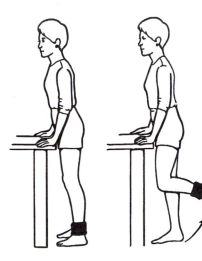
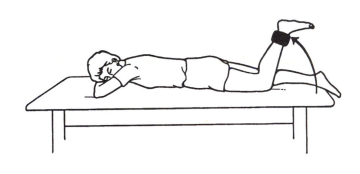

Knee Flexion

Foot and Ankle Stretching

Dorsiflexion

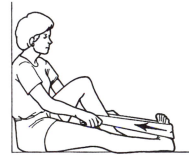
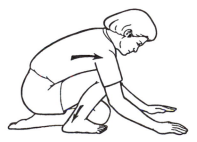
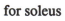
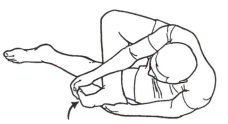

for gastrocnemius   for soleus   with toes extended for plantar fascia

Foot and Ankle Stretching
continued

Plantar Flexion

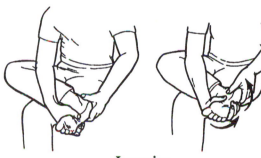

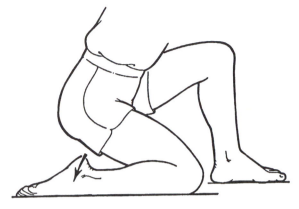

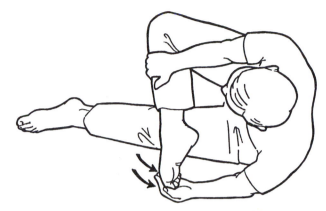

without toes flexed

with toes flexed for extensor tendons

Inversion/Eversion

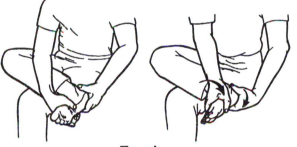

Inversion

Eversion

Foot and Ankle Strengthening

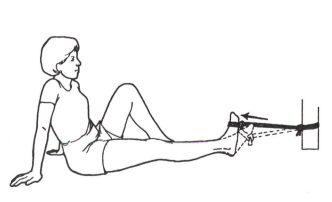

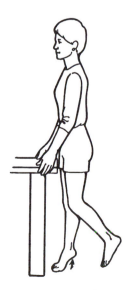

Dorsiflexion

Plantar Flexion

Foot and Ankle Strengthening
continued

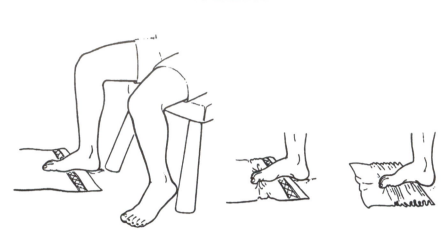

Toe Flexion

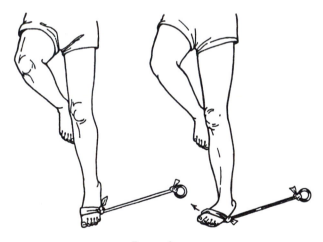

Inversion

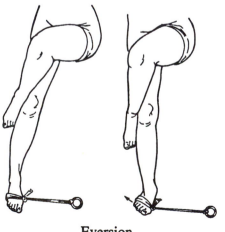

Eversion

Combination Lower Extremity Strengthening and Proprioception Exercises

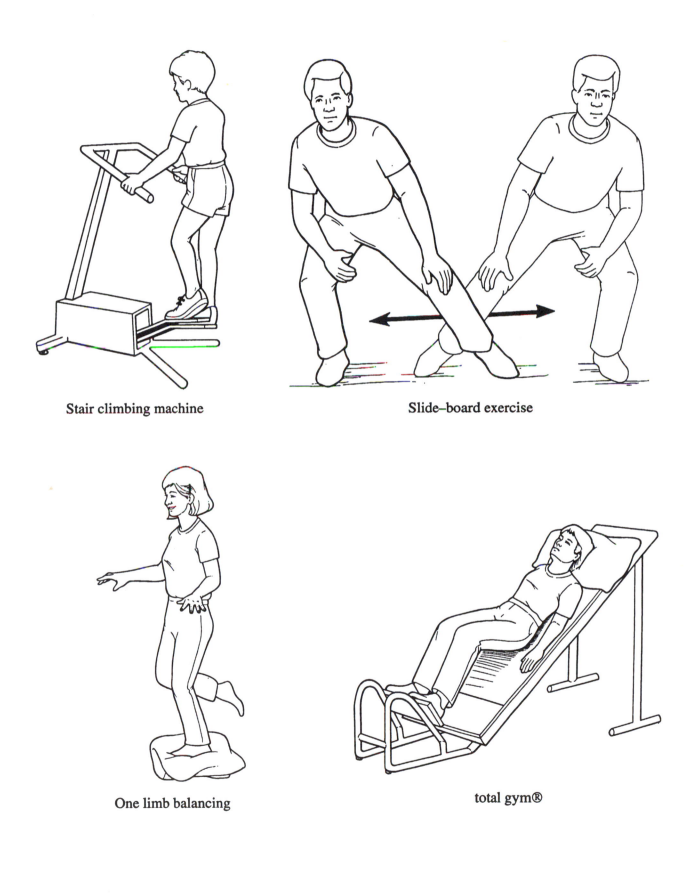

Stair climbing machine

Slide–board exercise

One limb balancing

total gym®

CHAPTER 13

PREVENTION OF EXTREMITY INJURIES

INTRODUCTION

A detailed discussion of the medical provider as an industrial back injury prevention consultant is found in *Evaluation, Treatment and Prevention of Musculoskeletal Injuries*, Volume I—Spine. Many of the same prevention concepts will be presented here but are condensed and modified where applicable for the extremities. Our discussion of industrial preventive techniques will focus on upper extremity injuries because of the relatively small incidence of lower extremity cumulative trauma problems in industry.

The upper and lower extremities can suffer acute injuries and cumulative trauma disorders. The mechanism of injury is often a single traumatic incident related to sports or other vigorous activities. The classic example is the football player's anterior cruciate ligament (ACL) tear, where the knee joint was normal at one moment and severely injured a moment later. Conversely, sports injuries can be related to cumulative trauma that either directly causes a problem or predisposes the athlete to injury. An example here is the rotator cuff tear. Repetitive microtrauma weakens the tendon, predisposing the athlete to tendon rupture during vigorous use or a fall. Prevention of both types of sports injuries will be discussed.

THE MEDICAL PROVIDER AS AN INDUSTRIAL CONSULTANT

The severe economic problems caused by industrial cumulative trauma injuries have made way for the industrial injury prevention consultant. Industrial injury prevention consultants can come from many different backgrounds, including fitness, medical, ergonomics, and business. The most qualified consultant, however, is one who realizes cumulative trauma solutions do not lie in any one specialty area. Medical providers can be very effective consultants, as long as they become competent in traditionally non–medical areas, or direct their clients to resources that can help them develop a comprehensive prevention and management strategy, of which the medical provider is only a part.

As medical providers, we have the opportunity to work with industry in two ways. First, since many cumulative trauma disorders appear as intermittent, acute episodes, we often find ourselves involved as the clinician treating a patient with one of these episodes. Our involvement may end when the patient's symptoms resolve; however, experience shows that this is often insufficient. The patient and employer may think that if there is no pain, there is no problem. Of course, this is often untrue. If the causes are left uncorrected, the patient will probably suffer another painful episode. Additionally, many patients never fully recover from a painful episode until factors at work are addressed concurrently with treatment. In these instances, the clinician may find his or her role expanding to that of "industrial consultant" to help that patient fully recover and prevent subsequent episodes.

Second, the medical provider may directly consult with industry to prevent injuries. Instead of working with a single patient, the therapist works with a whole department or company to develop injury prevention strategies. The first contact with an employer is often through a patient, but the clinician's role expands as the employer discovers that treatment concepts for an injured worker are often identical to prevention strategies for the whole company.

THE MEDICAL PROVIDER'S ROLE IN SPORTS INJURY PREVENTION

Patients can be injured while participating at any level of sports competition, from recreational leagues to professional teams. There are three main ways that medical providers can be involved in preventing of sports injuries: 1) primary injury care provider; 2) pre–participation screening; and 3) sports consultant.

Primary Injury Care Provider

The most common way for the clinician to be involved in preventing sports injuries is as a primary injury care provider. The patient is usually referred to the clinician by a physician. The patient may have an acute traumatic injury or a chronic problem caused by repetitive trauma. The clinician's involvement often ends when the symptoms resolve and the individual returns to sport activity; however, if the factors causing the onset or aggravation of the problem are not addressed, recurrence is likely. Causes include poor conditioning (e.g., poor flexibility, strength, or cardiovascular fitness), improper technique, or faulty equipment. Effective rehabilitation programs emphasize prevention principles and patient education as part of treatment.

Pre–participation Screening

Any athlete should obtain medical clearance before participation in sport activities. The examination should be performed by qualified physicians and physical therapists or athletic trainers who have experience evaluating and treating patients with sports injuries. The examination should take place at least 4–6 weeks before sport participation to allow the athlete time to prepare for the activity based on the findings screening.[2]

Sports Consultant

Physical therapists can also be involved in sports injury prevention as sport consultants. This can include working as a personal fitness trainer or with a team as a strength and conditioning specialist or athletic trainer. The goals are to teach the athletes techniques to prevent injury while training or participating in sports.

INDUSTRIAL CUMULATIVE TRAUMA INJURY PREVENTION

Many of the neuromusculoskeletal disorders discussed in this text are not caused by a single traumatic event but by a combination of cumulative factors. Many disorders develop from environmental and ergonomic factors, while others are related to predisposing physical factors such as disease, obesity, emotional stress, and fatigue. There is much controversy about the role each factor plays in injury. A variety of solutions are offered in the literature, many of them in direct conflict with the others. For example, some authors advocate certain upper extremity stretching exercises as a preventive technique,[1,14] while other authors warn of the dangers of performing such exercises.[5,15] In the midst of such controversy, it is more important than ever to apply common sense and clinical reasoning to each situation. The best solution is always one that involves a comprehensive, customized approach.

A Comprehensive Industrial Injury Prevention Approach

Cumulative trauma injury prevention strategies encompass four main areas that overlap: 1) management practices; 2) ergonomics; 3) education and training; and 4) fitness. If a prevention consultant addresses any of these areas without considering the other areas, he or she has provided the client with a short term solution at best and has caused new problems at worst. For example, if a prevention consultant gives employees ergonomics awareness training without making sure management is willing to make changes in the workplace, frustration or even open hostility may result.

Management Practices

Management practices are very important. If management does not support the prevention process, attempts to take proactive steps in other areas will be futile; therefore, it is paramount to help management develop a comprehensive, prevention–oriented philosophy and a way to handle injuries when they do occur. Three management issues will be discussed: 1) administrative management; 2) medical management; and 3) claims management.

Administrative Management

A company's upper management must be involved in creating an environment in which active and effective injury prevention can thrive. Not all the actions that are presented here are easy to implement. Many companies may initially resist the consultant's efforts to take a serious look at the effect management's policies and attitudes have on their workers' compensation costs. Many companies want a "quick fix," such as a work habits training session or an ergonomic analysis.

It has been our experience that successful injury prevention involves detailed consultation with management about a comprehensive plan to decrease the incidence and severity of injuries. This may require a willingness to change the way the company operates.

Here are some of the more common steps progressive employers are taking to decrease their injury and severity rates and the effect injuries have on their bottom lines.

Job Rotation

Employees "trade" jobs with other employees, increasing variety and reducing exposure to repetitive actions or sustained, awkward positions.

Job Enlargement

Employees perform more and different tasks in the manufacturing process, again promoting variety and reducing exposure to repetitive actions or prolonged positions.

Job Enrichment

Employees are given job goals, but are allowed more choices in how to accomplish those goals. This promotes teamwork, problem solving, shared responsibilities, and increased control over pace.

Reduced Pace

Employers reduce the required production pace.

Work Place Exercise

Stretch breaks or exercise breaks are incorporated into the work day.

Disability Accommodation

Employees with disabilities or injuries are truly accommodated and become productive members of the workforce.

Early Injury Reporting

Employees are encouraged to report symptoms early when they are easiest to treat.

Modified Duty Programs

Injured employees are provided with productive, temporary jobs that encourage early return to work.

On–the–job Work Hardening Programs

Employees are provided with progressive return to work programs that gradually ease them into unrestricted duty while maintaining coworker relationships and support.

Gaining Support

For injury prevention to succeed, management must support it. This fact seems simplistic, but companies often need to be persuaded that they really can influence the rate and severity of work related injuries. It is frequently necessary to convince them that a proactive, organized effort on their part will pay dividends.

Upper management is motivated by bottom line profit. If they can be convinced injury prevention will increase the profitability of the company, they will support it. There is good evidence that cumulative trauma injury prevention procedures, as described in this chapter, can reduce workers' compensation costs. It will be necessary to present this information to the management team to help them make the decision to implement effective interventions.

Getting department managers and supervisors to buy into the program may be a different story. Managers and supervisors often live within their own departments and have somewhat misguided ideas of their ultimate role with the company. A production manager or engineer, for example, may think his or her job is to produce a certain product as quickly and as efficiently as possible. If a new assembly line design or work procedure improves efficiency by 5%, he or she will, of course, think it is a good idea and want to implement it as soon as possible.

What if the new design or procedure also increases the risk of upper extremity cumulative trauma injuries? Who will pay for the injuries?

One of the goals of a comprehensive prevention program is to get department managers and supervisors to see the same bottom line as top management. A good start is to charge the workers' compensation costs back to the individual departments where they originated. They become an expense item, the same as raw materials. They will be factored into the efficiency formula and department managers and supervisors will see health and safety issues *are* production issues.

Thus, if the health and compensation department at corporate headquarters pays for the injuries, the production department manager may not see the same bottom line effect that the company president would. But the production department manager will immediately see that improving efficiency that simultaneously creates another expense is not necessarily a good idea *if he or she is held accountable to a safety or workers' compensation budget.*

Top management must show support by approving funding, clearly communicating policies, and providing written directives.

Above all, however, all levels of the management team must be vocal and visible in their efforts to decrease and manage injuries. In other words, management cannot simply give "lip service" to injury reduction but must be seen as an active champion and facilitator of the entire prevention process.

Providing Authority

In addition to supporting the injury prevention process, top management must provide authority for implementation, establish accountability, and delegate the responsibility for implementing recommended policies and procedures to appropriate team members.

This may require a major shift in the corporate culture; however, if management has done a good job of selling the program to department managers and supervisors, then establishing accountability and creating new responsibilities for certain team members can be a smooth process.

Changing Attitudes Toward Work Injuries

Making the department managers and supervisors accountable for the injuries in their departments will go a long way to change all employees' attitudes from reactive to proactive. In particular, the direct supervisor's attitude should be addressed because he or she is the most visible representative of management in the injured worker's environment. If the supervisor has misconceptions about the cause and effect of cumulative trauma injuries, misunderstandings can easily occur and undermine the success of upper management's policies.

For example, many upper extremity injuries occur gradually without any definite precipitating incident. If a supervisor is not informed about the nature of cumulative trauma and is not aware of the implications of his or her attitudes, an atmosphere of suspicion can develop when such an injury is reported. In a work environment where the supervisor and employee do not have mutual trust and respect, and the supervisor has negative opinions or experiences with upper extremity injuries, the following thoughts may cross his or her mind:

- Why wasn't the injury reported when it happened?

- How do I know this injury didn't occur at home?

- How do I know the employee isn't trying to get out of work?

- How do you know a tendinitis or a carpal tunnel syndrome is real? I can't see any evidence of harm.

- Doesn't everyone's arms hurt at one time or another? Mine sure do, but I don't miss work because of it.

Verbal and nonverbal communication may convey to the injured employee that he or she is not trusted and that the supervisor does not care about his or her welfare. Without support and training, this supervisor may turn a minor problem into a major confrontation that will cost the company a lot of money and will start the injured worker down a long path that will eventually lead to disability. In the end, everyone will lose.

Establishing Work Procedures and Rules

During the investigative process, problems contributing to injury and possible solutions to them will surface. It is imperative that each of these specific problems and solutions be documented and that someone has the authority and responsibility to communicate the resolutions to all employees. All companies have work rules and procedures, but they are not always fully understood or enforced. It is essential to clarify safety rules and work procedures, to gain consensus and support, and to make sure everyone understands what is expected.

Medical Management

Business and industry can rapidly improve their work injury statistics through medical management. Much of this change can be accomplished simply by teaching the workers themselves about upper extremity cumulative trauma injuries and which treatments are effective and ineffective. This same information will help management and supervisors counsel the injured worker to make sure he or she is receiving proper care and support from the organization in a timely fashion. Equally important is the active involvement of management with the medical providers who actually treat the injured employees. Management can be proactive in the following ways:

1. Encourage early, aggressive treatment of reported injuries.

When an employee reports an injury or the first symptoms of a cumulative trauma problem, management should encourage early, aggressive conservative care. Acute injuries are easier to treat than chronic ones.

2. Find competent physicians and therapists.

A company must find competent physicians and therapists with whom to work if they are going to implement an effective medical management program. They must actively seek physicians and therapists who practice the principles of treatment and management described in this textbook (an emphasis on common sense, clinical problem solving, and early return to function). They must then make clear to these medical providers their expectations of them.

3. Encourage employees to see designated medical providers.

Employers cannot afford to allow their employees to be treated by physicians and therapists who do not support their injury prevention and management philosophy. Workers' compensation laws vary from state to state, and a company does not always have complete control over this situation. Our experience has shown that companies with an organized, positive, proactive medical management system are able to direct most injured workers to the selected providers.

4. Provide modified duty and on–the–job work hardening and make sure medical providers understand it

The company's medical providers must do everything possible to return the injured workers to appropriate work. Some experts believe return–to–work is the single most effective thing that can be done for the injured worker. There is considerable evidence of the cost effectiveness of early return–to–work programs.[3,13,19,20] Management and all employees must understand that return–to–work is a treatment issue, not a production issue. Returning injured workers is cost effective even if little or no productive work is accomplished.[3,13,19,20]

A common mistake with return–to–work programs is using them in isolation—that is, as the only method of treatment or rehabilitation. In such cases, the injured worker is likely to stay in a status quo situation for weeks or months. One should never think of return to modified duty as the sole means of treatment or rehabilitation. The return–to–work process should always involve patient education and an exercise or Work Hardening program. It should always have time limits and involve weekly or biweekly reassessments and updates by the physician and therapist. An appropriate on–the–job Work Hardening program is preferred to a clinical Work Hardening program.

5.   *Make sure medical providers consider ergonomic factors in the treatment plan*

The medical provider must have a basic knowledge of the interaction between the work setting and the employee's abilities. An ergonomic change may be the most important "treatment" of all. Even if the patient has symptom relief, return to the same job without ergonomic changes may cause the problem to recur.

Claims Management

A corporate claims management philosophy should emphasize the following objectives:

- regular contact with an injured employee

- effective communication with medical providers

Companies should have specific, written claims management policies. The policies should clearly outline a sequence to be followed every time there is an employee incident that may result in lost work time.

Injured workers need to be managed as well as treated. The medical providers treat the individual, but the company manages the case. It is no longer appropriate to rely entirely upon the doctor's opinion about the injured worker's care and management. Obviously, the workers' compensation insurance company will be involved in case management to some degree, but company management still needs to know medical management principles (if for no other reason than to make sure the insurance carrier is doing a good job).

Injured workers must not be allowed to continue ineffective treatment. If progress is not being made with a certain treatment approach, the Claims Manager must be proactive and ask the treating physician if other methods of treatment and rehabilitation should be considered.

Eventually, the injured worker will achieve maximum benefit from medical treatment. Too often, cases go on and on from one physician to another, with very little, if any, progress. If the employee has had adequate evaluation and appropriate treatment and rehabilitation; has had multiple medical opinions; and an unusual amount of time has lapsed since injury, he or she has probably achieved maximum benefit from available medical care. The case should be settled. The employee may return to a permanent job within his or her restrictions at the present employer or may have to be placed outside the company. Even so, the case should be settled because an open case that is not progressing and has no end in sight is damaging for both the employee and the employer.

Another case that must be settled is the uncooperative employee. When the employee refuses to cooperate with the treatment and rehabilitation plan, the case must be moved to a conclusion. Good communication between the company, the insurance adjuster, and the medical providers is critical to identify and manage these cases.

The key to long term success in managing injured employees is developing a positive, open line of communication between the supervisor and the injured worker. If the employee genuinely feels management cares about his or her well being, it is more likely that he or she will cooperate. A positive atmosphere is extremely important. The objective is to make the employee feel secure and welcome. Without this feeling, an employee is far more likely to seek legal counsel, which will only result in higher costs and increased frustration.

Ergonomics

Ergonomics is a crucial concept in upper extremity injury prevention and management. Ergonomics is the science of designing workplaces, machines, and tasks with the capabilities and limitations of the human body in mind. By applying the basic principles of ergonomics, the company and its employees can take many steps toward a safer, more productive work environment.

Providing a safer, more productive workplace is important in the overall prevention process. Ergonomics, education, and management practices overlap significantly. For example, training employees in proper work practices often makes them aware of needed ergonomic changes, but it will not be possible to implement the changes successfully unless management provides the means to do so.

The best ergonomist is the employee doing the job; therefore, a major part of an ergonomics program is teaching the workers and front line supervisors the basic principles of ergonomics. Once these basic principles are understood, the employees can return to the workplace and recommend corrections.

Worksite evaluation and redesign can also be performed by experts who are trained in industrial engineering and ergonomics. If specific problems are found that cannot be corrected by application of the basic principles of ergonomics, a company may want to hire an ergonomic consultant to redesign a particular job or machine; however, even if major worksite redesign is impractical, the company can often make simple and inexpensive modifications to greatly reduce the risk of injury.

When conducting the ergonomic survey, it is important to note good examples as well as bad. Most of the information gathered in the ergonomic survey will be incorporated into the education sessions later. Positive information will be just as important as negative information as the process unfolds.

Purpose of Ergonomic Survey

A worksite evaluation or ergonomic survey of the work area should be performed early when undertaking cumulative trauma injury prevention. It is done for two reasons: 1) to familiarize the prevention team with the work tasks and work procedures so any educational programs presented can be customized to address specific problems; and 2) to identify problem areas that can be redesigned or modified to prevent injuries.

The prevention team should be familiar with the company's injury records before the worksite evaluation begins. This helps focus attention on possible problem areas.

Performing an Ergonomic Survey

Some basic design principles must be understood before performing a worksite evaluation. With these principles firmly in mind, the consultant should begin the worksite evaluation by reviewing an activity or job believed to be more physically stressful than others. All jobs in the work area should then be carefully reviewed. The consultant should examine the positions employees assume or maintain as work is performed. Several common problems contributing to upper extremity disorders are discussed below.

Work too low (Fig 13–1)

If the work is too low, an employee will be forced to stand or sit with the head and neck forward, shoulders slightly rounded, and the low back in a forward bent position. Rounded shoulder postures may shorten muscles in the front of the shoulders and chest and reduce blood flow to the arm, wrist, and hand. Can the work be raised or tilted toward the worker? Ideally, the work station should be adjustable. The right work height also depends on the type of work. Regular work should be at elbow height; light, precision work above elbow height; and heavy work below elbow height. If the work level is not adjustable, the fixed work height should be biased toward taller individuals (36" for regular work). This may be accomplished simply by placing boards under the legs of a table.

Work too high or far away (Fig 13–2)

Continuously working at a height requiring excessive wrist flexion or extension can be very stressful. Working too high usually causes excessive wrist and shoulder flexion and elbow extension. The problem can be compounded by a flat work surface or one that is angled away from the worker. Ideally, work should be performed in the worker's "swing space" (Fig 13–3). The consultant should look for tasks that make the elbows exceed a 45° angle away from the sides or front of the body and try to lower the work height or raise the worker. This can often be accomplished by using raised work areas, tilting the work toward the worker, rearranging storage areas, or by providing stair platform ladders, which are safer than stepladders.

Repetitive, forceful, or sustained wrist and finger movements

Forceful contraction of muscles causes tendon stretching, possibly leading to ischemia, fibrillar tearing, and inflammation.[2] Frictional damage to the tendon sheaths can also occur.[4] Repetitive loading without adequate rest causes progressive lengthening and "creeping" or sliding of tendon fibers through the ground substance matrix, resulting in inflammation.[17] These factors have been correlated with higher incidence of carpal tunnel syndrome and other cumulative trauma disorders.[21,24]

Mechanical pressure on soft tissue

Direct pressure on soft tissue can cause ischemia and inflammations. Common examples include pressure on the median nerve from using a screwdriver, pressure on the volar forearm from the sharp edge of a desk, or pressure on the elbows from improperly adjusted armrests. Tool redesign, padding or rounding the edges of tables, and proper adjustment of armrests can alleviate these risk factors. Tight watchbands, gloves, or clothing can also be problematic and workers should be taught to avoid these situations.

Vibration and cold

It is difficult to separate the effects of vibration and cold from the other ergonomic factors listed above. For example, several studies indicate that the intensity of a worker's grip increases with handle vibration.[12] Other studies have shown that grip increases with low temperatures, presumably because of the loss of tactile sensitivity and manual dexterity.[16] Poorly fitting gloves may further decrease tactile sensitivity and dexterity, leading to increased grip. At any rate, vibration and cold have been correlated with increased upper extremity disorders,

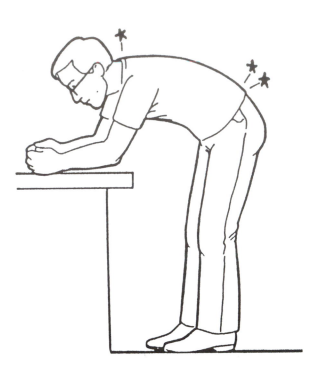

Figure 13–1. Work too low.

and devices that decrease these effects while minimizing loss of sensitivity and dexterity can be helpful. Tool redesign and improved environment are recommended where possible.

The Role of Splints and Supports in the Workplace

Using splints and supports on the upper extremities is controversial. Opinions range from discounting them altogether to advocating them in the workplace as a preventive measure. Research is scant in this area, and most opinion is based on anecdotal evidence. We have seen instances where supports have been helpful and other occasions where supports have actually caused more harm than good.

Splints or supports are ineffective in isolation and without careful consideration of all four preventive factors discussed in this chapter. Our experience has shown prophylactic splinting is successful *only* when all other factors have been considered. If ergonomic conditions are suboptimal, e.g., repetitive work is performed too high, where excessive wrist flexion is encouraged, using a wrist support is unwise. The employee may actually "fight against" the forces of

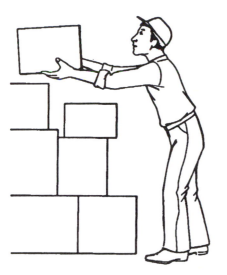

Figure 13–2. Work too far away.

the support, fatiguing the wrist musculature, winging the elbows out away from the body, or making other unacceptable compensations.

In another example, the employee may tend toward excessive tightness of the wrist muscles. If a wrist support is prescribed, and the individual uses it without frequent stretching breaks, the employee's wrist musculature becomes tighter, predisposing him or her to soft tissue problems.

On the other hand, we have seen instances where post–injury, on–the–job splints have contributed to a successful return–to–work. In other instances, companies have made wrist supports available to their employees as part of a comprehensive prevention effort; employees have responded favorably and indicate fatigue is lessened and productivity is improved.

When splints or supports are prescribed prophylactically or for long term use post–injury, the employee must be taught to use them properly. Proper use includes frequent stretch breaks; use only when heavy or repetitive work is performed; and concurrent optimization of ergonomic principles. If common sense principles are adhered to, splints and supports do have a role in the workplace.[9,12]

Education and Training

Education and training spans all other areas of cumulative trauma injury prevention. It is the vehicle for implementing effective intervention. Everyone in the company—hourly employees, supervisors, and upper management—must be part of the educational process. The information on management policies and attitudes is just as important to present as the traditional prevention program for the hourly employee and must not be forgotten.

Both the method and the content of education and training are critical to its effectiveness. This chapter will not discuss the content of educational programs in detail. There are excellent training resources available to the educator that provide the needed content, including actual presentation materials.[5,6,7,8] This chapter will focus instead on the method and process of delivering information to the appropriate personnel in an organization, including the basic information that must be presented to the management team.

Education for Employees

Effective dissemination of information is essential if policies addressing ergonomics, fitness, and management are to succeed. There is, however, basic background information about upper extremity cumulative trauma injuries with which everyone must be familiar so that all education is enhanced.

All participants of a cumulative trauma injury prevention program, whether they are managers, employees, or patients who already have a problem, must first have a basic understanding of certain facts, including the common causes of upper extremity

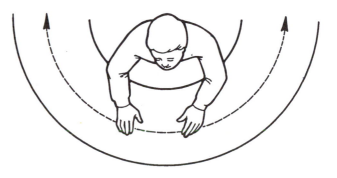

Figure 13–3. Swing space.

problems, what to do when an injury occurs, and the importance of a healthy lifestyle, good work practices, ergonomics, and fitness.

Although an educational program must be flexible and meet the individual needs of companies and institutions, a standard or model program should be developed. The basic program should consist of 2–4 hours of instruction by a qualified and experienced instructor. Ideally, a maximum of 30 participants should be included in each course. Instruction should be carried out by means of an audiovisual program, instructor demonstration, and active class participation. Open discussion should be encouraged.

The participants should be taught the anatomy and function of the major anatomical structures. The mechanical strain in different positions and during different movements should be discussed. Unfavorable working postures should be analyzed in detail.

The pathology of the major upper extremity cumulative trauma disorders (carpal tunnel and tendinitis) should also be discussed in relation to the above mentioned stressful postures. Various methods of treatment should be talked about and the body's natural capacity for healing should be emphasized.

The program should teach individuals what to do when a cumulative trauma disorder occurs. Participants should be taught that what they do to manage their injuries is almost always more important than what their physician or therapist does.

Even when a company makes every effort to eliminate ergonomic stressors, there will still be times when the employee's choice of technique will make a big difference; therefore, employees must be taught proper technique, safe work practices, and how to reverse stressful activities through positional changes and exercise.

Many workers do not take proper work procedures seriously. Instruction should be directed toward attitudes, forcing the worker to recognize his or her obligation to perform work tasks properly.

The worker should be encouraged to review his or her standards of fitness, nutrition, and stress control. Participation in various types of physical activities and sports should be encouraged. Exercise improves psychological and physical tolerance to pain and stress. The participant should be informed that proper nutrition is a foundation of good health. Obesity has been shown to be a risk factor for carpal tunnel syndrome.[10,23] It should be pointed out that stress directly affects emotions and muscle tension. The participant should be told how relaxation exercises can help in stressful situations.

At the conclusion of the program, participants should be provided with examples of proper and improper work practices and postures and take part in active problem solving sessions. Each participant should receive a booklet or pamphlet outlining the main points of the course. The booklet should also contain a section of general flexibility and strengthening exercises for the upper extremities and related areas such as the upper back and neck. Each of the exercises should be demonstrated and discussed in the class.

Education for Management

Many concepts about management's role in overall prevention have already been discussed. A company should never present an injury prevention program to hourly employees without making sure management's issues are addressed concurrently and management personnel have received aggressive training in needed areas.

Additionally, all management personnel should take part in the same program presented to hourly employees. This will make sure everyone in the company is receiving consistent information and will also underscore management's commitment to injury prevention. The management team should be seen as active participants and facilitators of prevention rather than passive observers.

A representative from the company's workers' compensation insurance carrier should participate in any educational programs presented to management and employees so that the insurance adjusters handling the company's claims are well informed about company philosophy and policies.

Exercise and Fitness

A serious look at both specific exercises and general fitness is important to overall preventive strategy. No matter how well a company performs in other areas, injuries will still be a problem if the workers are not fit to perform the critical physical demands of their jobs. Fitness is often a difficult area to address because how well individuals take care of themselves is usually outside company control; however, there are many things employers can do to facilitate on–the–job fitness and to motivate and educate workers to practice healthier lifestyles away from the job.

General Fitness

There is considerable evidence to indicate people who are in poor physical condition and who practice other unhealthy lifestyles are at a greater risk of injury;[16,19,21] therefore, it seems logical that any prevention program should help individuals identify deficiencies and try to help them improve their levels of physical fitness, thus reducing their risk of injury. It is important to emphasize that many work situations are like athletic events: they require a certain level of physical fitness, strength, and flexibility. Many people try to work at jobs that require considerable physical labor and involve stressful positions, but they make little or no effort to keep their bodies in the physical condition required to do these jobs.

It is true that most individuals work hard at their jobs, and it is sometimes difficult for them to think that they should exercise when they are already tired from work; however, hard work and exercise are not always accomplishing the same thing. In most work situations, we get too much of one type of activity or exercise and usually not enough of another. Many people work hard all day, yet are still very stiff and are in poor cardiovascular condition. Fatigue and stress can contribute to injury. An exercise program should emphasize the type of exercise that is lacking at work. For example, if an employee sits or stands all day, he or she should make sure aerobic activity is performed on the "off" hours.

Business and industry have a lot of options when it comes to fitness. The importance of exercise and other healthy lifestyles can be incorporated as a part of an educational program. A certain number of individuals will indeed be motivated to exercise on a regular basis through such a program, but it is unrealistic to expect every employee to be motivated to participate on their own in a home exercise program. A company can take the issue of fitness much further than simply teaching about it in an educational program. Some companies are encouraging on–the–job exercise programs.

On–the–job exercise as an important component of the total injury prevention process is just beginning to create interest in industry. Many companies begin by helping start voluntary programs. In such cases, the company may provide a place to exercise and then hire an instructor to organize and lead the exercise sessions. Once a group gets started, participants from the group often volunteer to lead the sessions and the paid instructor is no longer needed. Voluntary exercise classes are usually offered before or after working hours or during break times. Exercise classes during lunch are often popular, and companies sometimes extend break times or the lunch hour a few minutes longer for participants. On–the–job strength and flexibility exercise programs can be very effective if offered 3–5 times per week in 10–20 minute sessions.

Mandatory exercise during work is attracting some interest. Companies are trying mandatory exercise programs on a limited or experimental basis. If these programs prove effective, mandatory exercise during work may become a popular and effective way to reduce cumulative trauma injuries. The obvious advantage to mandatory exercise is that those who are in poor physical condition and lack motivation to exercise on their own can be required to participate. It is often easier to get these people to participate willingly after they have attended an educational session.

A mandatory exercise program can backfire if it does not have the grassroots support of the employees. Companies should move with caution if they plan to implement a program of this sort without emphasis on participation in the decision making process.

Specific On–The–Job Exercises for the Upper Extremities

Many stressful or repetitive movements will be unavoidable. If the worksite cannot be modified, workers can be taught specific stretches to counteract stressful movements or positions. These stretches can be performed during short breaks that take place naturally in most jobs. The role of specific stretching and strengthening exercises for upper extremity injury prevention is highly controversial. Studies have both supported and strongly condemned wrist flexion and extension stretching exercises as a preventive, on–the–job technique.[1,5,14,15,22] This is another place where common sense clinical reasoning must apply.

It is commonly assumed that soft tissue tightness is a predisposing factor for neuromusculoskeletal injury. Clinically, we often see patients with wrist or elbow tendinitis presenting with tight wrist extensors or flexors. In many cases, it is obvious the tightness has been present for a long time, certainly before onset of symptoms.

It is an accepted fact that stretching before and during sports activities helps prevent soft tissue injury. Why then, have some "experts" proclaimed wrist flexion and extension stretches are contraindicated? Presumably, it is because repetitive wrist flexion and extension are causes of upper extremity disorders. Common sense tells us, however, that a gentle, prolonged stretch is not the same as repetitive overuse. This principle is clear in sports medicine. Furthermore, Hansford, et al,[14] have shown that on–the–job exercise breaks increase blood flow at the wrist more than regular rest breaks. Increased blood flow is thought to be a positive factor in prevention.[1,11]

When suggesting exercise for prevention of upper extremity injuries, the consultant should not neglect related body parts such as the neck and upper back or shoulders. For example, stretching the arms overhead while pumping the hands may promote improved blood flow and increased upper back and shoulder flexibility. Retracting the scapulæ and stretching the neck will help prevent rounded shoulder posturing and tight anterior chest muscles.

SPORTS INJURY PREVENTION

The Pre–participation Screening Examination

Preventing sports injuries starts with a pre–participation screening. The primary goal of this examination is to identify factors that may predispose the athlete to injury. There are **six components** of a pre–participation examination:[2,4,17]

1. medical history

2. general medical examination

3. musculoskeletal examination – including posture and general alignment, flexibility, strength, percent body fat, girth measurements, and ligament stability

4. cardiovascular endurance

5. physical examination specific to the athlete's sport (or position)

6. review of all medical information by a physician to determine if participation should be allowed, disallowed, or modified based on all examination findings

The primary role of the physical therapist in the pre–participation examination is in the musculoskeletal screening examination.

The extent of the musculoskeletal examination depends on the number of athletes to be examined, the number of clinicians available, and the athletes' sports. The aim of the musculoskeletal screening examination is two–fold: 1) identify physical findings that may predispose the athlete to injury; and 2) document baseline measurements for comparison with follow–up tests in case of injury. School athletes who participate in screenings year after year will have multiple baseline measurements for comparison.

A common method for screening examinations is to have examination stations for the upper and lower extremities. Testing at each station should include: a) observation of any structural abnormalities; b) anthropometric measurements; c) range of motion; d) ligamentous stress testing; e) palpation of muscle and joints; and f) gross strength testing (similar to an upper or lower quarter screening examination).

Other tests that may be included in the screening examination include balance and agility; isokinetic strength testing; calculation of percent body fat; and sport specific testing. The entire examination should be closely related to the athlete's sport. Normative isokinetic strength values are available for some sports. These normative values can be useful in the screening examinations. Sport specific skills should be considered in functional tests to measure the athlete's potential to play a certain sport or position.

Some tissues are more commonly injured in certain sports and should be examined in all athletes who play that sport. For example, shoulder and ankle injuries are common in softball players, so athletes participating in this sport should have thorough shoulder and ankle examinations. Ankle injuries are common in basketball, so basketball players should have close screening of this joint. Ankle, knee, shoulder, and cervical spine injuries are common in football players, so these areas should be examined in depth.

Other Considerations for Sports Injury Prevention

General Fitness

Athletes need a balance of aerobic and anaerobic conditioning to safely and effectively participate in sports.[21] Continuous and interval training can be used to improve an athlete's aerobic capacity and energy reserves.[24] These types of training help build resistance to fatigue, which can be a major cause of injury due to a breakdown in proper body mechanics and technique. Anaerobic conditioning is also necessary, especially for athletes who participate in anaerobic sports like hockey. For both aerobic and anaerobic training, the athlete should participate in activities that functionally re–create the demands they will be facing during their specific sport.

Mobility

Sufficient mobility reduces the risk of injuring muscles, joints, and nerves during sports. Flexibility may be one of the most important parts of athletic conditioning.[24] Both acute and chronic injuries to the muscle–tendon units can be caused by decreased flexibility.[21] Full range of motion of the muscles, joints, and nerves is necessary for the movements needed during most sports; however, excessive flexibility should be avoided, since unstable joints are more prone to subluxations and dislocations.[12] Static stretching, hold–relax proprioceptive neuromuscular facilitation techniques, and active stretching can be used to increase flexibility.

Strength

The body is subjected to tremendous stresses during sports. The muscles function to accelerate movement through concentric contractions, decelerate movement through eccentric contractions, and stabilize joints through isometric contractions. Muscle weakness, poor muscle endurance, and muscle imbalances can make an athlete susceptible to sports injury.[21,24]

When designing a resistance training program, the clinician should consider the type of muscle contractions that occur during the sports and the particular muscle groups involved. Stabilization of joints with ligamentous laxity is critical to proper muscle and joint interaction. Resistance training should be performed functionally to mimic the movements and activities necessary to participate in sports. One of the most important principles to consider in resistance training is the application of the specific adaptation to imposed demands (SAID) principle.[16] According to the SAID principle, the training must be specific to the athlete's sport, position, age, and sex.

Healthy Attitude

Athletic injuries can be particularly devastating if they detract from the athlete's physical capabilities to such an extent that self–image and self–identity are altered.[2] Most athletes are highly motivated and will do whatever is needed to return to their sport activity;[10,14] however, an athlete with too much motivation to excel may overtrain and cause cumulative trauma problems. It may be necessary to monitor the highly motivated athlete closely to help prevent reinjury. A healthy and balanced attitude is essential to injury prevention after injury and while training.

Dietary Needs

A proper, well–balanced diet is necessary for both the athlete and non–athlete. The ideal diet should consist of 15% protein, 25% fat, and 60% carbohydrates.[17] During sport participation, fluid and caloric requirements change. The athlete must adjust accordingly to have adequate energy stores and fluids needed for the stressful environment of sports.

Proper Equipment

Using improper equipment has been linked to increased susceptibility to injury in young athletes.[2,11] All athletes should have equipment that fits, from pads and helmets to clothing. Proper fitting of racquets and golf clubs is also important. Sports equipment is continually modified and improved, particularly for those sports in which injury is common.[25] Special equipment to protect the head, face, eyes, ears, teeth, and hands has been developed for many sports.

Appropriate Footwear

Most sports have specific footwear, and the athlete should use the appropriate footwear for the sport. The footwear should have the proper fit, cushion, stability, and flexibility for the specific sport, the surface to be played on, and the athlete's foot type.

Environmental Risks and Rules

The rules and the environment the sport is played in should be considered when addressing athletic injury prevention. Adverse weather may increase the chance of injury, especially when rain or snow makes playing surfaces slippery. Some weather can be life–threatening (e.g., lightning). Excessively hot and humid conditions will increase the chance of injuries from heat prostration. Sport participation at high altitudes can present problems for the athlete unaccustomed to it. The rules regarding protective equipment, on–the–field treatment, and injury re–entry should be studied and enforced.[2]

Training Errors

Athletes often make errors in training for sports. These may include overtraining, undertraining, and inappropriate training. Inadequate rest and fatigue from overtraining can lead to poor performance and overuse injuries such as stress fractures and tendinitis. Clinical studies of runners have shown that 60–80% of overuse injuries of the lower extremity are attributable to training errors.[1] Inappropriate training methods that do not mimic sport function or that involve poor sport technique may also contribute to injury.

One method of preventing training errors is varying the type and intensity of exercise throughout the year, called "periodization" or "cycling training."

Preventative Braces and Taping

Using taping and braces to prevent athletic injuries is quite common. Combining high–top basketball shoes with ankle taping has decreased ankle sprains in intramural basketball athletes.[18] A retrospective study of college football players showed those who combined low–top shoes with a lace–up ankle brace had the lowest incidence of ankle injury when compared to other combinations like taping and high–top shoes.[5] Although taping is used extensively, its exact indications and specific effects need more research.

Preventive knee braces have been used since the late 1970's. At first, the braces were considered a panacea for injury prevention; however, this has been unsupported by laboratory or clinical data. Many studies have been done to try to demonstrate the preventive value of knee braces during sports. An excellent literature review article summarizes 24 studies and reports on the efficacy of prophylactic knee bracing.[15] In recent years, prophylactic knee brace use has decreased because some research has shown they do not protect and are potentially harmful.[15] Prophylactic bracing clearly needs well–controlled studies of large populations to provide a rationale for its use with any joint.

SUMMARY

In this chapter, we have discussed both industrial and sports preventive principles. The four areas that must be addressed in industrial cumulative trauma injury prevention were detailed. The specific roles of the physical therapist in sports injury prevention were outlined. The components of the pre–participation examination were presented. Finally, additional considerations to preventing sports injuries were discussed.

REFERENCES

1. Arnheim DD: <u>Modern Principles of Athletic Training</u>. Times Mirror/Mosby College Publishing, St. Louis MO 1985.

2. Bates BT, Osternig LR, Mason B, James LS: Foot Orthotic Devices to Modify Selected Aspects of Lower Extremity Mechanics. Am J Sports Med 7:338-342, 1979

3. Centineo J: Return-To-Work Programs: Cut Costs and Employee Turnover. Risk Management 44-48, Dec 1986.

4. Donatelli R, Hurlbert C, Conaway D, St Pierre R: Biomechanical Foot Orthotics: A Retrospective Study. JOSPT 10:205-212, 1988.

5. Faris GJ: Psychologic Aspects of Athletic Rehabilitation. Clin Sports Med 4(3):545-551, 1985.

6. Gardenswartz A: Equipment for Sport. In <u>Sports Medicine</u>. D Appenzeller and R Atkinson, ed. Urban and Swartzenberg, Baltimore MD 1981.

7. Garrick JG, Requa RK: Role of External Support in the Prevention of Ankle Sprains. Med Sci Sports 5:200-203, 1973.

8. Garrick JG: The Frequency of Injury, Mechanism of Injury, and Epidemiology of Ankle Sprains. Am J Sports Med 5:241-242, 1977.

9. James SL, Bates BT, Osternig LR: Injuries to Runners. Am J Sports Med 6(2):40-50, 1976.

10. Kibler WB, Chandler TJ, Uhl T, et al: A Musculoskeletal Approach to the Preparticipation Physical Examination. Am J Sports Med 17(4):525-531, 1989.

11. Kroll WA, Stone WJ: <u>Sports Conditioning and Weight Training</u>, 2nd ed. Allyn and Bacon, Boston MA 1986.

12. McCulloch MU, Brunt D, Vanderlinden D: The Effect of Foot Orthotics and Gait Velocity on Lower Limb Kinematics and Temporal Events of Stance. JOPST 17(1):2-10, 1993.

13. McReynolds M: Early Return to Work. Clinical Management 10:10-11, Sept/Oct 1990.

14. Moyer JA: Rehabilitation Goals in Sports Medicine. In <u>Rehabilitation Techniques in Sports Medicine</u>. WE Prentice, ed. CV Mosby/Yearbook, St. Louis MO 1990.

15. Moyer JA: Unique Factors in Rehabilitating the Young Athlete. In <u>Advances in Sports Medicine and Fitness</u>. WA Grana, JA Lombardo, BJ Sharkey, JA Stone, ed. Yearbook, Chicago IL 1990.

16. Moyer-Knowles J, Capelli Calibey T: Prevention, Treatment and Rehabilitation of Sport Injuries. In <u>Prevention Practice – Strategies for Physical Therapy and Occupational Therapy</u>. J Rothman and R Levine, ed. WB Saunders, Philadelphia PA 1992.

17. Novick A, Kelley DL: Position and Movement Changes of the Foot with Orthotic Intervention during the Loading Response of Gait. JOSPT 11:301-312, 1990.

18. O'Donoghue DH: <u>Treatment of Injuries to Athletes</u>, 3rd ed. WB Saunders, Philadelphia PA 1976.

19. Ratzliff J. and Grogrin T: Early Return to Work Profitability. Professional Safety 11-17, Mar 1989.

20. Ritzel D. and Allen R: Value of Work. Professional Safety 23-25, Nov 1988.

21. Rodgers MM, LeVeau BF: Effectiveness of Foot Orthotic Devices Used to Modify Pronation in Runners. JOSPT 4:86-90, 1982.

22. Rovere GD, Clarke TJ, Yates CS, et al: Retrospective Comparison of Taping and Ankle Stabilizers in Preventing Ankle Injuries. Am J Sports Med 16(3):228-233, 1988.

23. Samples P: Mind Over Muscle: Returning the Injured Athlete to Play. Physician Sports Med 15(10):172-180, 1987.

24. Smith LS, Clarke TE, Hamill CL, Santopeitro F: The Effects of Soft and Semi-rigid Orthoses upon Rearfoot Movement in Running. J Am Podiatr Med Assoc 76:227-233, 1986.

25. Wilmore JH: <u>Athletic Training and Physical Fitness</u>. Allyn and Bacon, Boston MA 1977.

Index